P9-DUP-226

RENEWALS 458-4574

DATE DUE

NOV 1 2			
NOV 2 9			
JUL 2 6			
DEC 1 7			
MAY 0 6			
GAYLORD			PRINTED IN U.S.A.

WITHDRAWN
UTSA LIBRARIES

Computers in Health Care

Kathryn J. Hannah   Marion J. Ball
Series Editors

Computers in Health Care

Series Editors:
Kathryn J. Hannah   Marion J. Ball

Marion J. Ball   Donald W. Simborg
James W. Albright   Judith V. Douglas
Editors

Healthcare Information Management Systems

A Practical Guide

Second Edition

With 39 Illustrations

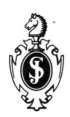

Springer-Verlag
New York Berlin Heidelberg London Paris
Tokyo Hong Kong Barcelona Budapest

Marion J. Ball
Information Services
University of Maryland
Baltimore, MD 21201, USA

Donald W. Simborg
Medicus Systems Corporation
1301 Marina Village Parkway
Alameda, CA 94501, USA

James W. Albright
Rex Hospital, Inc.
4420 Lake Boone Trail
Raleigh, NC 27607, USA

Judith V. Douglas
Information Services
University of Maryland
Baltimore, MD 21201, USA

Cover photograph © D. Chmielewski/Westlight

Library of Congress Cataloging-in-Publication Data
Healthcare information management systems : a practical guide / Marion
  J. Ball . . . [et al.], editors. — 2nd ed.
      p.   cm. — (Computers in health care)
    Includes bibliographical references and index.
    ISBN 0-387-94477-X (alk. paper)
    1. Health services administration—Data processing.
    2. Information storage and retrieval systems—Medical care.
    I. Ball, Marion J.   II. Series: Computers in health care (New York,
    N.Y.)
      [DNLM: 1. Health Facilities—organization & administration.
    2. Management Information Systems.   WX 26.5 H4345 1995]
    RA394.H45   1995
    610′.285—dc20
    DNLM/DLC
    for Library of Congress   95-6682

Printed on acid-free paper.

© 1995, 1991 Springer-Verlag New York Inc.
All rights reserved. This work may not be translated or copied in whole or in part without the
written permission of the publisher (Springer-Verlag New York, Inc., 175 Fifth Avenue, New
York, NY 10010, USA), except for brief excerpts in connection with reviews or scholarly
analysis. Use in connection with any form of information storage and retrieval, electronic
adaptation, computer software, or by similar or dissimilar methodology now known or here-
after developed is forbidden.
The use of general descriptive names, trade names, trademarks, etc., in this publication, even
if the former are not especially identified, is not to be taken as a sign that such names, as
understood by the Trade Marks and Merchandise Marks Act, may accordingly be used freely
by anyone.
While the advice and information in this book are believed to be true and accurate at the date
of going to press, neither the authors nor the editors nor the publisher can accept any legal
responsibility for any errors or omissions that may be made. The publisher makes no warranty,
express or implied, with respect to the material contained herein.

Production coordinated by Chernow Editorial Services, Inc., and managed by Laura Carlson;
manufacturing supervised by Jacqui Ashri.
Typeset by Impressions, a Division of Edwards Brothers, Inc., Madison, WI.
Printed and bound by R.R. Donnelley & Sons, Harrisonburg, VA.
Printed in the United States of America.

9 8 7 6 5 4 3 2 1

ISBN 0-387-94477-X Springer-Verlag New York Berlin Heidelberg

Library
University of Texas
at San Antonio

*To the father of medical informatics,
Morrie Collen, for bringing theory
into practice, and his wife, Bobbie,
for supporting him and his work*

Series Preface

This series is intended for students and practitioners of the health professions who are seeking to expand their knowledge of computers in health care. Our editors and authors, experts in their fields, offer their insight into innovations and trends. Each book is practical and easy to use.

Since the series began, in 1988, we have seen increasing acceptance of the term "informatics" and of the innovations it brings to health care. Today more than ever we are committed to making this series contribute to the field of healthcare informatics, the discipline "where caring and technology meet."

MARION J. BALL
KATHRYN J. HANNAH

Preface

In the four years since the publication of the first edition of this book, we have witnessed the introduction of a complete new generation of information technology. During this same period, we have seen powerful market forces transform the buying and selling of health care from insurance-dominated fee-for-service medicine to a path leading inexorably to capitated managed care reform. Both of these powerful forces—technology change and market-based healthcare reform—have stimulated the need for the revisions in this second edition of *Healthcare Information Management Systems: A Practical Guide.*

Many of the fundamentals of information management remain unchanged; hence, some chapters from the first edition remain as relevant as before and were revised and retained. Still others have been replaced by chapters covering new ground.

In 1991, we did not have a public awareness of an emerging "information superhighway." Today, with over 30 million users of the Internet and daily reference to the opportunities this technology brings, we have become almost casual in our expectation of universal worldwide access to countless products and services for every aspect of our lives. The healthcare industry will be a major component of the national information infrastructure (NII), as the "information superhighway" is formally called. We already have business-oriented services, such as claims submission, insurance verification, and electronic payment, as well as clinically oriented services, such as results reporting, prescription ordering, and x-ray image communication that utilize the healthcare NII. Clinician access to reference materials and knowledge bases has been in place for years and is growing steadily. Even more exciting is the beginning of consumer access to similar sources of health-related information. In September 1994, a report[1] was published en-

---

1. "An Architectural Framework for the National Information Infrastructure Cross-Industry," Working Group, Corporation for National Research Initiatives, 1895 Preston White Drive, Suite 100, Reston, Virginia 22091-5434. Reprinted with permission.

titled "An Architectural Framework for the National Information Infra-structure," in which various scenarios were described to illustrate the future use of the NII. One of those scenarios was as follows:

"Thank you very much, Dr. Robinson. I appreciate your call," said Frank, placing his wireless videophone into its charging stand in the kitchen. Gazing out the window and sighing deeply, Frank tried to digest the news that he had cancer. A fit and trim 62-year-old, Frank had planned for an active retirement. Yesterday's physical exam was supposed to be routine, but Dr. Robinson had spotted something suspicious. Additional test data bore out these suspicions.

Frank remembered an advertisement he'd encountered when browsing his news service. It described a commercial service, MedAssist, which integrated a wide variety of information for people seeking to participate in their health care. Using the desktop communicator in his home office, Frank opened a secure link to MedAssist.

First, Frank sought basic information about his condition. He described verbally what he knew to queries made by the automated MedAssist intake manager. His responses quickly led him to be linked to a human diagnostic reference specialist, and they discussed what sort of reference materials might be most useful to him. Together, they selected several reports and informative multimedia presentations. MedAssist quickly gathered these for Frank from its network of professional and popular sources.

After working his way through the materials, Frank understood the general nature of his illness somewhat better. He then browsed through several anatomical simulations and presentations about treatments from a local university's medical library. High-resolution images, treatment simulations, and the accompanying audio "footnotes" created a customized one-time "performance" of this material.

Dr. Robinson had advised Frank to get a second opinion. He followed up on this by opening a communications window on his screen, conferring with both his insurance provider and Dr. Robinson's office, and making an appointment using his electronic scheduling agent with a specialist he had identified through MedAssist. Frank then sent permission for Dr. Robinson to release the relevant medical records to this specialist.

His new doctor examined the records with colleagues located at her group's satellite offices and with Dr. Robinson. They all agreed that Frank's disease suggested treatment along several paths. The specialist placed a visual call to Frank to introduce herself and lay out possible treatment options so Frank would be well prepared for his examination.

Frank linked to MedAssist again to learn more about the treatment plans and outcomes based on other men of his age and physical condition. He was referred to an on-line service of a state health agency, which offered both statistical information and analytical assistance through MedAssist. Through an easy-to-use automated query manager within the database, Frank learned about medical outcomes and patient levels of satisfaction for various treatment paths. He asked some questions, responded to other questions, and was guided to look at his illness in some interesting ways. He began to feel more comfortable with the likely options for treatment and the prognosis his doctors had indicated.

This scenario was meant to be futuristic, but much of it is already here. As the readers of this edition will discover, our contributors describe the technologies and services of the sort the fictional Frank and his caregivers turn to as they deal with his diagnosis and treatment options—from consumer technologies to physician workstations, from health information networks to consumer resource centers, and much, much more.

The rapid changes affecting our industry are not driven solely by technology. Healthcare reform, regardless of its pace at the federal level, is happening at the state and local level. Most states today have some form of managed care option for their Medicaid patients. Employer and consumer healthcare buying coalitions have already begun to show their power in numerous markets. In some areas, capitation contracts are the fastest growing form of healthcare purchasing. Competition is here. Healthcare provider organizations are responding by forming vertical organizations, or integrated delivery systems (IDSs) as they are known, in order to survive this competition. The independent community hospital as we know it will become a cost center to an IDS rather than the center of our delivery system.

But survival will require more than changes in ownership and relationships. It will require an information underpinning that will stress the limits of our impressive technology changes. The IDSs of tomorrow must cope with an incredibly complex environment in which the financial incentives will continually be changing and often in conflict. Although capitation is growing, it will be a decade or longer before it dominates most markets—if ever. Fee-for-service, which rewards providers for doing more, will coexist with capitation, which rewards providers for doing less. Both the consumer and the provider must seek out that value point in health care where a reasonable balance between costs and outcomes can be determined. The key to doing this well will be the information management system.

This is the challenge facing our current information management systems. This is the challenge we, as editors, have put to the contributors of this edition. We believe they have responded. As was the case in the first edition, this edition speaks to healthcare practitioners. Our look into the future is not a fantasy ride, but a practical analysis of the short-term directions of the industry and the technology. For the here and now, the practitioner is exposed to the full spectrum of issues involved in moving into the future and managing that move. At the current rate of change, we very well may need a third edition four years from now.

We believe we have put together an edition which responds to the forces at work in our industry. We hope you will enjoy reading it as much as we have enjoyed preparing it.

MARION J. BALL
DONALD W. SIMBORG
JAMES W. ALBRIGHT
JUDITH V. DOUGLAS

Contents

SECTION 1   MOVING INTO THE FUTURE

Unit 8   Developing and Purchasing Expertise

Healthcare Information Management Systems

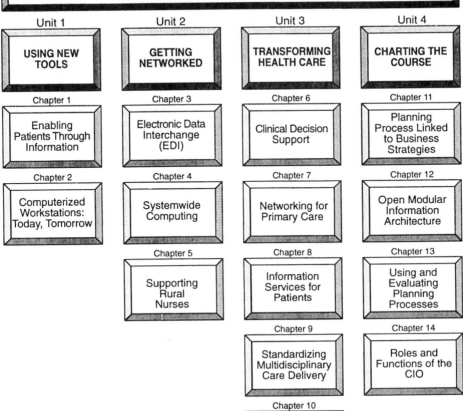

Unit 1

USING NEW TOOLS

Chapter 1

Enabling Patients Through Information

Chapter 2

Computerized Workstations: Today, Tomorrow

Unit 2

GETTING NETWORKED

Chapter 3

Electronic Data Interchange (EDI)

Chapter 4

Systemwide Computing

Chapter 5

Supporting Rural Nurses

Unit 3

TRANSFORMING HEALTH CARE

Chapter 6

Clinical Decision Support

Chapter 7

Networking for Primary Care

Chapter 8

Information Services for Patients

Chapter 9

Standardizing Multidisciplinary Care Delivery

Chapter 10

Performance Measurement and Quality Improvement

Unit 4

CHARTING THE COURSE

Chapter 11

Planning Process Linked to Business Strategies

Chapter 12

Open Modular Information Architecture

Chapter 13

Using and Evaluating Planning Processes

Chapter 14

Roles and Functions of the CIO

A Practical Guide

Unit 5	Unit 6	Unit 7	Unit 8
ADDRESSING THE IMPACT OF INFORMATION TECHNOLOGY	**CHOOSING AND WORKING WITH SYSTEMS**	**CHANGING THE PROFESSIONS**	**DEVELOPING AND PURCHASING EXPERTISE**

Chapter 15	Chapter 17	Chapter 20	Chapter 24
People Aspects of Change Management	Connectivity and Open Architecture	Integrated Systems for Nursing	Improving Personal Productivity

Chapter 16	Chapter 18	Chapter 21	Chapter 25
Moral Obligations in the Information Age	Systems: from Vision to Evaluation	Resources and Needs in Nursing Informatics	Designing a Computer Course for Clinical Nurses

	Chapter 19	Chapter 22	Chapter 26
	Establishing Good Vendor Relationships	Pathology Department Systems	Understanding the Marketplace

		Chapter 23	Chapter 27
		Imaging and Picture Archiving Systems	Consultants: Tasks, Benefits

			Chapter 28
This contents array presents the architecture of the book in reader-friendly terms. Use it to get a feel for the thrust of the units and chapters and to quickly select what you want to study in more depth.			Client Advice on Using Consultants

Section 1
Moving into the Future

Unit 1
Using New Tools

Unit Introduction

What were visions of the future in 1991 are now becoming realities in the healthcare setting. Forward looking projects are putting power in the hands of consumers and providers alike, from fax-on-demand and interactive laserdisks, to the computer-based health professional workstation.

Anderson discusses healthcare information systems designed for consumers. Such systems can improve care by supporting shared decision making, gathering data for outcomes-based research, and enhancing the content of knowledge repositories. Programs he describes rely on a variety of tools, ranging from "electronic house calls" to interactive laserdisks, broadband video services, and fax-on-demand.

Afrin and Del Bene focus on the computer systems supplanting the telephone as the physician's workstation of choice. They offer experiences at their own institution to illustrate the evolution of data availability and user interface design, most recently with Open Architecture Clinical Information Systems (OACIS). For them, data security and confidentiality remain issues, and computer systems are marked by an inherent complexity—as is the practice of medicine itself.

1
Technology for Consumers and Information Needs in Health Care

EDWARD L. ANDERSON

The New Paradigm

Healthcare information technology designed specifically for the healthcare consumer offers enormous opportunity to improve the efficiency and outcome of healthcare services. Existing healthcare information systems have developed a high level of sophistication to meet the accounting and some clinical requirements for the delivery of medical services. However, systems that deliver integrated, comprehensive interaction with the healthcare consumer are severely underdeveloped. Only recently has the importance of the healthcare consumer been appreciated. The consumer shares an equal role, along with the provider, as a critical decision maker who drives the entire healthcare enterprise. We have entered into an era of healthcare informatics that empowers consumer decision making through the use of emerging interactive and multimedia technologies. These technologies can be distributed to virtually anyone, anywhere, at anytime.

This new focus is the result of a paradigm change in the delivery of health care. Consumers want to actively participate and partner with healthcare providers and become an integral part of the decision-making process. They are no longer satisfied to passively accept whatever is directed by physicians and other healthcare professionals. Healthcare consumers are seeking resources that can give them the knowledge and tools to more effectively interact with providers and credible information that validates provider recommendations. Outcomes research has shown that there is enormous waste in the healthcare system because many services that are delivered offer no demonstrable benefits and may actually be harmful. Research on medical appropriateness done at the Rand Corporation of Santa Monica, California, estimate that between one-fourth to one-third of all medical care is either inappropriate or offers no benefit to the patient (Brook, 1989). Unfortunately, consumers have not been able to participate with their providers in determining what is best for their specific situation because they do not have access to healthcare information systems that have been designed with that purpose in mind.

This paradigm change also impacts on providers because they must find more effective ways to collect *and* communicate outcomes-based research to their patients. In the near future, "electronic house calls" and concurrent feedback from patients during their course of treatment may emerge as the current standard of care. Not only will concurrent education and instruction be communicated from the health professional to the consumer, but interactive feedback and data collection will occur directly with the patient during treatment and will be used to influence decision making. Decision making will be shared between the provider and the patient. These types of data, collected concurrently during treatment, will also contribute to an expanding clinical and functional outcomes knowledge base that will help establish, along with clinically acquired data, best practices and critical clinical pathways.

The challenge of healthcare information management is to create an information environment that melds the consumer with providers and systems of care. This information architecture is the foundation for continuous quality improvement in health care and it is this interface where caring and technology meet.

Information That Improves Employee Productivity

Two of the most important concerns that face corporations today are the cost of health care and the cost of lost productivity. Strategies can be implemented to improve employee productivity and attendance while reducing the direct costs for employee medical care. This occurs because employees who are productive are less likely to use additional or unnecessary healthcare services.

The cost of lost productivity due to health-related absenteeism is two to three times as much as a corporation spends on employee medical expenses. These costs include lost revenue, replacement worker costs (including overtime for coworkers), inefficiencies brought on by employee absence, and wage and salary replacement costs paid to employees during their absence. These figures have been supported by our own experience at Bell Atlantic and confirmed as valid for other large corporations by healthcare consultants including Mercer, Inc., and The Medstat Group.

Because of the enormous financial impact of lost productivity, corporations must find ways to reduce lost time while improving the health of their employees. Consumer-focused health information systems offer an excellent approach in assisting in the management of a corporation's human capital. A more participative consumer is likely to better use the healthcare delivery system and avoid services that are unnecessary (Greenguard, 1992). Immediate information that directs appropriate care reduces delays in seeking the appropriate level of care and early intervention is likely to reduce the severity or complexity of a health condition. Self-care is also an important educational component of consumer-based health promotion because, with better knowledge, healthcare consumers can decide when it is necessary to seek advanced medical care. This avoids unnecessary utilization of healthcare delivery services for minor clinical conditions. These approaches can improve employee productivity and reduce the cost of medical care to the corporation.

Technology Requirements: Interactive Voice Response Systems, Fax-on-Demand, and Inbound Fax

The technology required to deliver consumer-based information services to employees does not have to be complex, nor does it require broadband, multimedia systems. The requirement for consumers is that information must be delivered at the time and point of need. Narrowband services such as fax-on-demand and interactive voice response systems (IVRs) are excellent ways to deliver consumer-focused information. Because the basic telephone network is used, information services can be delivered to virtually anyone at any location in the world. Application of this technology with health promotion programs supports the corporation's need to improve productivity, contain healthcare costs, and invest in its human capital.

At Bell Atlantic, we have implemented these technologies with excellent employee acceptance and participation.

IVR System

An IVR presents a caller with a selection of choices from a prerecorded menu of services. Using a key tone-based phone, the caller responds to these options and navigates through a series of branching questions and responses. The system ultimately directs the call to the desired service. The caller can be directly connected to an online counselor or the caller's keyed-in responses can be used to collect data or activate additional IVR-based outputs. One such output sends data to a fax server and requests that it transmit a document directly back to the consumer's fax machine. This service is referred to as fax-on-demand.

Fax-on-Demand

Fax-on-demand is simply using this IVR gateway to direct the faxing of specific documentation to the consumer's individual fax machine. During the IVR session, the voice prompts the user to enter his fax phone number, along with the requested document number. If the user does not know the correct document number, then a catalog of all available documents can be requested, initially, to be faxed back to the caller. After reviewing this document, the user then reenters the IVR gateway and selects the desired document(s).

Inbound Fax: Data Entry from a Fax

Through the use of fax technology, this system also offers the consumer the opportunity to interact with the information system and populate a database using "inbound fax." In this instance, a form is requested by the user that is faxed back immediately for completion. This form is actually "intelligent" and contains specifically defined regions that require filling in a bubbled response similar to those contained on traditional, optically scanned forms. Special software is required to create this "intelligent," fax-read form. After the consumer has filled in this "intelligent" form, it is then faxed to the health information system where the user's responses are read and converted into data elements that populate industry standard databases. Because this form is returning to the fax server, it is referred to as "inbound fax." A commercially available software product that delivers this application is TeleForm, developed by Cardiff Software, Inc. in Solana Beach, California.

Using this inbound fax technology, each fax machine essentially becomes a graphical-based entry terminal and consumers can interact with the health information system for a number of useful applications.

Health Promotion: The Bell Atlantic Experience

How can corporations address the need to improve employee productivity, contain the cost of medical care, and implement preventive health programs while downsizing (or eliminating) their corporate health and medical departments? This problem faced Bell Atlantic in 1992 and continues to be a challenge for other corporations. We recognized the advantage of using information systems that enable employees to participate in health promotion anytime and anywhere. The real product of health promotion is information and education. Furthermore, this information must be available on demand when it is critically needed. Programs also need to be available that solicit enthusiastic participation by employees and that support personal accountability. These assumptions formed the basis for our Bell Atlantic[SM] HealthFit[SM] program, which made health promotion immediately available to participants, anytime and anywhere. It emancipated health promotion from limitations imposed by a "hands-on" clinic or site-based program through the use of information technology.

The employee, dependent, or retiree enters the information gateway through an IVR. After selecting the health promotion option, the consumer is able to navigate through voice menus to choose various products. One choice refers the employee to select a health assessment profile. This profile will be available in the near future, through a fax-on-demand basis. The employee completes the profile and mails or faxes this back for mechanized scoring and interpretation. Based on the results, the employee can request additional information through fax-on-demand or through direct discussion with a master's prepared nurse counselor.

An additional choice through the IVR is to be directly connected to this nurse health counselor. This encounter permits better patient understanding of her health condition and how to best use the healthcare delivery system, avoiding inappropriate or unnecessary care. This service is used by employees and their dependents while they are still working; however, it has additional value to those who are absent for medically related reasons and need health information support. This facilitates improved productivity by offering informational services to those who are actively utilizing the healthcare delivery system and ensures efficient and appropriate use of medical care. Services can be expanded to include the capture of functional outcomes data; these data can be related back to specific health plans and individual providers.

Another important part of health information is the ability to get written content on demand. Using the IVR voice menu and fax-on-demand, the healthcare consumer can request a variety of health-related topics that are immediately faxed back to the user. A complete menu of topics can also be requested for immediate fax back. New topics can be quickly added or existing content can be rapidly modified, thereby assuring that all information distributed to consumers is current and accurate.

One of the additional advantages of using this topic-based fax-on-demand system is that our corporate health professionals can determine patterns of need or interest, based on the number of requests made for specific topics. Utilization of these services can be tracked against employee demographics in order to most efficiently use corporate resources. Statistical analysis of fax-on-demand utilization can assure that this information is reaching the targeted populations within a corporation, based on age, sex, and job assignment demographic distributions. Our experience at Bell Atlantic has shown that fax-on-demand for health information is extremely well accepted and reaches all age populations equally, based on employee demographic distribution. Deployment of risk reduction programs can be based on actual consumer needs or interest reflected by employee utilization, rather than being based on assumptions and speculation about these needs.

The IVR also offers a selection for consumer participation in physical activity programs. The participant is able to enter the amount of time spent performing aerobic activities and the system tracks each individual's achievement. Incentives and recognition are provided, based on the user reaching certain milestones of activity. This facilitates continued participation because of concurrent feedback, incentives, and coaching provided by the information system.

Future Directions Using Fax-Based Technology

The great flexibility of this system is that new programs can be rapidly introduced to anyone who has a telephone and access to a fax machine. Here are some examples:

- Consumers can enter results of a health assessment profile (health risk appraisal), receive immediate scoring, a report, and interpretation using inbound fax and fax-on-demand.
- Consumers supply information about their functional status that can be used for outcomes studies (such as responses to the SF-36, which is an industry standard for measuring an individual's functional status). This can be used to track the rate of functional recovery following medical procedures and link these data to specific providers and medical treatment.
- A health provider can obtain a patient's medical history and a review of systems prior to an individual's visit to a clinic or for preadmission for inpatient/outpatient treatment.
- Health providers and healthcare delivery organizations can perform patient satisfaction surveys to measure perceptions of quality of care.
- Consumers can request the generation of customized reports or information that is faxed-on-demand, based on a user-defined query (an example might be to provide a list of all participating providers within 10 miles of the patient's home who are female, board-certified gynecologists, and completed training within the past 15 years).

Until interactive video services to the home or office are widely available, fax-on-demand and inbound fax, coupled with IVR, will serve as inexpensive, readily available, and powerful technologies that deliver consumer-based health information services.

Information That Permits Shared Decision Making

Whatever type of information technology that is deployed, it is essential that it supports the consumer's need for immediate access to knowledge bases that permit shared decision making. Patients must be able to rapidly gain understanding of their health conditions and appreciate the risks and benefits of various treatment alternatives. This requires that the information is balanced, concise, and delivered to consumers on an educational level that is easily understood.

Better outcomes of care are likely when there is good patient compliance to a provider's treatment plan. Personal involvement by the consumer in healthcare decision making leads to a greater personal accountability and this supports better compliance (Taylor, 1993). This patient/provider partnership delivers a greater personalization of medical care. It puts the patient in control and makes medical care more "person-centered" (Reiser, 1993). What has been missing in the traditional healthcare paradigm was a partnership between the provider and an informed healthcare consumer who shared in the decision-making process. Providers have told patients what kind of and how much care they need while the patient has remained passive.

Shared Decision Making

Dr. John Wennberg, director of The Center for Evaluative Clinical Sciences at Dartmouth Medical School, and his colleagues have pioneered the concept of shared decision making using interactive laserdisks. They formed the Foundation for Informed Medical Decision Making in Hanover, New Hampshire; using a PC-based interface, they are developing a number of interactive educational programs that allow shared decision making between the patient and the provider. Dr. Wennberg, who is a recognized expert in outcomes-based research, realized that, for decades, physicians have dictated to patients the type of care or treatment that they should receive without ever asking the patient about personal preferences. Consumers have not been given the opportunity to understand the alternatives and the outcomes of these choices. These interactive programs begin by asking a number of patient-specific questions and then presenting the educational content that is unique for that patient, based on his/her responses. The content is presented as interviews between actual patients and a health professional as well as graphic and animated displays. The educational content is reinforced for the consumer by computer-generated printouts, following an interactive session.

The strength of this technology is in its ability to customize the delivery of health content while concurrently collecting patient-specific data that can be integrated with other clinical and functional data. The concept of shared decision making has been extremely well accepted by consumers. Patients are better prepared to discuss treatment options and ask more intelligent questions to their providers after participating in this interactive program (Greenguard, 1992). This leads to more efficient use of the physician's time and expertise, while giving patients more personal esteem and control in deciding their care. Better informed patients are more likely to remain compliant to treatment recommendations; this leads to better outcomes of care (Blossom & McCann, 1990).

From a legal perspective, this system consistently documents informed consent, which reduces provider liability. The content of the information is comprehensive and ensures that patients are well informed of the risks and benefits as well as alternatives to care. It also can clearly document a patient's preference and understanding of the educational content.

In two HMOs (Group Health Cooperative of Puget Sound, Seattle; and Kaiser Permanente of Denver), this product was tested on patients undergoing treatment for benign prostatic hyperplasia that results in urinary tract obstruction. In the Kaiser group, surgery dropped by 44 percent the first year without a subsequent rebound (Greenguard, 1992). At the Seattle HMO, prostate surgery dropped by 60 percent. In both instances, men chose medical management instead of a surgical approach after participating with the interactive laserdisk product. CIGNA has used this program at seven staff model HMOs. Outcomes-based research was used as the source for the educational content in these interactive videos. Wennberg's approach offers great opportunities for healthcare cost containment associated with improved quality of care because care is based on consumer-induced demand, not provider-induced demand (Rice, 1993).

Currently, the consumer must interact with this product at a specific office site; therefore most users have been patients in staff model HMOs and large group practices. The hardware required to deliver this program to a single station costs approximately $8,000. This type of technology used by Wennberg could be offered to the consumer's home or multiple clinic locations through video information networks, thus greatly expanding the opportunities for consumer participation, especially in nonstaff model HMOs. Using an interactive device similar to a wireless mouse, consumers could respond to the program at remote locations, including their homes, whereas their responses could be stored in a database and forwarded to the designated healthcare provider(s). Printouts could be generated and faxed back to the nonoffice-based user. A technology currently exists called ADSL (Asymmetrical Digital Subscriber Loop), using ordinary twisted pair copper wire and the telephone line. Bell Atlantic has already delivered video-on-demand to the home, using regular telephone lines, to hundreds of employees during field tests and will shortly be offering interactive video services to thousands of regular customers using this technology.

In the future, HMOs and other healthcare delivery systems will be able to deliver video programming to each member's home. This opens the opportunity for extensive patient education about preventive health topics, explanations of pending surgical or diagnostic procedures, clinical shared decision-making programs, disease treatment education, and health plan-related information. Patients will be able to interact with these video programs to schedule appointments, ask questions, see specific content on demand, and even choose a physician by "meeting their doctor" through a short video vignette. These informational video services will give these HMOs competitive advantage in the marketplace. Members will be attracted to HMOs and healthcare delivery systems that enhance their opportunity to actively participate in their care. These HMOs will also benefit by having more informed consumers who will have realistic expectations of care and an appreciation of treatment alternatives.

Information That Improves Patient Care

The physician/patient encounter has been recognized as fundamentally essential in establishing a therapeutic relationship. Unfortunately, the time spent during most of these important encounters is limited, and patients frequently complain that they have difficulty remembering important questions they meant to ask and what was said to them by their provider. From the provider's prospective, this encounter is also often too short to effectively communicate information to their patient about health conditions and treatment, including risks and alternatives. Recent research also suggests that patient compliance is dependent on an effective physician/patient communication that solicits direct patient decision making (Blossom & McCann, 1990).

Consumer-based information systems allow for an extension of the physician/patient encounter, and in the near future, this extended encounter will occur in the patient's home or other locations far removed from the provider's office. The effect of these opportunities will be to increase the intensity and content of information that can be shared between the physician and patient. This leads to greater patient/provider partnering, better patient compliance, and improved provider clinical decision making.

The Importance of Consumer Compliance

Improved patient compliance is better achieved through more effective provider/patient communications, using educational strategies. Studies that have measured patient compliance to treatment have shown nonadherence to physician's recommendations occur from 50 percent to 92 percent of the time (Blossom & McCann, 1990). This extraordinarily high rate of nonadherence is alarming and constitutes a major failure of the healthcare enterprise to achieve desirable outcomes of care.

Investigators have identified that the traditional physician/patient interaction is responsible for this high rate of nonadherence. It occurs because physicians have not facilitated patients in the decision-making process. Patient education has been based on the model applied to teaching children in which the teacher's (physician's) relationship is authoritative. The learner (patient) is passive and cooperative. However, what is more effective in ensuring compliance is the model used to teach adults in which the learner is participative and interactive in the educational process. This type of education places the physician in the role of a facilitator or coach, and promotes the patient to partner with the provider (Blossom & McCann, 1990).

The opportunities afforded to the consumer through shared clinical decision making and interactive clinical care establish precisely the kinds of behaviors that lead to better patient compliance because they are based on the adult model of learning.

The "Electronic House Call"

In the future, electronic house calls will be possible using video and multimedia interaction. The home television will become an interactive terminal for the healthcare consumer. A patient will be able to return home following a clinical encounter or recent hospitalization and interact concurrently with their provider during recovery. Instructions given to the patient by the provider can be viewed using interactive video with the advantage that the patient can replay the instructions until they are clearly understood. An instructor can actually show the patient or family member how to do basic care, such as change bandages, irrigate catheters, etc. Video programmed education delivers a richer content than can be provided through traditional printed material. Similarly, information about prescribed medications and their side effects can be reviewed by patients with improved educational content delivered by video rather than paper media.

Interaction between the consumer and provider is not limited to broadband, video-based content. A terminal located in a patient's home can offer electronic mail exchange of information with their provider. Many questions can be answered quickly and without the need for an office visit. Prompt advice at the time of need can prevent unnecessary health care because the patient is able to make the right decisions initially, as soon as symptoms appear. An even more primitive example of this type of exchange occurs today through the use of voice mail. Large group practices and staff model HMOs use voice mail as a way of rapidly responding to patient inquiries, thereby avoiding unnecessary office visits.

Complications to treatment can be monitored through a series of interactive sessions with the patient. Examples of patients with various levels of complications can be displayed in full motion on the patient's home television and the patient can respond to screen prompts that request his current status. Patient responses are transmitted to secured databases that are accessible to his healthcare provider. This allows for concurrent monitoring of a postoperative or treatment course while the patient is still at home. If serious conditions develop, then the information system alerts the provider and the patient is seen in the office. Based on expected patterns of healing, the interactive information system continually compares the patient's status with the expected status based on norms, and any variations will trigger an alert to the provider. This information system provides for early intervention should complications develop. In the current healthcare delivery system, many patients delay seeing the provider until their next scheduled appointment or until the complication becomes worse. This interactive system encourages early, appropriate intervention.

Concurrent patient feedback allows the tracking of a patient's progress and responses to therapy, while following critical treatment pathways as well as patient compliance. It also provides the clinical and functional outcomes data that will collectively contribute to continuous refinement of "best treatment practices." When poor patient compliance occurs or when conditions develop that predict a likely poor outcome, the information system can alert the provider and the patient.

Patients with chronic conditions such as diabetes or hypertension that require periodic monitoring also greatly benefit from this type of interactive "house call." The advantage of this technology is that very detailed patient education can be offered without utilizing limited (and costly) resources delivered directly by the provider. Concurrent tracking of a patient's clinical and functional progress can occur remotely, without intense, direct provider interaction. Patients can enter data from self-administered tests performed at home and this can be transmitted to their providers. This reduces the cost and number of visits to the clinic for care while improving the quality of information about the patient. The provider has acquired almost as much information as if the patient had been seen in the clinic setting on a daily basis. When actual patient visits do occur, the provider will have immediate access to timely and comprehensive information that directs better clinical decision making.

Consumer-focused technology supports better patient/provider partnering. Improved patient/provider communication also ensures greater patient satisfaction. Healthcare delivery systems, such as HMOs, that offer this type of consumer-based information exchange are more likely to achieve higher member satisfaction rates and member subscription. Furthermore, quality metrics required of health plans that indicate outcomes of care must include consumer-based data. These data can be more efficiently collected directly from consumers using these types of systems because the data are generated concurrently during an episode of care.

Harvard Community Health Plan and InterPractice Systems

Although no health information system exists today that offers all of these services and benefits, a system recently tested by Boston's Harvard Community Health Plan serves as an excellent example of applying some of these concepts. Terminals were placed in nearly 200 member's homes during an 18-month study and patients interacted with the system to obtain health information, health assessments, and self-diagnostic protocols (Gareiss, 1994). This system, known as Triage and Education Systems, used at the Harvard Community Health Plan was built by InterPractice Systems (IPS). IPS was formed as a joint venture by the Harvard Community Health Plan and EDS (Electronic Data Systems). Current plans call for this system to be made available to all members of the health plan.

Not only was information available to the healthcare consumer on demand, but personal health data were recorded and used to update the member's personal health record. When a serious health condition existed, the system alerted the patient to call the physician and concurrently paged the doctor. When the patient arrived at the clinic for an assessment, much of the history had already been acquired from this interaction, thereby improving the quality of the physician's time spent with the patient. Patients are extremely pleased with the fact that they do not have to wait for a call back from their physician. They can interact immediately and become active participants in their health care.

This trial showed very high patient satisfaction with over 90 percent rating the service quality as "high." Economic analysis showed that outpatient visits to the clinic decreased by 5 percent for those in the study compared with patients in the health plan who did not use the home terminals (Gareiss, 1994).

One of the nonmeasurable advantages of this type of home-based system is the personal effect it has on the consumers' perspectives about their personal role in health care. Patients expressed a feeling of satisfaction knowing that health information was immediately available and accessible (Gareiss, 1994). This knowledge creates an environment that drives behaviors toward greater personal health accountability. It gives the consumer a sense of control. Information technology generates a healthcare environment that supports consumer behaviors that drive personal health enhancement. For both providers and consumers, health care *is* information management.

Opportunities for Cost Reduction

A study conducted in 1992 by the Cambridge, Massachussetts-based Arthur D. Little Company concluded that widespread use of home-based consumer access to healthcare information had the potential of reducing health costs by $15 billion a year ("Telecommunications: Can it help," 1992). This included a savings of $8.3 billion due to fewer visits to clinics and hospitals, $1.9 billion savings due to self-help and early intervention, and $5 billion savings due to improved communications of health results. Many factors account for the magnitude of these total savings. Unnecessary medical care, such as visits to emergency departments and clinics, is prevented; appropriate, timely care prevents increased costs due to delays in seeking care. A decrease in professional time spent directly with patients answering questions and monitoring chronic conditions also accounts for a large amount of this cost reduction.

Building Knowledge Bases That Direct Health Care

These transactions are important because they establish communication between the provider and consumer. The ultimate value of these interactive transactions lies in the ability to build knowledge bases that support continued improvement in provider and consumer decision making. These health information encounters each generate data that collectively contribute to an expanding knowledge repository.

This process has been referred to as "practice-based research" because it collects the experiences of many patients in community-based settings who have common health problems. This type of research is different from controlled studies where only select groups of patients that meet rigid criteria for inclusion in a study are examined. Practice-based research has the potential to be of great value because of the direct involvement of the consumer in choosing alternatives of care. Furthermore, practice-based research can examine multiple outcomes of care with a focus on the quality of life and functionality (Alexander & Clancy, 1994). Controlled studies are more often focused on mortality and individual interventions.

From this knowledge repository, critical pathways of care can be developed and applied to patient care. Networking of numerous local knowledge bases forms a health information architecture that supports a rational, efficient healthcare delivery system. For clinical guidelines to be successfully applied, the consumer's needs, preferences, and participation are essential. Patients have almost universally been left out of the process of developing guidelines, yet patient preferences should be incorporated into developing guidelines, according to a recent Institute of Medicine report (Howard et al., 1994). Patients vary as to the value of a particular outcome of treatment and display wide variation, based on individual preferences.

Conclusion

Information systems must offer consumers the opportunity to tap into knowledge repositories at the point of time and need and partner with their providers to enhance the quality of health care. Delivery of health information services directly to the consumer through IVR, fax, terminals, and broadband video services will also facilitate the capture of consumer preferences, values, and behaviors. These data support outcomes-based research and enhance the content of knowledge repositories. Prevention, education, and personal accountability are additional benefits of these consumer-focused health information services.

Health care begins and ends with the patient. The patient shares in defining care and it is the patient who ultimately decides if a treatment is successful (Reiser, 1993). Integrated health information management systems designed for the consumer are essential to transform our healthcare system and reaffirm our commitment to excellence in improving the quality of life.

Questions

1. Describe the changing role of the healthcare consumer.
2. What benefits can consumer-focused health information systems offer to employers?

3. Briefly describe how Bell Atlantic is using the following technologies for health promotion:
   Interactive voice response (IVR),
   Fax-on-demand,
   Inbound fax.
4. List additional possible uses of fax-based technology in health care.
5. Describe the role of consumer-focused information systems in shared decision making.
6. Explain how patient-focused information systems can improve patient care, with attention to the following:
   Patient compliance,
   Electronic house calls,
   Cost reduction.
7. Defend or dispute the author's statement, "For both providers and consumers, health care *is* information management."

References

Alexander, G., & Clancy, C. (1994). Practice-based research: Laboratories for health care reform. *Journal of Family Practice, 38*(4), 428–431.

Blossom, J.H., & McCann, D.P. (1990). The physician as patient educator: From theory to practice. *The Western Journal of Medicine, 153*(1), 44–50.

Brook, R.H. (1989). Practice guidelines and practicing medicine; are they compatible? *The Journal of the American Medical Association, 262*(21), 3027–3031.

Gareiss, R. (1994). Electronic triage. *American Medical News, 37*(16), 37–41.

Greenguard, S. (1992). The physician's new care companion: Interactive videodiscs expand the patient's role in making treatment decisions. *American Medical News, 35*(25), 9–11.

Howard, M.O., Lambert, M., Suchinsky, R., & Walker, R.D. (1994). Medical practice guidelines. *The Western Journal of Medicine, 161*(1), 39–45.

Reiser, S.J. (1993). The era of the patient: Using the experience of illness in shaping the missions of health care. *The Journal of the American Medical Association, 269*(8), 1012–1018.

Rice, B. (1993). Giving patients a bigger say in choosing treatment. *Medical Economics, 70*(19), 138–145.

Taylor, K.S. (1993). Shopping for surgery: Consumers want to talk outcomes and have a say in their care decisions. *Hospitals and Health Networks, 67*(14), 42–45.

Telecommunications: Can it help solve America's health care problems? (1992). Cambridge, MA: Arthur D. Little, Inc.

2
Physician Workstations

LAWRENCE B. AFRIN AND VICTOR E. DEL BENE

The Paradigm Is Shifting

What exactly *is* a physician workstation? In a broad sense, it is a device for collecting medical and related information and delivering that information to a physician. The information may come from one or more sources, such as laboratory, radiology, or medical records facilities. Some workstations may provide mechanisms for physicians to not only retrieve but also enter information, such as physical examinations. More advanced workstations may also provide tools for analyzing data.

Upon reflection, most physicians would consider the telephone to be the original physician workstation. Certainly this device remains by far the most widely used workstation. The telephone allows retrieval and entry of information. By eliminating physical distance as a barrier to obtaining information, the telephone has had a profound effect on practice management efficiency. The typical modern physician could not handle the multitudes of patients and problems encountered in an average workday were it not for the telephone. The modern physician considers the telephone as essential a tool as a writing instrument (perhaps more so).

Yet the telephone is not the ideal physician workstation. Information usually can be communicated by telephone to only one destination or from one source at a time. The telephone has no capabilities for data analysis, and it has almost no clinically useful information indexing resources. In fact, most physicians would agree that the greatest inefficiency in the telephone system lies usually not in the device itself but in the person whom the physician is calling. That person (a) may not be available to talk, (b) may not be able to understand the purpose of the physician's call, (c) may not know who else in his or her department could help understand the purpose of the physician's call, (d) may not be able to retrieve the information the physician needs, (e) may not be able to communicate the retrieved information to the physician, or (f) may mistakenly communicate erroneous information to the physician [an old computerese acronym, GIGO (garbage in, garbage out) applies to people as well as computers].

17

Computer systems have obvious theoretical advantages over telephone systems as mechanisms for communicating information to and from physicians. Perhaps most significantly, there is the elimination of the person at the other end of the line. Speed of data communication is usually greatly enhanced by a computer system. A computer can gather and distribute information from and to many sources and destinations simultaneously. Compared to the telephone's ability to handle only voice-range audio, a computer can handle information of many different types—text, still and moving images, full range audio, and any other conceivable energy pattern (for example, EKGs, EEGs, pressure readings during cardiac catheterization and spirometry). Computer systems are much better than telephone systems at indexing information resources, an issue that is becoming increasingly important as the sheer quantity of available information multiplies yearly at an overwhelming rate.

Still, telephone systems, having been commercially available nearly 50 years longer than computer systems, have certain advantages inherent in their maturity and relative simplicity compared to computer systems. Until recently, the telephone network connected the physician to a far greater number of information resources than could his computer. Indeed, until the last decade or so, the idea of a physician owning his/her very own "personal computer," unlike a personal telephone, was a Jules Verne-ish fantasy. However, with the birth of the microelectronics industry in the 1970s (a direct result of the American space exploration program in the previous decade), the idea of the personal computer soon became very real.

The telephone still very much has the advantage over the computer in terms of the human interface: no civilized person today does not know how to dial a telephone, but only a distinct minority of current humanity understands how to use a computer to retrieve, enter, or process information. Both the layman and the physician are significantly hindered in their use of computers by the plethora of vastly different computer systems currently in use, whereas successful use of a telephone anywhere in the world requires knowing only how to dial a telephone number and how to use a telephone directory or, at a minimum, how to call the telephone operator.

Computer systems are maturing and catching up with telephone systems at an almost dizzying pace and promise to be the workstations of choice. This change in the physician's *modus operandi* is so significant as to qualify as a genuine paradigm shift. The physical expanse of the global computer network is just beginning to approach that of the global telephone network, and computers are just beginning to be as pervasive in First World cultures as telephones had become decades ago. Thus, information available previously only by paper or telephone is just now in this decade becoming available by computer. It is anticipated that in the near future the global telephone, cable television, and computer networks will effectively merge into a single network through which all information is transmitted in digital form. (It is this network that is currently referred to in the popular press as the information superhighway.) The year 1994 saw the arrival of the first personal computers that can not only perform all the usual computing tasks but can also act as a telephone/answering machine/fax machine *and* display any desired cable TV channel.

Other advantages of computers help further to explain why they will be the workstations of choice. First, with each passing year, user interfaces (the methods by which users give instructions to and receive responses from their computers) are becoming more standardized, requiring less investment of the user's time to learn a new system and start using it productively. (The telephone, a far simpler device, never had to face this issue to any significant degree.) The standardization of computers—or at least the standardization of their interfaces to humans as well as to other computers—is now being recognized as a critical feature required for a new computer system to be successful. Second, elimination of the human at "the other end of the line" significantly reduces information retrieval delays and also can reduce significantly (but probably never entirely eliminate) the GIGO problem. Third, the computer can not only collect data from multiple sources simultaneously but can analyze data for hidden significance. These abilities to collect and analyze data from multiple sources, combined with the computer's speed, will make it as easy for the physician researcher to sift through an entire nation's collective clinical database to unearth important public health trends as it will be for the private practitioner to sift through the complete biomedical literature of the last five decades for information he needs to help in establishing a treatment plan for a patient afflicted with a rare disease. Both of these physicians will accomplish these tasks and a multitude of others via the personal workstations at their workplaces.

Despite the benefits to be reaped with the use of computer systems in the practice of medicine, one must remember that new technologies are always accompanied by new problems, and medical computer systems are certainly not exempt from this fact of life. Infrastructure and security are likely to be the two biggest concerns in this area. First, the investment in the infrastructure (computer equipment, networks, computer programming) needed to establish standard interfaces among medical computers and between medical computers and humans is staggering, likely to be several orders of magnitude beyond that required for establishing telephone system standards. The obvious corollary is that as the investment in the standard architecture grows, so will grow the reluctance in the future to upgrade to another standard that may be proposed in order to take advantage of the improvements that are certain to come in data processing systems. This observation implies that during the design of standards for medical computer systems, extreme effort should be placed on anticipating future developments and designing the standard to be able to accommodate upgrades as easily as possible. The well-designed physician workstation will bear the marks of such efforts.

Second, data security becomes a frighteningly Medusan problem with the transition of medical data from paper databases to computer databases. In general, as barriers to legitimate information access (such as access time) fall with electronic systems, so do barriers to illegitimate access. The challenge becomes the retention of barriers to illegitimate access without burdening legitimate access methods with safeguards to a degree that completely negates the efficiency gain otherwise realized by having instantaneous access to information. Certainly, different environments in which information is accessed will require different solutions. A simple user-identification/password system may be quite sufficient for a private practitioner's office, whereas much more rigorous user-identification methods, such as fingerprints or magnetic strip-encoded data access cards (similar to credit cards), may be necessary for large institutions. Can a consultant make a patient encounter note in his office's database accessible to the referring physician but no one else? Can a patient in a multispecialty practice or large institution truly receive confidential psychiatric treatment without other healthcare personnel being able to find any scraps of online information that would even suggest the patient is receiving such treatment? Will an AIDS-infected politician be able to trust his physicians' (and pharmacists', and third party payors') computer systems to keep his diagnosis confidential and inaccessible to all except those who truly need to know? Will interphysician electronic mail, in which patient matters will be routinely discussed, be considered as confidential as the electronic patient medical record? But in such an environment of data secrecy, how can one conduct clinical research? Can provisions be made to allow access by authorized users to all data except identifying information? Standard solutions for these and many related problems must be developed and implemented as computer systems penetrate further and further into the physician's daily life. The design of the physician workstation will of necessity be heavily influenced by the manner in which these problems are addressed.

To be sure, the paradigm shift described above will have little to no impact on the essence of the doctor/patient relationship—the hands-on physical examination or the face-to-face discussion of various matters of the patient's health. But as physicians find it necessary in the coming years to stay abreast of more and more information and to process this information more and more efficiently, the computerized physician workstation surely will play a steadily increasing role in the physician's daily practice.

Physician Workstations: The State of the Art

The original computerized physician workstations provided only one significant advantage over the telephone: elimination of the inherent delays caused by the person at the other end of the line. Were it not for this being such a significant advantage, the problems with early computers clearly would have prevented their penetrating as far as they have into clinical practice today. First, the early computer workstations were nothing more than simple keyboard/video units called "dumb" terminals because they had no built-in microprocessors (and thus no ability to analyze data). All of the actual processing of data was performed in a large, central computer, or mainframe. This arrangement required an expensive network of cable be laid throughout the institution's false ceilings for the exclusive purpose of connecting the computer to the terminals. Changing a terminal's location (or, perish the thought, changing the central computer's location!) was discouraged in view of the cable rerouting expense. A second problem was that usually only one type of data, typically lab test results, was available, because separate computers for management of separate types of data would obviously require separate networks of cabling and terminals. Early computers were reasonably well suited for managing numerical data such as lab results, but text management capabilities (e.g., for patient encounter notes) were primitive, and image management was something that would eventually come in the next century. Also, early computers had little flexibility to handle more than one type of data. A third problem was that user interfaces were almost universally cryptic, requiring an entirely new vocabulary of codes and commands to use the system. A fourth problem was to be found behind the scenes: programming the early computers to perform even the simplest tasks was relatively difficult, usually making the team of computer caretakers appear to be inadequately responsive to the data processing needs of the users.

The modern era dawned for most large institutions in the 1980s due to three principal technological advances: (1) improved mainframe computers that were easier to program, (2) the introduction of the personal computer, and (3) the redevelopment of the cable network as an entity apart from any one computer. Each successive generation of central computers has shown a substantial improvement in the ability to handle a wide array of data types, and with each new generation has also come an ever more sophisticated set of programming tools that make it easier for the computer caretaker to manipulate data in ways requested by the users. Replacement of the dumb terminal with a personal computer as a physician workstation opened the door to an entirely new paradigm of data management, one in which the central computer finally could be focused on what it does best— storage, processing, and output of data—whereas the outlying terminal could be focused on translating the cryptic output into a form easily understood by the user, and vice versa on the input side. Previously, it had been too much of a burden on the central computer to accomplish both of these tasks. Finally, establishing the cable network as an independent entity made it possible to not only link multiple central computers to a single system of cables but also have the personal computer (PC) workstation act as a single interface (conceptually, at least) between the human and the central computers (Figure 2-1). In the early years of this transition, the PC

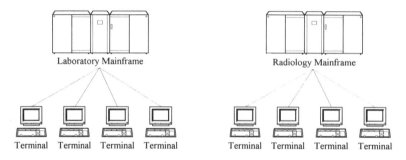

A. Before the network, separate computer systems required separate cable systems linking them to dedicated terminals. Input commands and output formats are different for each system.

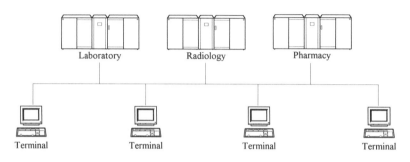

B. The network eliminates redundant cabling (and excessive terminals) and enables each terminal to access multiple types of data. Each central computer still has unique input commands and output formats.

FIGURE 2-1. Impact of the network on data accessibility.

still presented to the user a different interface for each central computer, thus continuing to require a forbidding amount of user education and complicating efforts to make new central computers available to the user community. However, at least physically distinct terminals were not required for access to different types of data—in theory, anyway. In practice, application-specific terminals (such as digital radiology display stations) continue to haunt even the institutions at the vanguard of today's ongoing medical informatics revolution. The much vaunted concept of the so-called universal workstation is much closer to reality today than it was a decade ago, but it will be years yet before the technology for such a panacean interface spreads beyond but the largest institutions.

With these developments, a steadily increasing number of types of data have become available online in the last decade. It is not uncommon at a large institution today for the physician to have access via his or her workstation to laboratory test results, radiology reports (sometimes even the actual images!), pathology results, other specialized testing reports, transcribed physicians' dictation, nursing information, physicians' orders, patient demographic information and encounter histories, and a wealth of data from the institution's pharmacies. Although the availability of such an expanse of clinical data may seem attractive to today's private practitioner, a critical review of most "state-of-the-art" physician workstations finds a substantial drawback: a different user interface for nearly every central computer, the problems of which were discussed above. Slowly, both central computer systems and physician workstations are being redesigned to present a common, intuitive interface regardless of the type of data being requested by the physician. As the speed and other capabilities of the PC improve, user interfaces are evolving from text-based interfaces (text user interfaces, or TUIs) requiring substantial keyboard input (a problem for most physicians who are not proficient typists) to image-based interfaces (so-called graphical user interfaces, or GUIs), which only require the physician to recognize, for example, that pointing the mouse at the miniature chest x-ray icon will call up radiology data. The rest of this decade and much of the next will continue to see an evolution toward a common, intuitive GUI for the universal physician workstation, but this development will mainly alleviate problems with data retrieval. Designing a system to accept physician input in a practical, efficient manner opens a Pandora's box of problems, and this matter is considered in detail in the next section.

One Institution's Experience

The above-mentioned evolution in data availability and user interface design is amply demonstrated at our institution. Prior to 1988, the only clinical data available online to the physician at our institution were laboratory test results. A central mainframe computer in the hospital laboratory was hard wired to dumb terminals located chiefly at the hospital's nursing stations. No security codes were required to achieve access, and most users were able to retrieve data in only one fashion: request all available data on the specified patient, in reverse chronological order—usually sufficient for routine daily work, but highly inefficient for retrieving the result of the erythropoietin level ordered two weeks previously or of the tuberculosis cultures submitted six weeks ago. Technically, the system could handle such specialized requests, but no user could make such a request because the command vocabulary necessary was too cryptic to learn or remember. Much time was spent by physicians scrolling through page after page of unneeded data to get to the desired results, but they spent the time anyway because it was still faster than calling the main laboratory, only to be transferred to a specialty laboratory and wait for a technician (who also had a terminal available but could not remember the necessary commands either) to wade through a hardcopy log book to find the results.

StatLAN

In 1988, after substantial investment in upgrading the cabling system and other network paraphernalia and obtaining a critical mass of PCs, our institution rolled out the new StatLAN data retrieval system to all clinical areas of the hospital. StatLAN, a product of Simborg Systems Corporation, embodied many of the concepts of the new era in clinical computing that were discussed above in the abstract. StatLAN acts as a translator or "gateway" between a workstation and an array of widely different central computers—the user identifies a particular patient and then requests a type of data from that patient's record. StatLAN passes the request through the network to whichever central computer harbors the desired data. The central computer retrieves the data and presents it back to StatLAN as fast as possible so that it (the central computer) can then be freed to respond to other requests. Because the central computer is not presenting the data directly to the user, it is relieved of the burden of processing the data into a format suitable for display on the user's workstation. That task is handled by StatLAN. StatLAN assesses the returned data and then turns around and retransmits the data to the workstation, this time with formatting instructions included. The program running on the workstation's microprocessor receives the data and shows the data in an easily understood format. Some sample StatLAN displays are shown in Figure 2-2. Some security is provided in that access to StatLAN does require the user to enter an assigned user identification and password, and the system will automatically log a user off the system after a period of inactivity. The user interface in a StatLAN workstation is a TUI using a simple menu driven by single keystrokes. StatLAN itself does not store any data, nor does it provide any analytical tools. Principal types of data currently available on StatLAN are patient location, basic patient demographics, and laboratory, radiology, and pathology reports. The hospital's central bed tracking system is also interfaced, or gatewayed, to StatLAN so that ward clerks can perform all ADT (Admission, Discharge, or Transfer) functions through the StatLAN workstation. A primitive electronic mail system is also integrated into the product. Workstations are physically located at essentially every site on campus where health care is delivered (nursing stations, physician workrooms, outpatient clinics, specialty units such as dialysis, pre-op, and post-op) but generally not in administrative areas. Our institution currently has approximately 225 StatLAN workstations and 5200 StatLAN users. The computer novice physician can be taught the essentials of the system in approximately five minutes. A novice StatLAN user who is a poor typist can access the system, request some testing results, and see the requested data appear on the screen in approximately 30 to 60 seconds. An experienced StatLAN user who is a good typist can perform the same operation in less than 10 seconds.

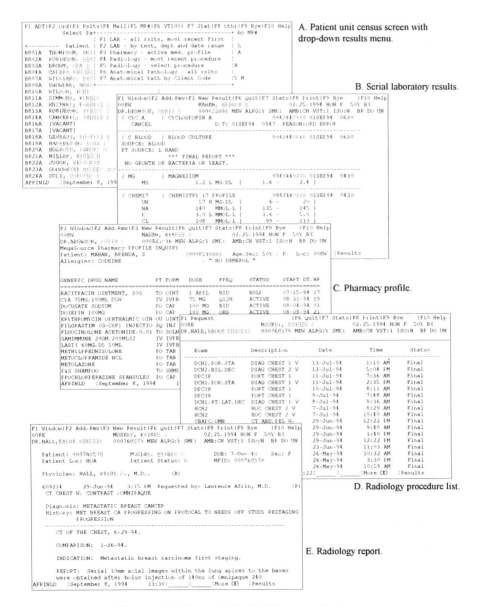

A. Patient unit census screen with drop-down results menu.

B. Serial laboratory results.

C. Pharmacy profile.

D. Radiology procedure list.

E. Radiology report.

FIGURE 2-2. Sample StatLAN screen displays.

Practice Partner System

On another front, certain of our institution's ambulatory care clinics use the Practice Partner system from Physicians' Micro Systems, Inc. (PMSI) to collect point-of-care information. Like StatLAN, the Practice Partner user interface is a TUI and is heavily dependent on the user pressing various function keys to accomplish desired operations. Also like StatLAN, Practice Partner is interfaced to our institution's laboratory and radiology computer systems, allowing retrieval of these important elements of clinical data. However, there the similarities end, as Practice Partner's chief function is actually to maintain a longitudinal medical record. Practice Partner stores in a central database a variety of clinical data including problem lists, histories and physicals, progress notes, medication profiles, and reports from laboratory, radiology, and other ancillary systems that may be interfaced. Although physicians are certainly allowed to type their own progress notes into the system, most still choose to dictate, and a transcriptionist then enters the notes for subsequent physician review and electronic signature (essentially, entering a password). In practice, the only type of data that most physicians routinely enter themselves is medication data because of the ease of having the system print prescriptions. Included in the laboratory chart functions is a capability for basic graphing of laboratory test values to help in trend identification. Although an elementary figure drawing program is included, the system is not capable of displaying actual images such as x-rays. However, image display admittedly is an exceedingly difficult task to accomplish well in the TUI environment. Because GUI-based systems (such as those running under the Microsoft Windows or X environments) are inherently and easily able to manipulate images, it is doubtful that any significant imaging capabilities will ever be found in a TUI-based product for a physician's workstation.

Sample displays from the Practice Partner system are shown in Figure 2-3. Usually, cursor-movement keys on the keyboard (such as the up and down arrows) are used to move from one menu option to the next, although there are numerous function key-driven shortcuts for navigating around the system if one takes the time to learn such subtleties. Clearly, the system requires a significant amount of keyboard input. Thus, it is no surprise that the system has not found unanimous acceptance among the physician populations it serves—those physicians who type proficiently are more active participants in the system than their "two-finger, hunt and peck" counterparts. Still, its advantages are so obvious and conducive to providing efficient patient care that even poor typists will usually concede the system to be a significant improvement over the old paper-based system. Our institution currently has approximately 140 PMSI workstations and a similar number of users. Basic physician training time is typically 2 to 3 hours.

OACIS

As a final real-world example meant to illustrate the current leading edge technology in physician workstations, we will briefly describe the OACIS product (Open Architecture Clinical Information Systems), initially conceived and developed by Bell Atlantic Healthcare Systems and currently continuing development under the aegis of OACIS Healthcare Systems. Our institution has served as an alpha test site for this product since 1991.

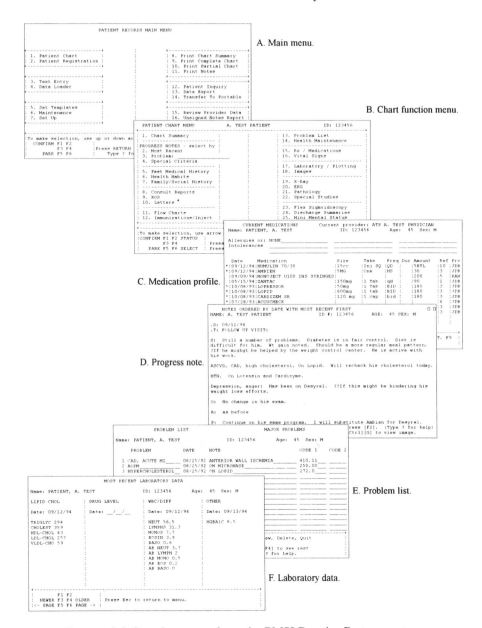

FIGURE 2-3. Sample screens from the PMSI Practice Partner system.

(The "alpha" stage of development essentially means the software is highly experimental, numerous bugs are likely to exist, and considerable modifications may be made to any aspect of the project before release of the software to any additional users.) The OACIS concept is similar to Practice Partner: to provide the practitioner with a longitudinal view of his patients' medical records as well as the tools to analyze the data in those records.

However, the design of OACIS is much more robust than Practice Partner, and the product requires substantially more powerful central computers and workstation computers to provide acceptable performance. Although Practice Partner can easily be adapted to a group practice, OACIS is clearly targeted more at sizable medical institutions, though certainly neighboring practices can be equipped with additional workstations to also participate in the system. Also, OACIS makes use of a sophisticated GUI rather than a TUI, an aspect that is not only highly attractive to keyboard-shy physicians but also provides considerably greater potential for displaying a diversity of clinical data.

OACIS has many facets. The most central one is the Clinical Database, which continuously and cumulatively acquires patient data as they are generated by all interfaced systems. Currently, all the systems available through StatLAN are also reporting data to the OACIS Clinical Database. Also, the hospital transcription system and certain ambulatory clinic transcription systems are interfaced to OACIS. Access to OACIS, like StatLAN, is controlled via a user identification and password unique to each user; OACIS also automatically logs a user off the system after a period of inactivity. OACIS, however, additionally requires the user to change his or her password each time a configurable interval (usually a few months) has elapsed. Upon gaining access to OACIS, the user is presented with a table called a patient "roster" (Figure 2-4). The user's current list of patients, from which

Practitioner LAWRENCE BRIAN AFRIN		Facility MUSC				User Roster clinic		
Location	Patient Name	LAB	RAD	MICRO	PATH	ENCOUNTER	TRNSCR	CHART
	ADAMS, ...	1mo			1y	1mo	1mo	*
010E B105 A	AILL., ...	1d	1d	17h	7mo	1w	1mo	*
	ANCRUM, ...	3mo	3mo		9mo	1mo	3mo	*
	BLACK, ...	3mo	4mo			4mo	2mo	*
	BOYD, ...	51mi	1w	3w	6mo	1w	3w	*
	BROWN, ...	1d	1mo	1y	1y	1w	1w	*
	CLEVEL..., ...	3h	5mo	1y	1mo	2mo	2mo	*
	COX, ...	4mo	4mo			4mo	4mo	*
	CUTSHAL..., ...	7mo				7mo	6mo	*
	DESROSI..., ...	3w	3w			4w	5mo	*
	DORITY, ...	1mo	7mo		7mo	1mo	1mo	*
	FLOYD, ...	5mo	5mo			5mo	5mo	*
	GIBSON, ...	3mo	1y	1y		3mo	2mo	*
	GILME..., ...	3mo	3mo			4mo	3mo	*
	GOURD..., ...	1mo	1mo		4mo	1mo	1mo	*

Close   Print...   Cleanup   Lookup Pat...   Pat. List...   Roster Menu   Help

FIGURE 2-4. Sample window from an OACIS display showing a patient roster. Time intervals in the grid indicate when the latest data was received. Intervals in bold type indicate data has been received that has not been displayed yet. The more darkly shaded box (solid arrow) is actually displayed in red, indicating a critical value that has not been displayed yet. Because the system also is interfaced to the hospital's bed tracking system, the user is automatically made aware of patient admissions, transfers, and discharges (outlined arrow).

he may add or delete patients at any time, is listed down the left-hand side of the table. Each table column is labeled with the name of a service such as laboratory, radiology, or any one of the other types of data collected by OACIS into its permanent clinical database. Some services can be broken into components. For example, microbiology can be separated out from laboratory into its own column. Each user can have multiple rosters (for example, an inpatient list, a Tuesday clinic list, or an AIDS patient list), and the columns can be easily custom configured by the user for each roster independently. At the intersection of any given row and column in the table is an elapsed time telling the user how long it has been since patient X has had a new result reported by service Y. No matter how long it has been since the user last reviewed a patient's data, he or she can instantly identify what data have not been reviewed because the elapsed times in those boxes in the table will be displayed in bold type. These "not yet reviewed" flags are maintained separately for each user; therefore, just because a consultant reviews newly available data on a patient does not affect the bolding of the appropriate elapsed time on the roster of the patient's primary physician. By moving the mouse pointer to a box of interest and clicking the mouse button, the user sees ("drills down to") more data in that area. These data may be, for example, a submenu of services, a report summary, or a detailed report. The general principle is that the system only presents the user with one level of detail at a time. The user can drill down to any level of detail needed (Figure 2-5). Any displayed data can be printed.

The user may also select from the roster that a particular patient's data be displayed as a table-like "chart." A chart in this sense is similar to an oncologist's flowsheet. Data from a variety of services (various labs, items of nursing information, pharmaceuticals, etc.) are listed down the left-hand side, dates and times across the top, and the boxes in the table are filled in accordingly. Any type of data can be included in a chart. If the actual piece of data (a radiology report, for example) cannot be conveniently fitted into the allotted box, the user is given an indication in the box that clicking on that point will allow retrieval of the full result. Most types of data can be displayed in a number of different ways, whichever suits the user's needs or tastes best. For example, an oncologist can set up his flowsheet to display a series of white blood cell counts either as the actual counts or as a line graph (with the area between lower and upper limits of normal being shaded), essentially giving a picture at a glance as to the patient's position in the chemotherapy/neutropenia cycle (Figure 2-6). Each user can establish multiple custom charts and change on the fly which chart is used to display a patient's data. For example, a pulmonologist may prefer one chart for his ICU patients and a separate one for his clinic patients, but for the critically ill leukemia patient in his care, it occasionally may be helpful to "flip" back and forth between an ICU chart and a leukemia chart.

The OACIS user interface is a fully windowed GUI running on a PC. Each click of the mouse sends the request through the campus network to

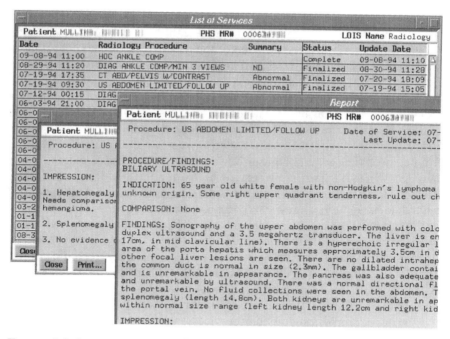

FIGURE 2-5. Sample OACIS windows illustrating the principle of "drilling down" to display greater degrees of detail.

the Clinical Database computer (typically a powerful minicomputer or mainframe). The Clinical Database returns the requested data to the program running on the Clinical Display workstation, which opens a new window and appropriately formats the display of this next layer of data detail. The quest for data need not be pursued in a strictly hierarchical fashion. The user can be buried six levels deep in windows of pharmacy information on one patient, then with a single click return the roster to the top of the stack of windows, select a different patient and/or service, and begin pursuing that path. "Clean-up" buttons exist on higher-level windows to permit the user to click but once to close all windows that followed from the one containing the "clean-up" button. Other capabilities of OACIS are too numerous to recount here. OACIS is currently being piloted in a few areas in our institution. Approximately 40 dedicated OACIS workstations are spread throughout these areas, together with about 60 additional nondedicated workstations, and over 500 users are registered. Basic physician training time is only 5 to 10 minutes, basically because of the simplicity of the graphical interface. Training in the more advanced features of OACIS requires an additional 15 to 30 minutes.

The chief advantage to systems like OACIS (and StatLAN and Practice Partner) is that whenever one wants to begin capturing a new source of

Horizontal Chart										
Patient MULLINS, ... PHS MR# 00063...						User TimeChart HonFlow2				
	Jun94		Jul94					aug94		aug94
	19	26	3	10	17	24	31	7	14	21
SODIUM (mmol/L)	newest		138	140	134				139	
POTASSIUM (mmol/L)	newest		3.4	4.7	4.1				3.9	
CHLORIDE (mmol/L)	newest		98	108	104				102	
CO2 CONTENT (mmol/L)	newest		28	21	24				29	
UREA NITROGEN, BLOOD (BUN) (mg/dL)	newest		8	8	9				10	
GLUCOSE, SERUM (mg/dL)	newest		126	91	141				133	
CREATININE (mg/dL)	newest		.9	0.9	0.9				.8	
MAGNESIUM (mg/dL)	newest			1.7						
CALCIUM (mg/dL)	newest			9.1						
PHOSPHORUS (mg/dL)	newest		2.7	3.0					4.0	
URIC ACID, SERUM (mg/dL)	newest		6.5	6.5					6.1	
TOTAL PROTEIN, SERUM (g/dL)	newest		6.1	5.5					6.3	
ALBUMIN, SERUM (g/dL)	newest		4.1	3.4					4.2	
BILIRUBIN, TOTAL (mg/dL)	newest		.8	1.0					1.1	
ALKALINE PHOSPHATASE(Inactive) (IU/L)	newest									
AST (SGOT) (IU/L)	newest		32	33					30	
ALT (SGPT) (IU/L)	newest		18	17					19	
LACTATE DEHYDROGENASE, SERUM (IU/L)	newest		254	449					185	
HCT 47.00 % 21.50										
HGB (gm/dL) 10.30 1.20	newest	9.8	9.8	8.9	7.7	7.6	8.2	7.4	8.0	9.7	10.7
WBC (K/cumm)										
NEUTROPHILS (%)	newest	66.8	60	58	48	55	48	41	38	36	40

Close Print... Save... Select... Make Data Time... Vertical Columns... Delete... Help

FIGURE 2-6. Sample OACIS chart demonstrating an oncology flowsheet generated from a chemotherapy patient's record.

data, one merely has to add the necessary translation functions into the system's front-end gateway and, if necessary, extend the workstation program to be able to display the new type of data. The potential for extending any of these systems to cover extra-institutional data sources is obvious (other hospitals, private offices, community pharmacies, etc.).

The chief problem to be faced by designers of all such systems will be query response time. Systems that do not themselves store any data (such as StatLAN) or that display only one type of data for one patient at a time (such as Practice Partner) do not face this problem nearly to the degree faced by systems that display multiple types of data for multiple patients simultaneously (such as OACIS). This holds true regardless of whether the user interface is text or graphical based, as systems such as OACIS by their very nature being asked to process far greater amounts of data in generating displays. Yet, it does not take a degree in psychology for one to realize that the typical user, usually a busy physician or nurse, will not wait for any response more than a few seconds before concluding, perhaps, that the system is too inefficient to be of any practical use.

Other major problems to be addressed by the designer of any physician workstation will include direct provider data input. Security will have to be substantially tightened, but specific policies will likely be different from institution to institution. The one constant to be expected is that the issue will likely become almost breathtakingly complicated. (For example, a surgeon should not be able to read his patient's psychiatrist's encounter notes. For that matter, the surgeon should not even be able to find out his patient is under the care of a psychiatrist if the patient has not authorized release of that knowledge to the surgeon.) User preferences for different personal computers (for example, IBM-compatible vs. Macintosh) will further complicate development of advanced workstations. Another issue to be of increasing importance (especially as networks start transmitting medical image data) is that of "bandwidth," a computer term referring to the maximum capacity of a computer data transmission line to convey data. A transmission line with a capacity of 10 million bits per second that served well in the 1980s will be completely inadequate by the mid to late 1990s, when data transmission traffic will have grown to the point where bandwidth of at least 100 million bits per second will be necessary.

The Future: Finally, the World at Your Fingertips

Advances in physician workstations in the coming years will be driven largely by advances in computer and network hardware. Tools exist today to develop most of the software that an ideal physician workstation should have. The problem is that with today's hardware, system response time would be totally unacceptable. This phenomenon is already being seen in some of the more ambitious clinical computing projects of late. A system that takes longer than a few seconds to respond to a physician's query will have that physician looking elsewhere for solutions to his information processing needs.

Today's most advanced commercially available microprocessors execute an admittedly respectable 10 to 100 million instructions per second, but the microprocessor in the physician's workstation of 2005 will beat this by at least an order of magnitude. Networks now moving 1 billion bits of data per second will need to outperform this rate by at least two to three orders of magnitude. This increase will be necessary in some part due to so many more people being connected to the network, all of whom will be entering and retrieving information via the network. The largest part of the increase, however, will be due to a huge increase in transmission of images. To put the matter in better perspective, one must appreciate that whereas a page of text can be represented in digital form in roughly 20,000 bits (a bit is the unit of all digital information), a color image requiring the same amount of printed space is represented in 2,000,000,000 bits, a difference of five orders of magnitude. Various technological skulduggery can reduce this difference to only two to three orders of magnitude, but not much more. Further, there is the matter of transmission of video information, which conceptually is nothing more than the transmission of a rapid series of still images. How rapid? The human eye must see at least 30 images per second for the mind to be convinced that the objects in the images are moving smoothly. The mathematical consequences are obvious.

Fortunately, the technology to achieve these higher processing and transmission speeds is already being developed and is fully expected to be available commercially by late this century or early in the next. If we presume such a technology base to be available, what form can we imagine the physician workstation will assume?

First, it will assume at least two different forms physically, the desktop workstation and the pocket workstation. Both will give the physician access to the same set of data entry and retrieval capabilities via an identical user interface. Indeed, so will any clinical workstation the physician uses (at the hospital, at the office, at home, consulting at an outreach clinic, etc.). However, the desktop unit will have advantages of a larger video monitor that can display more information at a time, greater capabilities for data analysis, and freedom from concerns of exhausting a battery pack. The pocket unit will have the same access to information as the desktop unit thanks to a wireless connection to the network. The pocket unit will make a physician's stack of index cards or other personal patient data filing system obsolete. Both units will integrate video, telephone, and fax services with all data processing services. Aside from the workstation itself, the network will make the location of a desired piece of data irrelevant. Whether a progress note is stored in the office computer, a lab result in a laboratory computer, an echocardiogram in a consultant's computer, or a dosage in a published research paper, the network will not only make it as easy to access the one as the other but more than likely will know automatically which computers or databases to query to access. The *data* will be all that is important; the behind-the-scenes *process* by which the data are obtained will be invisible, irrelevant, and ignored by the physician.

What clinical data will be available? Essentially all of it! And accessible in a near instant, too. Textual reports, still images, moving images, pressure curves, electrical tracings—indeed, any information-containing energy pattern imaginable.

A physician needs more than just clinical data, though. The average private practitioner may not think of it as such, but he is an avid researcher. One moment, he may need to consult a drug reference. A few patients later, he may need to review diagnostic criteria for a seldom-seen disease. Later, he may want to track down additional background information on a topic presented at the local medical school's grand rounds. At the end of the day, he may be reading a *New England Journal of Medicine* article and want to learn more about an intriguing aspect of cytokines discussed in the article. Then there is the academic physician, who might have all the same needs as the private practitioner and also could benefit from his computer keeping a constant watch on relevant databases for news of research developments and grant opportunities in his chosen field.

Fortunately, the information highway in its current form already provides the tools needed to accomplish such research missions. Information systems already available on the Internet, such as Gopher, WAIS, and the World Wide Web, provide the user with an inconceivable wealth of information. Unlike in the earlier, poorly indexed days of the Internet, when in order to retrieve a piece of the data one had to know its exact location, the user today is presented with a menu or page of information giving topics of interest. Figure 2-7 gives an example of this concept as implemented by the World Wide Web. Selecting a particular topic, or "link," causes the system to call up another menu or page giving more detail. Link after link can be pursued until the desired information is found, but no doubt along the way one will encounter other unexpected and intriguing items that also would be worthwhile pursuing. Tracking down specific information need not be a lengthy process, because this type of system encourages a high degree of cross-referencing. All the while, the location of each piece of information is irrelevant. Tracking down a piece of the data might require the user's computer to access a computer at the local medical school or pharmacy. On the other hand, the pursuit may require browsing through offerings

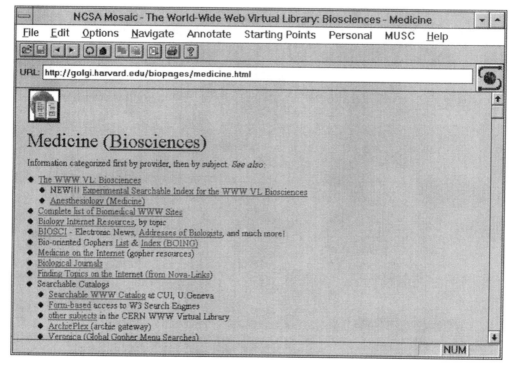

FIGURE 2-7. Sample screen from the NCSA Mosaic program, a software tool for accessing the World Wide Web.

contained in computers on five different continents. Regardless, the search requires only a few seconds of the physician's time!

These tools (which, we should remind the reader, are available today) are available for all the common user interfaces—Microsoft Windows, Macintosh, OS/2, and UNIX, to name a few. The recent migration of these tools to graphical user interfaces makes them far more accessible to the general population. Although in their usual form these tools are not crafted to ideally meet the specific needs of the physician, they can be configured fairly easily to meet such needs. Indeed, a single user can take advantage of multiple configurations. For example, the tools on an academic physician's clinic workstation can be configured to give rapid access to clinical databases, whereas the workstation in his office or lab can be set up to give rapid access to research databases. (Both configurations would still provide access to all other types of data as well.)

Beyond clinical and research data systems, though, are the mundane but logistically critical systems such as visit scheduling, third-party reimbursement processing, vacation and leave scheduling for employees, and many other such applications. All of these systems will be available through the same user interface, and all will be available through the network. The busy physician, finishing rounds at the hospital, can access (via the network) his office's computer and consult his appointment schedule for the day. Later in the day, when receiving a visit from his accountant, he can use his desktop workstation to analyze his office's performance in the last quarter in terms of billings and collections. When he receives a letter from the PPO in which he participates claiming he is hospitalizing too many of his patients for too long, he can independently investigate the PPO's contention by using his workstation to access the hospital's computer(s) and request the relevant statistics. Logistical support systems will be interfaced to clinical systems, too. Each day a "patient reminder" system could automatically search the office's clinical database and send reminder letters to patients who are due or overdue for a particular service or test. The conditions that trigger such letters would be definable by each physician. When a physician in a group practice decides to take vacation, the computer could send rescheduling notices to all patients scheduled for routine visits, and contact the computers at colleagues' offices to schedule visits for patients who must be seen while he is on vacation.

We have considered thus far in this section the physician's access to data already in "the system," but an equally important consideration is how the practitioner himself will get data into the system. Indeed, intuitive GUIs will make data *retrieval* a fairly simple task for those physicians without undergraduate computer science degrees, but it should be noted that with respect to *input* of data, even a well-designed GUI may not make the system sufficiently efficient for routine use by the physician if the system does not handle the input with some degree of artificial intelligence. From the outset, it is clear that voice will be the major mode of input. Not even professional transcriptionists can type at the speed necessary to keep up with fluent dictation; certainly, physicians can do no better. It surely will be necessary for all physician's workstations (desktop, pocket, or other type) to accept voice input as continuous speech, something that today's most advanced systems still cannot achieve. The leading products in the field of voice recognition still require the physician to pause briefly between each word, yielding an effective transcription speed of only 40 words per minute, or about as fast as the average typist. This would be an unbearable decrease in efficiency for the typical practitioner. Most voice recognition systems also require the user to invest substantial time in training the system to understand his or her speech. If physicians are to find the same interface regardless of which computer they are actually using, this voice-training requirement also will not stand. Beyond the requirement for continuous voice recognition, though, is the necessity for the system to understand the difference between spoken and written communication and to translate appropriately. The dictation of many physicians does not even begin to approach grammatical correctness. Such notes may be acceptable when intended for internal use only, but when a report needs to be sent out, the physician is typically (and silently) helped to a significant degree by the transcriptionist who rearranges wording, inserts punctuation, and creates a reasonable sentence structure on the page. Designers of computerized dictation systems must address and solve this problem before such systems are useful to any but a handful of specialized markets.

In addition to voice recognition, true artificial intelligence will play innumerable other roles in the future physician's workstation. For example, the physician who dictates (or even types) "Pen Vee-K 500 q.i.d. for 7 days" in the "Plan" section of a patient encounter note will not stand for a system that requires him to then switch to the system's pharmacy display and re-enter the same data to keep the patient's medication profile up to date. The system will have to make that logical connection for itself and will also need to determine itself that the actual dose is 500 mg, not 500 units. (Even better, perhaps, during the actual encounter the physician could use his pen or stylus interface to scribble such a prescription on his combination pocket digitizing tablet/wireless-networked computer, which would simultaneously notify the main office computer to add the prescription to the encounter note's Plan section, add the prescription to the patient's medication profile, print out the prescription for the patient to pick up at the front desk, notify the appropriate third-party payor of the new prescription, and notify the computer at the patient's regular pharmacy of the new prescription so the pharmacist can have it filled in short order. The office computer could even query the computers of all the area pharmacies to determine whether an alternative pharmacy has a substantially better price!) Similarly, when the physician is in a hurry, wants recent lab results on patient John Smith, and does not know offhand John Smith's medical record number, the system should be able to "figure out" which of the 53 John Smiths in its database this particular physician is referring to based on available data such as which John Smiths have had lab work ordered recently and which of these John Smiths have this particular physician as their doctor. To date, no system anywhere close to commercial release can demonstrate such intelligent processing of physician input.

Other problems, too, will confront the future physician's workstation. Although it must provide access to an incredible scope of data, the user interface must be designed to be essentially intuitive. Training time needed will have to be minimal. Yet, the interface must be supremely flexible so that it can be custom configured to accommodate the different needs of different physicians. The tools for such configuration must be equally intuitive, as it is only the physician who knows how best his workstation can be configured to meet his needs; thus, it is the physician himself who will be performing such configurations.

The issue of data security and confidentiality will likely be even more of a problem in the future than it is today. We have discussed many ramifications of this issue in the previous sections, and the increased accessibility to data provided by the future physician's workstation only amplifies the gravity of the problem. (Consider, for starters, the physician researcher desiring access to a multi-institutional database of clinical data. Before searching the database, need he first obtain security clearances from each of the participating institutions? How long would that take? What about the myriad issues involved with electronic signatures? How does one prove that an electronic signature is valid?) Solutions will of necessity be complex and will probably be computerized to an extreme degree—in an environment where access to data must be near instantaneous, security checks must also be performed equally fast.

Still another problem will be the hardware in the system. As capabilities for data storage and data transmission speed improve, software to take advantage of those capabilities will follow and ultimately stretch the hardware to its limits—at which point better hardware will be needed, leading to new software, and so on. The circle never ends.

Thus, when we take a step back from the wondrous potential of computerized workstations and see some of the problems yet to be solved, it is only realistic to have some concerns about the inherent complexity of such systems. Can any system so complex ever truly work well? The problem with this perspective is its failure to acknowledge just how complex and error prone are current noncomputerized systems of handling medical data. Also, the quantity of data to be handled in the future is virtually guaranteed to rise exponentially, regardless of what kinds of systems (automated or manual) exist to handle the load. Although the systems that are capable of handling this load may not be much, if any, simpler than today's, they certainly must be faster—much faster. A physician who fails to keep up with the data processing demands of his practice not only places his patients at increased medical and financial risk but also risks harming his own financial welfare. Computerization of clinical data and instant accessibility to this data will be key factors supporting the successful practitioner in the future.

It will probably be a rare reader who, upon reflecting on this vision of the future, does not dream wistfully of simpler times when issues of practice efficiency, third-party payors, malpractice, incomprehensible scientific advances, etc., were not issues at all. The typical physician endured the rigors of medical school and postgraduate training primarily because he or she wanted to help patients feel better, *not* to juggle mountains of paper or gigabits of electronic data. Indeed, we all dream, but we all wake from our dreams to face reality. For some, dealing with future reality will be an entertaining challenge; for others, a nightmare; and for most of us, somewhere between those two extremes. Regardless of our personal place in this spectrum, the computerized physician's workstation will be the key to coping with it all.

Annotated Bibliography

Consistent with the current pace of technological advancement, the most current reports in the field of healthcare information systems are generally found in symposia proceedings and other outlets with relatively short lead-times from manuscript submission to presentation or publication. For many years the annual Symposium on Computer Applications in Medical Care (SCAMC) has been a popular forum for reporting the latest advancements in clinical computing, explaining the large number of SCAMC *Proceedings* citations below. Judging by the program for SCAMC '94, there again will be many papers in the 1994 *Proceedings* addressing workstation and user interface design, alternative input technologies, multisystem integration, large database research, use of Internet information tools, and other issues mentioned in this chapter. Listed below are selected references on some of these topics.

1. Although few papers have addressed physician workstation design as an isolated issue, most discussions of the issue have occurred in the context of various institutions' descriptions of their own, inhouse-designed health information systems.

Clayton, P.D., Sideli, R.V., & Sengupta, S. (1992). Open architecture and integrated information at Columbia-Presbyterian Medical Center. *MD Computing, 9*(5), 297–303.
Dewey, J.B., Manning P., & Brandt, S. (1993). Acceptance of direct physician access to a computer-based patient record in a managed care setting. *Proceedings of the Annual Symposium on Computer Applications in Medical Care, 17,* 79–83.

Fafchamps, D., Young, C.Y., & Tang, P.C. (1991). Modelling work practices: Input to the design of a physician's workstation. *Proceedings of the Annual Symposium on Computer Applications in Medical Care, 15,* 788–792.

Frassine, R., Bertelli, S., & Innocenti, E.B. (1993). Developing a general practice medical workstation: The integration aspect. *Proceedings of the Annual Symposium on Computer Applications in Medical Care, 17,* 238–242.

Hammond, J.E., Berger, R.G., Carey, T.S., Fakhry, S.M., Rutledge, R., Kichak, J.P., Cleveland, T.J., Dempsey, M.J., Tsongalis, N.M., & Ayscue, C.F. (1993). Progress report on the clinical workstation and clinical data repository at UNC hospitals. *Proceedings of the Annual Symposium on Computer Applications in Medical Care, 17,* 243–247.

Hammond, J.E., Berger, R.G., Carey, T.S., Rutledge, R., Cleveland, T.J., Kichak, J.P., & Ayscue, C.F. (1991). The physician's workstation: An example of end user integration of information systems. *Proceedings of the Annual Symposium on Computer Applications in Medical Care, 15,* 970–972,

Hendrickson, G., Anderson, R.K., Clayton, P.D., Cimino, J., Hripcsak, G.M., Johnson, S.B., McCormack, M., Sengupta, S., Shea, S., Sideli, R., et al. (1992). The integrated academic information management system at Columbia-Presbyterian Medical Center. *MD Computing, 9*(1), 35–42.

McDonald, C.J., Tierney, W.M., Overhage, J.M., Martin, D.K., Wilson, G.A. (1992). The Regenstrief Medical Record System: 20 years of experience in hospitals, clinics, and neighborhood health centers. *MD Computing, 9*(4), 206–217.

O'Dell, D.V., Tape, T.G., & Campbell, J.R. (1991). Increasing physician acceptance and use of the computerized ambulatory medical record. *Proceedings of the Annual Symposium on Computer Applications in Medical Care, 15,* 848–852.

Roderer, N.K., & Clayton, P.D. (1992). IAIMS at Columbia-Presbyterian Medical Center: Accomplishments and challenges. *Bulletin of the Medical Library Association, 80*(3), 253–262.

Safran, C., Rury, C., Rind, D.M., & Taylor, W.C. (1991). Outpatient medical records for a teaching hospital: Beginning the physician-computer dialogue. *Proceedings of the Annual Symposium on Computer Applications in Medical Care, 15,* 114–118.

Turley, J.P., & Connelly, D.P. (1993). The relationship between nursing and medical cultures: Implications for the design and implementation of a clinicians' workstation. *Proceedings of the Annual Symposium on Computer Applications in Medical Care, 17,* 233–237.

van Mulligen, E.M., Timmers, T., & van Bemmel, J.H. (1993). Does an integrated medical workstation really help clinicians? A formal user evaluation. *Proceedings of the Annual Symposium on Computer Applications in Medical Care, 17,* 219–223.

2. Stanford University and Hewlett-Packard Laboratories recently have been collaborating on interesting work on improving physician workstation "intelligence."

Suermondt, H.J., Tang, P.C., Strong, P.C., Young, C.Y., & Annevelink, J. (1993). Automated identification of relevant patient information in a physician's workstation. *Proceedings of the Annual Symposium on Computer Applications in Medical Care, 17,* 229–232.

Tang, P.C., Annevelink, J., Suermondt, H.J., & Young, C.Y. (1994). Semantic integration of information in a physician's workstation. *International Journal of BioMedical Computing, 35*(1–4), 47–60.

3. A few papers have described early efforts with alternative input technologies. Maturation of these technologies will certainly be accompanied by a rapidly increasing number of corresponding reports.

Linn, N.A., Rubenstein, R.M., Bowler, A.E., & Dixon, J.L. (1992). Improving the quality of emergency department documentation using the voice-activated word processor: Interim results. *Proceedings of the Annual Symposium on Computer Applications in Medical Care, 16,* 772–776.

Lussier, Y.A., Maksud, M., Desruisseaux, B., Yale, P., & St-Arneault, R. (1992). Pure MD: A computerized patient record software for direct data entry by physicians using a keyboard-free pen-based portable computer. *Proceedings of the Annual Symposium on Computer Applications in Medical Care, 16,* 261–264.

McDonald, C.J. (1990). Observations and opinions: Input technology. *MD Computing, 7*(4), 201–204.

Wormuth, D.W. (1992). SCUT: Clinical data organization for physicians using pen computers. *Proceedings of the Annual Symposium on Computer Applications in Medical Care, 16,* 845–846.

4. The development of extremely large clinical databases may offer tantalizing promise in the clinical research arena, but such a wealth of data also introduces a new set of problems for the researcher.

McDonald, C.J., & Hui, S.L. (1991). The analysis of humongous databases: Problems and promises. *Statistics in Medicine, 10,* 511–508.

Tierney, W.M., & McDonald, C.J. (1991). Practice databases and their uses in clinical research. *Statistics in Medicine, 10,* 541–557.

Questions

1. User interface design is as much a blend of art and science as is the practice of medicine itself. Due simply to substantial physical differences between the physician's desktop and portable workstations (e.g., size of the video screen, ease of use of the pointing device, data transmission speed of the unit's link to the network, etc.), the all-important user interfaces of these two stations will likely also have substantial differences. Yet, a standard user interface across many different hardware platforms will be essential to increasing physician acceptance of computers and decreasing training requirements. How would you solve this paradox? That is, if you could design your own physician workstation user interface, how would it look? What would it be capable of doing, and how would you access each of its functions? To what degree does the design of the interface depend on specific hardware? How can the differences in the desktop's and portable's interfaces be minimized or eliminated? Is this even a feasible goal with current technology?

2. The physician's workstation hardware will doubtlessly undergo continuous evolution as new advancements in technology appear.

   a. Consider storage technology: currently it takes one or two compact discs (CDs) to contain the entire contents of a set of encyclopedias; any piece of information on the disc is available within 200 to 400 milliseconds. However, by the end of this century, there should be commercial availability of memory technology in which a single chip the size of one's thumbnail can store as much data as it now takes an entire CD to store, and access speed will be on the order of a few nanoseconds. How will such improved memory technology affect the capabilities of the physician's workstation? Will there be a differential impact on desktop vs. portable workstations? What new applications might be possible?

   b. Consider video technology: at the time of this writing, a French group has just announced a startling development in basic transistor technology: transistors engraved into a thin sheet of soft, flexible plastic. Because the video screen on a portable computer is nothing more than a grid of very closely spaced transistors, one can imagine the development of a paper-thin, plastic, flexible video screen. In fact, considering the possibility of using a transparent plastic as the basis for such a screen, one could even imagine lining one's eyeglasses (or contact lenses?) with an invisible plastic film that, when the computer is turned off, allows normal vision, but when the computer is turned on, the computer's display appears projected in space in the user's visual field. Again, what new applications might be possible? (And, as with any new technology, what new problems might arise from its use?)

   c. Consider input technology: this chapter asserts that voice input, along with a modicum of artificial intelligence, will be the primary mode of input from the physician, but new developments on the horizon may provide even better functionality for physicians either as distinct alternatives to voice input or in combination with voice input. For example, some early work has been done in using EEG signals to control a computer. Also, a miniaturized camera in the computer's video display could watch the user's eye movements and correspondingly move the onscreen pointer, effectively making the user's own eyes function as a mouse. What new applications might be possible with these technologies? How might the physician's home, office, and portable workstations differ in their use of the various present and future input technologies?

3. As mentioned in this chapter, electronic data security is and will continue to be a major issue. A few realistic security-related situations were depicted in that discussion. What situations touching on the security issue might arise in your day-to-day practice or work with clinical data? Would harder or easier access to data help you in your work? Would a colleague

in your line of work feel the same? What would a colleague in a different specialty think about this point? Would harder access to the patient's data (and, thus, improved privacy) help or hurt the patient? (Be sure to consider different patient situations: access to the record of a typical outpatient at a clinic visit may need different security restrictions than access to the record of a patient brought unconscious into the emergency room!) How would you design a single security system flexible enough to provide, in every conceivable situation, an "appropriate" degree of protection against "inappropriate" access? How seriously must you compromise ease of (appropriate) access to achieve such security? When a security breach does occur, how can it be dealt with? For example, how should one handle the physician who routinely gives his user ID and password to his medical students or residents? What actions should be taken when a physician loses his portable workstation, or has it stolen from him?

4. Research is an important part of every physician's professional life. What kind of questions would you routinely want to research? What kinds of databases and/or analytical tools might be required to carry out this research? Are these databases and tools available today? Another consideration is clinical research: in oncology, for example, currently fewer than 5 percent of all patients eligible for a clinical trial are actually enrolled in one, largely due to logistical difficulties with data collection and reporting at most physicians' offices. In what ways might the "information superhighway" facilitate your or your colleagues' participation in organized clinical research activities?

Unit 2
Getting Networked

Unit Introduction

Unit Introduction

Today we have the technologies to create and support vital networks. The challenge is not only to use those technologies, but also to address critical organizational and political issues.

Crowe and Eckstein discuss the fragmented nature of existing information systems and the move towards managed care. They explain how electronic data interchange (EDI) creates an informatics structure for networks and data traffic in health care and describe its benefits. In their view, systems integration forms the basis for enterprise development and community health information networks (CHINs).

Pickton and Seehausen review the information systems strategies taken by the EHS Health Care System, beginning in 1980. The 1994 EHS report highlighted infrastructure, information management, new technology, and support. Through its integrated delivery system (IDS), EHS acknowledges the need for system-wide computing, from transactional systems and multiple gateways to data warehouses.

Rizzolo and DuBois describe the network developed by the American Journal of Nursing Company to support rural nursing. The network provides content through forums, continuing education offerings, patient information, news, and databases. The project also focuses on process issues (education and training) and future plans (content expansion and design).

3
Health Information Networks

GLENN D. CROWE AND MICHAEL G. ECKSTEIN

Although health care has made astonishing gains in adopting advanced medical technology, the concern over accelerating costs has created a new imperative: treat more people at less cost. We are now in the fourth decade of the use of computers in the healthcare setting, and the need for more powerful and comprehensive systems for improved information management has never been more clear.

If, indeed, 24 percent of the healthcare dollar is spent on administration (including recordkeeping), and as much as 40 percent of medical testing is redundant, simple math would say that, added together, this is more than 50 percent of the healthcare dollar. It has been said that the holy grail of health care is to integrate administrative, financial, and clinical systems. This, in its simplest form, would allow correlation of costs to patient outcomes. Most believe that it is possible to reduce costs and improve quality through community-wide integrated networks. The inherent problems are not insurmountable, but as historians know so well, ". . . to know where you're going, you must know where you've been."

Historical Perspective

The healthcare system in the United States remains in the dark ages when it comes to information technology—5 to 10 years years behind other industries in automating. Expenditures for information technology in this industry have averaged a meager 2.6 percent, whereas manufacturing spent 5 percent, and the banking industry spent 7 percent.

There are a number of reasons for this. One is the fact that too many chief information officers (CIOs) are "techies" and are not business savvy. The "basement to board room" phenomenon is just now being understood by CIOs in health care. Typically, the number one priority of a hospital was to get those bills out. As a result, all too often, the information services people have been viewed as administration's people with no appreciation for the clinical needs. Typically, these departments have reported to the chief financial officer (CFO), creating even another perceived "fiefdom," as though the healthcare industry needs one.

Products/software in health care is fragmented and disjointed. The present system is broken. Ninety percent of systems currently in place have never been fully implemented or completely utilized. Whereas X. 12 may be a standard for communication with the outside world, HL7 continues to have as many flavors as that most famous ice cream store. This is not an indictment of anyone, just a statement of reality.

Over 90 percent of information systems companies in place today have revenues less than $100 million. This limits the investment in new technologies and real development. This problem is aggravated by the millstone they must carry in the form of an existing client base that has made a substantial investment in the current technology. The fear of losing both continuing software sales and new sales/contracts (by announcing any radical departure from the currently supported system) freezes these companies and prevents them from starting over with a blank sheet of paper. Their experience would be invaluable in designing new "open" systems. Regrettably, all too often, the harsh realities of the bottom line prevent them from being truly innovative, that is, revolutionary as opposed to evolutionary.

Again, this is not an indictment. The trail of information systems companies in the healthcare industry is littered with skeletons of those who "bet the company" on technology that was not accepted by the slow, prodding demands.

Strategic Success Factors

Health care, a trillion dollar industry that consumes one-seventh of the gross national product (GNP), is both imploding and exploding (Figures 3-1 to 3-4):

- Hospitals are shrinking in importance.
- Managed care plans achieve most of their economies by stressing preventive care.
- Health care is integrating organizationally from a "cottage" industry into large community health information networks (CHINs) encompassing doctors and hospitals, plus all new settings.
- Today's 6000 acute care hospitals will be part of 500 to 700 (maybe less) major regional CHINs by the end of the decade.
- Big CHINs will buy from big companies and will demand full service, "good hands" business relationships/partnerships.

From the perspective of the chief executive officer (CEO), problems/ requirements are as follows:

- Fragmented, disparate systems create what is in effect a mystique of information systems/processes.

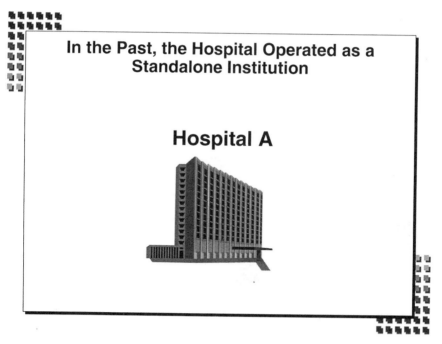

FIGURE 3-1. In the past, the hospital operated as a stand-alone institution.

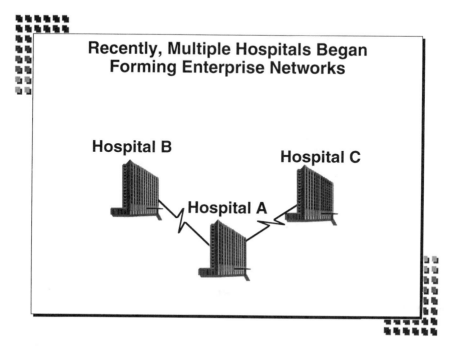

FIGURE 3-2. Recently, multiple hospitals began forming enterprise networks.

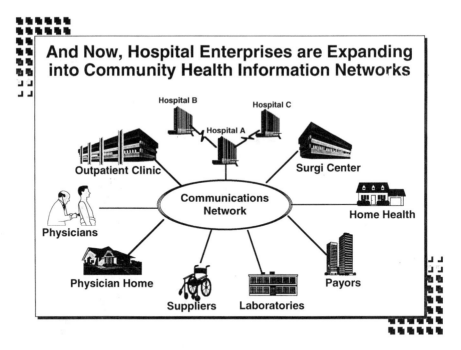

And Now, Hospital Enterprises are Expanding into Community Health Information Networks

FIGURE 3-3. And now, hospital enterprises are expanding into community health information networks.

- The transition from hospital to health system requires
  Process reengineering,
  Decision support for competitive information/contract management,
  Tools-scientific model,
  Cost reduction/outcome management,
  Mobile/adaptable computing (technology must follow the patient),
  Linking administrative/financial/clinical data to evaluate outcomes,
  Upgrading information technology, and
  Enhanced business functions.

Where We Are Today

The healthcare delivery system has radically and dramatically changed. The Bureau of Labor Statistics reflected in a November 1994 report the changes in types of medical care benefit plans for fulltime employees in large and medium private companies (Table 3-1).

As a result of these types of changes, the provider/payor relationships are very strained, but the alternate delivery models are growing rapidly. Managed care is here to stay—in a big way!

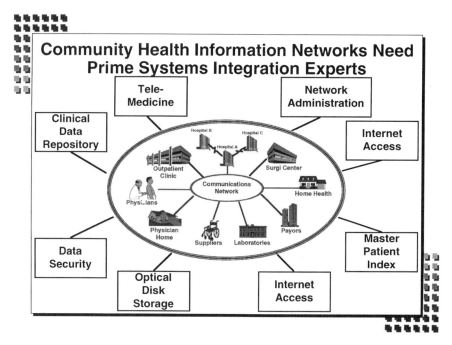

FIGURE 3-4. Community health information networks need prime systems integration experts.

The Market

The sum of all these trends is a healthcare system in dire need of help. Executives in these organizations are faced with figuring out how they might fit into a new system, as yet unidentified. The solutions are not easy or achieved without significant effort; and the decision makers have no one model that could allay their fears—yet. Experience has shown, however, that there are three key strategic issues for survival in this environment:

- Achieving a balance of specialization (today 70 percent of all doctors in the United States are specialists) within the overall organization,

TABLE 3-1. Medical Care Benefit Plans for Fulltime Employees, Large and Medium Private Companies

Type of Delivery System	1991	1993
Fee-for-service	67%	50%
Health Maintenance Organization (HMO)	17%	23%
Preferred Provider Organization (PPO)	16%	26%

Source: Bureau of Labor Statistics, November 1994.

- Guiding/controlling the physicians/professionals in managing the costs associated with providing healthcare services to the subsidiaries of the organization, and
- Having complete knowledge of the costs.

In short, you must be able to measure it if you are to manage it!

Managed Care

Managed care is a relatively new term coined to refer to the prepaid health-care sector, where care is provided under a fixed budget and costs therein are capable of being "managed." Originally descriptive of health mainte-nance organizations (HMOs), the term is now used to include preferred provider organizations (PPOs) and even forms of indemnity coverage that incorporate preadmission certification and other utilization controls. In a more global sense, a whole range of trends—sicker patients, more expen-sive treatment regimens, decreased reimbursement levels, more empty beds, and labor shortages—will force healthcare facilities to compete on the basis of cost as well as of quality, and to evolve into *systems of care* to ensure quality, appropriateness, and efficiency throughout the care delivery process. The system will encompass several care delivery environments. This linkage of all types and sizes of providers will develop to offer services in the lowest cost setting without detracting from quality or creating dupli-cate services, and provide smaller institutions needed access to high tech-nology and specialized expertise.

Electronic Data Interchange (EDI)

Standards

Any discussion of the healthcare informatics structure for networks and data traffic must include electronic data interchange (EDI) standards. As the disjointed islands of medical information slowly begin to communicate, the industry is developing respect for the standards process related to the generating, storing, retrieving, sending, and receiving of information. This is a mandatory business requirement as health care moves forward to be-come more cost effective and responsive to increasing demands for infor-mation at the point of patient care.

To better comprehend the cost/benefit economics of EDI, it must be understood that EDI is not a fax transmission, the rekeying of data, un-structured Email, etc. A look at the definition of EDI set forth by the Data Interchange Standards Association (DISA) sets the basic ground rules for defining EDI:

Electronic data interchange (EDI) is the transmission, in a standard syntax, of un-ambiguous information of business or strategic significance between computers of independent organization.

Application-to-application exchanges, without human intention, are the only true and effective use of EDI. Also, note the open systems philosophy of the technology; a standard syntax established between trading partners is the groundwork for an effective implementation work plan. This means no proprietary formats, so that any trading partner in any segment of the industry can implement an EDI business agreement with another third party without the fear of having to reinvent formats for the flow of business information.

There are three major reasons why EDI continues to gather momentum to the point of being the only way information exchange will be done in the future.

Reasons for Adoption of EDI

Cost Effectiveness

Providers and payors that have already embarked upon EDI programs re-port major reductions in costs associated with the processing of information. EDI invoices get generated, paid, and posted at $14 per transaction com-pared to the $70 expense for handling paper. Electronic remittance advices now get electronically uploaded into the A/R ledger as opposed to scores of data entry clerks rekeying the data from computer printouts. As more and more EDI transaction sets get put into production, the benefits of a truly integrated EDI program will fall straight to the bottom line.

Competitive Pressures

Acquisitions and mergers continue to accelerate in health care. By the year 2000, market pressures may have affected the industry to the point that less than 3000 acute care hospitals remain in business, as compared to 5500 today. The winners in these battles will be those organizations that can direct (and control) the flow of information within the different managed care environments. As the patient is now being viewed as a profit center, those that control the information relating to that profit center (whether it be on the payor or provider side) have the ability to negotiate from strength the reimbursement rates, levels of treatment, contractual discounts—in other words, drive profitability.

Medicare Mandates

Whoever thought that a government agency would be in the forefront of technology innovation and adaptation! Although the country may have to settle for healthcare reform bickering between the legislative and executive branches of federal government throughout this decade, the largest buyer of healthcare services in the United States is quickly moving to streamline its information flow and implement EDI. As one of the first proponents of electronic claims, the Health Care Financing Administration (HCFA) has a history of being an early adapter of automation to move and process incredible volumes of data. They have been quick to realize the power of the purse . . . to reward those who embrace electronic commerce with faster payments and a more convenient reimbursement process. This commitment to EDI permeates through the entire agency. Frequent news reports and Medicare bulletins point to the goals and objectives of HCFA to be 100 percent electronic within five to seven years. Given the major impact of Medicare on the economic structure of health care, the EDI direction of this powerful organization sends a very clear message about the role this technology will play in this industry.

Adoption of EDI

Technology is a weapon to decrease costs, operate more efficiently, and gain market share. However, technology for technology's sake is not only a waste of time and money, but it diverts the strength and focus of an MIS organization away from providing management the tools for an organization to grow, prosper, and flourish.

EDI is no different. Those organizations now implementing EDI plans have very strategic goals in mind for using this technology:

Reduce operating costs . . . increase productivity . . . send, receive, and analyze information as quickly as possible . . . link electronically with business partners for competitive advantage . . . be easy to do business with . . . create an EDI infrastructure to be adaptable and flexible as the marketplace and our corporate business charter changes.

The best examples today of early EDI adoption are the evolving community health information networks (CHINs) and managed care organizations (MCOs). In the 1980s, the word *bonding* was used to describe programs that attracted referring physicians to a particular institution for obvious economic reasons.

For the rest of the 1990s, EDI will be the glue to solve the connectivity problems in health care. No other option exists to have separate systems, incompatible machines, or diverse applications connect in a seamless manner. Done correctly, not one line of application code needs to be rewritten. Only through EDI translation software can provider sites (physicians, hospitals, labs, medical surgical centers, etc.), payor plans (indemnity sponsors, managed care organizations, self-insured entities), and employer initiatives (affecting human resource departments) be implemented with existing legacy systems and current technology assets.

Effect of EDI

EDI activities involving electronic claims, online lab results, electronic remittance advices, eligibility information, and claims status reports are already becoming common place with the more aggressive healthcare organizations. As plan structures continue to shift from indemnity fee-for-service to managed care in ever increasing numbers, work is now beginning to address the following data models:

- Electronic referrals,
- Electronic encounters,
- Formulary contacts,
- Treatment protocols,
- Medical certifications, and
- Practice guidelines.

The time is rapidly approaching where global registration, computer-based patient record files, and clinical data repositories will be commonplace throughout a medical enterprise system. To facilitate these applications working in a synchronized manner, strong EDI links will be the key part of the business and technical solution. The sharing of patient information—and a rapid, transparent yet secure manner—will be the cornerstone of the entire data infrastructure.

Once in place and utilized in the normal course of business, a fully implemented electronic commerce plan benefits all of those involved in the process. But most importantly, it permits and provides for better, faster, and more effective rendering of care to the patient population of the medical system.

The Future

The key to the future is building a system of care that takes responsibility for a defined population and focuses on the patient in terms of primary and preventive care and public health. Because every community is unique, no single example will provide the answer. One thing is sure: the benefit of information technology comes when the whole health care community is in an integrated network. Therein lies the opportunity. Health care is emerging as the largest single vertical market for information technology. Open systems and flexible computing will eliminate proprietary systems and host-based computing. In the future, the system with the most covered lives wins.

Incentives are the key to all healthcare finance. If there is any one key to the future of our industry, it is figuring out how to get the incentives in the right balance between physicians and hospitals. Those who cannot reengineer won't be around. Our information systems have been traditionally designed to meet the needs of a fee-for-service world. The new demands are coming on top of, rather than in lieu of, the old ones. The ability to provide the right information in an effective and efficient manner is the greatest challenge of all in our changing industry.

Taking some liberties with a famous Peter Drucker notion, the future will not just happen if one wishes hard enough. It requires decision—now. It imposes risk—now. It requires action—now. It requires allocation of resources and, above all, of human resources—now. It requires work—now.

Questions

1. Describe the forces behind the move from hospitals to managed care.
2. Discuss Electronic Data Interchange (EDI). Consider the forces for its adoption and what the effects of that adoption will be.
3. Provide your own vision of the integrated network.

4
Strategic Information Technology for an Integrated Delivery System

ROBERT J. PICKTON AND FRANCES C. SEEHAUSEN

Introduction

1980 Strategy for a Hospital System

The EHS Health Care System entered the 1980s with a self-developed hospital information system (HIS) that was unable to meet customer needs and took an ever-expanding staff to keep up with demands, both local and regulatory. In 1987, the information systems strategy turned the hospital system away from the mainframe and self-development philosophy. The five-year plan called for the development of a wide area network (WAN), linking individual facility local area networks (LAN) and building a distributed, open architecture platform. This design would enable EHS to select *best of breed* software, move to smaller and more economical hardware platforms, and utilize a model approach for the installation of selected products at each of the five hospitals owned at that time. The plan set up the infrastructure for EHS to act as a *healthcare system* as the demand for sharing and consolidation of information grew. This demand continues to grow more acute with the shift to managed care and the move toward reform.

1990 Strategy for an Integrated Delivery System

Healthcare in the 1990s has focused on the managed care approach, including emphases on wellness and preventive care—and the need of providers to survive in a capitated market. Integrated delivery systems (IDSs) have replaced hospital systems and must provide links between physicians, payors, and other community care providers. This is of crucial importance to allow any IDS to meet its objectives in providing quality, cost-effective care. The ability to do so lies in great part in information technology. No longer can the capital budget focus be on bricks and mortar, but on technology and how it can best serve a changing industry.

Strategy for the 1990s to 2000 and Beyond

In 1993, the EHS Health Care System based in Oak Brook, Illinois, undertook the effort to develop a three-year strategic plan and clearly identify the tactics required to make the plan a success. The published plan (EHS Health Care, 1994) was the basis for the information systems strategic plan.

Most information systems (IS) strategies are the result of weeks or even months of interviews with key administrators and managers throughout an organization. Given the clear direction set by the EHS strategic plan, this process was unnecessary. The IS plan took as its foundation the components of the EHS plan: six core strategies, core values, each operating unit's tactical plan, and the review of customer needs (Figure 4-1).

Within EHS, IS is positioned to impact the success of the total organization, as should every organization's IS department. The EHS IS department understands that organizations with strategic systems to support mission-critical business processes are those that will survive in today's and tomorrow's competitive marketplace.

With the emphasis on *wellness* and *lives,* information technology needs to support the full continuum of care. The EHS IS department and those of similar IDSs must provide centralized support, dependable transaction systems, seamless integration, and knowledge of the latest technology. IS departments are the architects of the information management strategy and are responsible for its successful implementation.

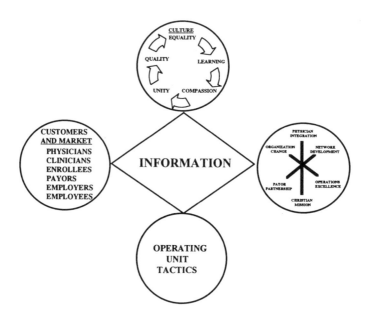

FIGURE 4-1. Health system integration.

There are four strategic competencies in the EHS information technology strategy:

* Infrastructure,
* Information management,
* New technology, and
* Support.

Each will be addressed separately in this chapter.

Infrastructure

Communication infrastructure is a key component to any information technology backbone. The use of this infrastructure to draw care sites together from a voice and data connectivity standpoint gives the EHS IDS and like IDSs a competitive advantage in their markets (Figure 4-2).

The EHS WAN links each of the major hospitals, home care facilities, and extended care sites. The challenge for the immediate future is to expand to ambulatory care sites and new acquisitions. It is absolutely critical to incorporate the offices of care providers affiliated with EHS, making it possible to share member information. Information sharing allows any IDS to meet its objectives in providing quality, cost-effective care. At EHS, it helps us meet our customers' expectations of convenience, quality, and satisfaction when attending to their healthcare needs.

EHS capitalized and developed its own WAN, but many smaller hospitals and healthcare systems have not yet done so. For many facilities it may still be beyond the reach of their available capital, but the need to share and obtain information is just as great. Many communities with multiple healthcare facilities and even systems with communication infrastructures, such as EHS Health Care, have undertaken efforts to develop Community

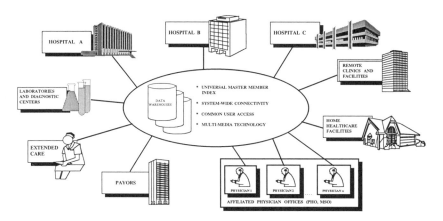

Figure 4-2. Integrated delivery system (IDS) network.

Health Information Networks (CHINs). The development of a CHIN as a collaborative effort seeks to avoid creating multiple, redundant, and costly networks in the same geographic region.

The collaborative approach, in addition to providing considerable cost savings by creating a purchasing group, provides a setting in which users can exercise considerable influence over the development and deployment of a CHIN. Payors must be included in this effort, for without their involvement the successes realized will be of a lesser magnitude.

Information Management

Health care is struggling with the challenges faced by retailing, banking, and manufacturing not so very long ago. Less than 10 years ago, banks required customers to fill out applications and duplicate data they had supplied in obtaining other services, whether savings, mortgage, credit card, or investments. Those same banks treated each department separately, and the customer was inconvenienced during each transaction. Today, most major banks have a centralized database about customers. Rarely is information gathering duplicated. Customer information is available to each department because customer service is a key business focus.

Today IDSs face the same challenges that other industries confronted in the recent past. In fact, our need for knowledge is even greater for we are responsible for the health of our customers. In *Post-Capitalist Society,* Peter Drucker (1993) defines the new society as a

post-capitalist polity. The basic economic resource—"the means of production," to use the economist's term—is no longer capital, nor natural resources (the economist's "land"), nor "labor." It is and will be knowledge. The economic challenge of the post-capitalist society will therefore be the productivity of knowledge work and the knowledge worker. The social challenge of the post-capitalist society will, however, be the dignity of the second class in the post-capitalist society, the service workers.

The service workers, who constitute the other class of workers, do and will continue to offer managers the greatest challenge to meet the business needs set before them.

Health care as an industry will not escape dichotomy between knowledge and service workers. Managing the needs of both groups poses a significant challenge and requires the use of information to meet those needs.

The information management model for EHS depicted in Figure 4-3 recognizes the importance of transactional systems. These systems require ongoing support, enhancement, and expansion in response to business decisions, including operational improvement initiatives. These systems facilitate collecting and processing data that enhance normal activity. Each

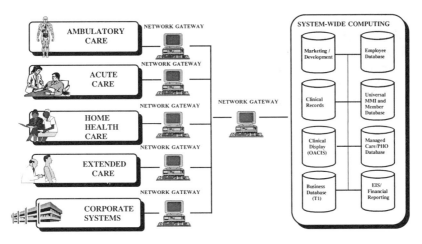

FIGURE 4-3. Information management model.

IDS must integrate all of the inpatient and outpatient systems to provide for a smooth flow of information. The challenge each IDS will face as it merges with, affiliates with, or acquires other institutions is whether to replace the transaction systems immediately with common systems, replace them using planned obsolescence, or maintain them with multiple interfaces and common data dictionaries.

Second, the model addresses the development of multiple gateways. Gateways are designed to move data between transactional systems and a warehouse or warehouses depending on the need. The software for the gateways will be composed of various tools and will require management of both the data required and the network to avoid "traffic jams" inconveniencing users and customers.

The last component of the system-wide information management model will be a mix of central and virtual warehouses. A central data warehouse is one populated with historical data. These data are not highly dynamic and can be downloaded from the transaction systems on a predefined time frame (e.g., daily, weekly, monthly). However, the virtual data warehouse supports dynamic data. These data need real-time updating and require continual access.

These concepts are better explained using examples. Consider the decision support system made by Transition Systems, Inc. This product is a central warehouse of data from the following areas: general ledger, payroll, patient accounting, patient management, and medical records. The data are organized and allow decision makers to query using individual preferences. All EHS facilities are implementing the product to enable EHS to perform top/down budgeting, contract modeling, and *best practice* prototyping as an example of a few of the uses for a warehouse.

The member warehouse with the universal master member index (UMMI) will be interactive. Data in this warehouse will be accessible to a variety of users, including physicians, ambulatory care facilities, and wellness facilities, to name a few. The data in this warehouse or repository will be drawn from systems such as benefits administration, clinical displays, and patient management systems. An enterprise-wide member management index will be necessary for easy access. The UMMI and its integration across all points of care will eliminate the redundant collection of information by each area for our members.

New Technology

There is no end to technology and the multiple applications used and suggested for use in health care. EHS supports new technology as its third strategic competency; thus, the IS department must be diligent in separating proven applications of technology from those only suggesting success.

Capital is at a premium and is a constraining resource. Payback and value will be of increasing importance when setting priority on purchase and use for a project. IS departments must identify the level of risk comfort, review choices, and use a business problem/alternative/solutions approach to select technology to support the IDS.

The EHS IS department becomes business partners with its customers to provide the solution to technology issues. As partners, the IS department worked with the management of a high tech outpatient facility to develop a five-year technology plan. The information and costs in the plan were used in conjunction with other data to support the purchase of the unique facility. The plan was comprehensive and addressed connectivity, model transaction systems, links between radiology machines and systems, and decision support needs. The process yielded a map utilizing risk free technology, cost benefit analysis that clearly outlined a payback, and valuable insight into how to successfully link other ambulatory sites into our continuum of care strategy.

Reimbursement for IDSs will not increase. As capitation gains momentum, the business approach gains even greater importance. EHS supports technology capital spending, but results are expected and will continue to be important as the IDS expands.

Support

Over the last three years, the IS department has reevaluated its approach to support. Four issues surfaced as key components to our support strategy: "systemness," design, vision, and business growth.

"Systemness"

As a corporate-based function, the IS department worked to develop leadership and to articulate a shared vision of what an IS organization is chartered to provide the IDS. Both the IS staff and its customers have stopped treating implementations as "IS projects" and necessary evils. IS staff and system users have stepped up to ownership of a process that, if done right, provides management with a vehicle to reengineer their daily processes.

Education of staff and system users has been a process of immersion and refinement. An aggressive implementation schedule across a broad spectrum of projects required transitioning away from a very traditional environment to an environment demanding a whole new base of skills. These skills were required to address increased technical complexity and to accommodate new business partnerships with our users. Communication, project management, facilitation, and planning took on new importance. Education of users focused on a "super user" approach, one that emphasized functional, technical, and troubleshooting training on a reasonably small, but very proud, set of users.

Design

The cost pressures being exerted on an IDS have forced every department to reevaluate the design of the support organizations. The IS department has a new imperative to identify all components of their support costs and rethink, reevaluate, and/or restructure their architecture. The need to be captive to technology is over. Henceforth all efforts must focus on implementing strategic solutions to gain competitive advantage in the healthcare market. IS will develop key vendor partnerships and move away from the traditional ones. IS will focus on system-wide versus facility implementation. The market and environment dictate that IS respond consistently in the most cost-effective means possible.

Vision

This vision moves the IS department in EHS and other IDSs closer to the customer using techniques fundamental to continuous quality improvement. IS will continue to build the business and technical skills of the staff to enable greater satisfaction and customer support. Better planning is required to know how IS resources have been committed and what processes will improve the outcomes. It is crucial to respond to business growth issues efficiently and effectively.

Business Growth

The demand for solutions will continue to grow, but IS will be under the same cost-containment pressure that every department is feeling. To opti-

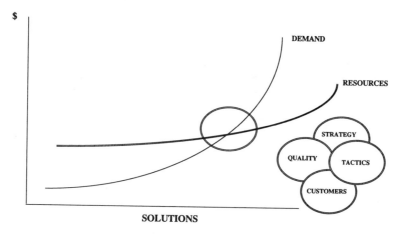

FIGURE 4-4. Information technology solutions.

mize the project requests with the available resources, it is necessary for the system-wide management to maintain the balance. Solutions will be optimized based on strategy, tactics, quality, and customers. A committee must prioritize the IDS's needs and expect to see the benefits and payback noted in a business plan. IS must be as accountable as its customers to the business plan and meet its commitments (Figure 4-4).

Summary

As shown in Figure 4-3, the new information management model for EHS Health Care acknowledges the need for system-wide computing and highlights

- Transactional systems as they relate to operations initiatives, and
- Multiple gateways designed to move data between transactional systems and warehouses.

Thus, the model supports the Vision 2000 strategies outlined in the system-wide strategic plan.

The EHS model will be a living model and supply the information that management needs to respond to the formidable challenges the future holds. The model will be evaluated regularly to validate its value and support to the growth and direction of EHS Health Care.

Change is the only certainty of the current environment, and Information Services must be ready to meet the challenges it presents.

Questions

1. Describe the evolution of an information strategy for EHS, from 1980 to 1990 and beyond.
2. Discuss briefly the four strategies competencies identified by EHS: infrastructure, information management, new technology, and support.
3. Describe the EHS Health Care model.
4. Is the EHS experience generalizable? What lessons might other health-care organizations draw from EHS?

References

Drucker, P.F. (1993). *Post-capitalist society.* New York: HarperCollins Publishers, Inc.

EHS Health Care. (1994). *Information systems plan.* Oak Brook, IL.

5
American Journal of Nursing (AJN) Network

Mary Anne Rizzolo and Karen DuBois

Introduction

In September 1993, the American Journal of Nursing Company (AJN) was awarded a three-year special projects grant from the Division of Nursing, Department of Health and Human Services, to develop an electronic information service to provide continuing education and information to nurses in medically underserved rural areas. AJN *Network* went "live" in March 1994. Using a train-the-trainer approach, over 150 trainers in our pilot states of North Carolina, Nevada, and Wisconsin were taught to use the network. This core group is now going out to rural hospitals to train other nurses on the system. During the first year of operation, AJN *Network* was available through a dial-up service. In September 1994, AJN established an Internet node so that the *Network* could be offered over the Internet, an international network linking hundreds of smaller computer networks throughout the world. This project makes use of the federal High Performance Computing and Communications (HPCC) initiative that provides a backbone extending across the country, capable of transmitting data at tremendous speeds.

This chapter includes a brief history of the AJN Company and its resources, traces the development of the grant proposal, describes the processes and procedures essential to project initiation, the services currently available on AJN *Network,* and plans for future development.

History of the AJN Company

Since the turn of the century, when the first issue of the *American Journal of Nursing* was published, the AJN Company's goals have been to disseminate and provide information to advance health care and spur progress in nursing practice, service, education, and research. The company has always been owned and operated by nurses. In 1912, AJN Company shares were given to the American Nurses Association; they continue to be the sole stockholder of the company.

In the early 1950s, the company began to expand its products and services, developing new journals and other publications, sponsoring workshops and conferences, and establishing an Educational Services Division (ESD) to develop and distribute multimedia materials. In recent years, ESD's videotapes, computer-assisted instruction, and interactive videodisc programs have won national and international awards.

Evolution of the Idea for an Electronic Resource

With a history of educational service to nurses spanning more than nine decades, the company is a repository of a large and ever increasing amount of clinical content and other valuable information for nurses. In fact, most nurses throughout the country view AJN Company as an information resource. In 1990, the author of this chapter, then director of videodisc development, encouraged the company to consider the feasibility of providing information to nurses in an electronic format. A steering committee was formed; CompuServe, a major online computer service, was contacted to explore the possibility of using their service to deliver information and foster discussion among nurses. At that time, costs were prohibitive. The idea was tabled, but corporate consciousness had been raised, and key administrative personnel carefully watched the evolution of health-related electronic services.

By 1993, there were more than 300 health-related bulletin boards, several of them created by and for nurses. These included

- Educational Technology Network (E.T. Net) at the National Library of Medicine's Lister Hill Center for Biomedical Communication, Educational Technology Branch,
- American Nurses Association's Workplace Advocacy Information System (which has now evolved into ANA*NET),
- Sigma Theta Tau's Electronic Library,
- FITNET run by the Fuld Institute for Technology in Nursing Education,
- The "Healthcare Building" of the Denver Free-Net,
- Nurses Corner (Florida),
- Nurses Station (Kentucky),
- PC Nurse (Delaware),
- Trilogy (Maryland), and
- SON*NET (Texas).

Besides bulletin boards, Internet options specifically for nurses began to expand. For example, there are "LISTSERVs" that allow all members of a mailing list to post and read messages; "Usenet" groups—bulletin board type areas for posting messages; and Gopher servers that use a menu structure to find, view, and retrieve files from other Internet nodes.

The proliferation of all of these electronic resources, although generally limited in scope, indicated that there were growing numbers of nurses who were willing and able to use the new communication technologies. In addition, the costs of computers, modems, and communication software continued to plunge, making new hardware technology more readily available. All of these factors indicated that the time was right to institute a national information service for nurses.

Grant Proposal Development

In the search for funding to support a project of this type, the special projects grants from the Division of Nursing immediately came to mind. These grants have traditionally supported innovative projects. AJN Company had previously been awarded a special projects grant to develop interactive videodisc programs for continuing nursing education. When the 1993 purposes for grant support from this agency were examined, the section earmarked for grants designed to provide continuing education to nurses serving in medically underserved communities seemed uniquely appropriate for the type of resource we envisioned. We knew that nurses working in rural areas have extremely limited access to information and continuing education, so they seemed to be an ideal group to target for a project of this type. A search of the literature and a needs assessment were undertaken to test our assumptions.

Literature Search

Our literature search focused on healthcare needs of rural Americans, the scope of practice of rural nurses, and their continuing education needs.

Health in Rural America

The literature revealed that the health of rural Americans has been steadily declining. Increasing poverty, loss or lack of insurance coverage, and difficult transportation needs all combine to significantly limit rural residents' access to the health care that is available to them. In this environment, it is not surprising that rural residents experience consistently higher rates of chronic illness, disability, and maternal and infant mortality compared to urban residents (Bigbee, 1993). In addition, the increase of the geriatric population with related health problems and the increase in new illnesses, such as the 37 percent increase in AIDS cases in rural areas from 1988 to

1989 (Carwein, Sabo, & Berry, 1993), have placed a serious burden on the already stretched rural healthcare system. All of this has increased the demands made of rural nurses.

Rural Nursing

The rural environment places special demands on the rural nurse. Isolated geographically, rural nurses are affected by the factors of excessive autonomy, lack of adequate staffing, lack of organizational resources, and limited technology (Muus et al., 1993). Clinically, rural nurses need to be proficient in all aspects of care. The rural nurse is often the lone practitioner and the generalist, having to meet any need presented by a patient. Yet recent employment data reveal that rural nurses have less professional education than their urban counterparts (Bushy, 1990).

The nurse in a rural community has both opportunities and limitations for development and fulfillment. The nurse can be a community leader and decision maker in health policy and community projects, but must deal with low salaries, longer hours of service and being on call, less time off, and less access to continuing education (Turner & Gunn, 1991).

Continuing Education Needs of Rural Nurses

The demands of handling a variety of healthcare situations and of keeping up with the latest information and technology have increased the needs of rural nurses for continuing education. New graduates, inactive nurses returning to work, nurses expanding into new roles, and experienced nurses all need educational programs offered at frequent intervals to meet the need for keeping up to date with healthcare advances. Currently, 22 state boards of nursing require that nurses and/or nurse practitioners acquire a defined number of continuing education hours to renew their licenses to practice. With or without a legal mandate, the rapid changes in health care now mean that nurses must stay current in order to practice safely.

Access to the necessary continuing education for rural nurses remains difficult, however. The factors of distance, travel and course cost, and the lack of personnel to provide coverage all contribute to reducing the ability of rural nurses to pursue continuing education (Anderson & Kimber, 1991). In addition, in-house educational programs that can cost as much as $5,000 per nurse have been the first to be cut as rural hospitals struggle to remain financially viable. Furthermore, there is not enough time for rural nurses to devote to education purposes when hospitals cannot cover the costs of replacement staff and cannot even spare senior staff for on-the-job mentoring. To our delight, we found that several experts in rural nursing recommended the use of electronic media to disseminate information and education to rural nurses (Parker et al., 1991).

Needs Assessment

A questionnaire was developed and administered to key personnel in area health education centers (AHECs) and to other individuals and organizations serving the continuing education needs of rural nurses across the country. Both the telephone and electronic networks (Health Alaska, Virtual Medical Center in Montana, ALF, the Rural Information Center electronic bulletin board, E.T. Net, and the Internet) were used to collect data. We assembled information from 25 sites in 22 states representing all geographic regions of the United States. The survey revealed that the major concern of rural nurses was access to continuing education and information. We learned that nurses isolated in extremely rural areas have problems traveling to conferences when swampy roads are covered with water and mountain passes are filled with snow. We heard about small rural hospitals without any library facilities or access to recent books and journals. Although access to computers and modems is limited in some rural areas, when nurses were asked if they would use computers for continuing education, their answer was "yes."

Three states were approached and asked if they would be willing to participate as pilot states if the project was funded. All three agreed. These states were selected because they had expressed the most interest in the project during the needs assessment and were willing to support our "train-the-trainer" approach to reach nurses in rural hospitals. These states also had access to technology. In North Carolina, for example, every rural hospital had a computer with a modem. Nevada has an electronic bulletin board system called CAMEL that includes email and literature search capabilities. In Wisconsin, a rural hospital cooperative had a long-standing relationship with the University of Wisconsin at Madison that involved them in many state-of-the-art distance learning projects. Our contacts in all three states were eager to participate.

Another aspect of needs assessment involved talking with a variety of experts in computer science and rural nursing for advice on various aspects of the project. Many of these same people were asked to serve on our advisory committee if the project was funded. Our final advisory committee consisted of Michael Ackerman, PhD, Acting Director, Specialized Information Service, National Library of Medicine; Elizabeth Bolyard, MPH, RN, Chief, Prevention Activity, HIV Infections Branch, Centers for Disease Control; Nancy DiMauro, MA, RNC, Director of Continuing Education at AJN Company; Stephen Erde, PhD, MD, Information Systems, Cornell University Medical School; K. Sue Kwentus, MSN, RN, CNAA, with an extensive background in administration in rural hospitals; Judith Nierenberg, MA, RN, Vice President for Educational Services, AJN Company; Diane Skiba, PhD, Director of Informatics and Associate Professor of Nursing at the University of Colorado Health Science Center; and Susan Sparks, PhD, RN, FAAN, Manager of E.T. Net and Educational Research

Specialist at the Educational Technology Branch of the National Library of Medicine's Lister Hill National Center for Biomedical Communication.

Project Objectives

Based on the information gathered, the objectives of the project were developed as follows:

1. To develop a computer network system, reachable through personal computer modems, that will serve the needs of nurses on a national level.
2. To provide access for nurses to information that will assist them in providing effective nursing care, including direct patient care, management, and promotion of community health by
    a. Establishing a nurse consultant helpline with expert nurses who will respond to specific inquiries from nurses;
    b. Establishing a bulletin board system for nurses to ask their peers for answers to specific nursing care and management questions and to share information;
    c. Making available AJN Company's library of patient information so that nurses can print this information directly for patients;
    d. Establishing a special consultation service on HIV/AIDS that will provide prevention information and increase the knowledge and skill of nurses caring for persons who are HIV positive or who have AIDS;
    e. Establishing a special consultation on sociocultural diversity for nurses to gain cultural competence, which will assist them in providing care to members of diverse cultural groups.
3. To provide greater access for nurses to continuing education by
    a. Offering computer-assisted instruction (CAI) programs on topics relevant to (and selected by) the users;
    b. Establishing a feature article of the month and a time during which nurses from anywhere can talk to the author through synchronous conferencing—the author can also respond to questions posted through the bulletin board;
    c. Offering on the network continuing education articles and tests that are available on a monthly basis in the *American Journal of Nursing,* the *American Journal of Maternal Child Nursing (MCN),* and other publications;
    d. Creating new continuing education course offerings from user input on the bulletin board.
4. To provide assistance to nurses in accessing the large, existing resources of healthcare information already available by
    a. Converting information from a variety of sources that currently exist in print format to searchable digital databases;
    b. Providing access to or information from existing digital databases available on the Internet and elsewhere;

c. Establishing a special feature section that provides national and international news affecting nurses and healthcare in medically underserved areas.

Project Implementation

The project was approved and funded in September 1993 in the amount of $746,187 over a three-year period. Mary Anne Rizzolo, the designated program director, began immediately to recruit personnel. Karen DuBois, MSN, RNC, was hired as project coordinator. Learie Pomesamy was named as network manager, and a secretary was hired. Project implementation began in full force.

Software and Hardware Selection

Financial support to develop a computer network that can provide nursing resources is only the beginning. Purchasing hardware and software requires comprehensive knowledge of what is available and a realistic view of future uses of technology. Time spent by the development team conceptualizing the final product cannot be underestimated during this process. The project director, project coordinator, and network manager joined with the director of information services and system operator, Jack Peterson, and the vice president for administration, Susan Krause, to make up the AJN *Network* development team.

Following an extensive two-month review of commercially available software, five bulletin board software packages emerged as potential choices. With additional input and guidance from our advisory committee, Res Nova software and a Macintosh server platform were selected. This hardware and software allow us to serve both PC and Macintosh environments. RIPterm, a shareware terminal emulation program, was chosen as the communications package we would provide to our users. It was selected because it is available in Macintosh, DOS, and Windows version, and has a user-friendly customizable graphical user interface.

Content Development

To select content that would be responsive to the needs of rural nurses in our pilot states, we developed a learning needs assessment that was mailed to our sites in North Carolina, Nevada, and Wisconsin. The results of this assessment, along with suggestions from the advisory committee members, were used to plan initial offerings on the AJN *Network*.

Forums

One of the first, and still most active, sections set up for our users was the forums area. In forums, nurses can post messages and respond to messages posted by other users. This area is intended to be used for professional support and informal peer education. The original forums included typical clinical areas like medical/surgical and maternal/child nursing. Others were devoted to trends and issues in healthcare. Additional forums will evolve based on user input. Nurses and other professionals with experience in the topic areas have volunteered to act as forum moderators. Forum moderators encourage participation, stimulate and give direction to new topics, organize responses, and monitor messages for appropriateness.

Nurse Consult

The goal of the nurse consult forum area is to provide consultation on clinical care problems. In preparation, a database of nurse experts was created and installed on AJN Company's local area network. The editors of AJN Company journals are in contact with authors on virtually every nursing subspecialty. The convention manager has an extensive list of speakers who have expertise in a wide range of nursing areas. These nurses entered their list of nurse experts into the database. It now contains over 2000 names. The nurse moderating the nurse consult forum will first attempt to answer questions by searching the literature. If the answer is not found, the moderator will contact the project coordinator, who will locate appropriate nurse experts in the database. Legal advice is under consideration regarding policies and procedures that would govern information that is provided in the nurse consult section.

Continuing Education

Continuing education (CE) offerings currently on AJN *Network* consist of CAI programs and CE print products that have been converted to text files for downloading.

Computer Assisted Instruction

Several producers and distributors of quality CAI programs agreed to provide their programs for rural nurses in our pilot states to download and use on their own computers. The project coordinator needed to educate appropriate company representatives on this concept of product delivery, but once they understood they were willing to make their programs available in return for feedback from users and usage reports. Negotiations are underway with other companies to provide demonstration copies or mini-versions of their programs (one case study, for example). This area of AJN

Network can evolve into an area that software developers could use to beta test programs under development. Eventually a "software store" will be set up where companies can advertise and provide demos of their programs and buyers can enter a credit card or purchase order number and download the software.

CE Articles

The project coordinator meets regularly with the AJN director of continuing education to identify CE offerings in print that are relevant to our users. These are converted to text files that can be downloaded and printed at the user's site. Conversion procedures and instructions on downloading and printing are posted with the articles to help users through this process. Those CE articles from both the *American Journal of Nursing* and the *American Journal of Maternal Child Nursing (MCN)* that are within the time frame for CE credit are available. Plans are underway to add articles from other journals. The systems operator is researching new software that will allow articles to be displayed and printed just as they appear in the journals, complete with photographs and graphics.

Journal Club

Project personnel have always understood that it is not sufficient to just convert print materials to an electronic format. Each medium has its own characteristics and strengths that should be matched to the content. Journal club was created to put this concept into practice. Journal club has two areas: one is a forum where authors will respond to questions about their article over a one-month period after the article has been posted on the network; a second area uses the "chat" feature of the system software, which allows users to log into the system and participate in a real-time discussion, or synchronous chat, with the author at a specific date and time. The editors of each journal work with the AJN *Network* staff to identify authors who will participate in this area.

The AJN director of continuing education is considering ways to provide CE credit for participation in the journal club. Our software can track the amount of time each individual user spends in the synchronous conference with the author as well as time spent posting and reading messages about the journal club article. If the amount of time equals 50 minutes or more, we should be able to grant CE credit. As learning needs are identified in the journal club and other forum areas, new CE course offerings will be created.

Another plan to provide innovative, timely, and responsive continuing education offerings involves using our forum moderators and project coordinator to monitor bulletin board messages for topics and themes that generate interest and discussion. The project coordinator will then work with the program director, the director of continuing education, and editorial staff to create a new CE course offering. As an example, we might pull questions and answers on HIV/AIDS from various parts of the network and create an article on "Rural Nurses' Major Questions and Concerns About HIV/AIDS." This objective will be developed more fully as our user base expands.

Patient Information

A sampling of patient information sheets has been converted to text files that can be downloaded and printed at the user's site. We plan to set up an area where nurses can dialogue regarding patient information and identify needs for new products. Other patient education material and lists of other patient resources are planned. Eventually an area where patients can communicate directly with nurses regarding healthcare questions may emerge.

News

Initial news offerings on AJN *Network* include segments from Nurse Executive News Scan, a monthly audiotape distributed by AJN Company, that are posted for discussion. Because the company has access to a variety of news feeds and a news editor, this area will expand and include such features as "EXTRA" bulletins when important news items that affect health care and nursing occur, and real-time simultaneous chats regarding nationwide television broadcasts about healthcare issues.

Databases

Several databases are presently available on AJN *Network:*

- Nursing conferences, which contains information about more than 400 national and international conferences, is updated weekly;
- Nursing organizations;
- Health-related organizations;
- Certification requirements of various specialty boards;
- Licensure and continuing education requirements for every state board of nursing.

All include the name of a contact person, address, and phone number in addition to relevant information. A full text Apple search engine is used to search for entries. A forum was also set up in the database area so nurses can dialogue with a professional indexer about search strategies. Future additions to this area will include bibliographic databases.

User Support

There is a voice helpline that users can call for personal assistance in logging on or using the *Network*. A database is used to log problems that users encounter and responses to common questions and problems are included in the user manual and in a "frequently asked questions" area online. The user manual and the frequently asked question areas are constantly revised to reflect changes in the network.

Process Issues

Although considerable effort has been devoted to selecting appropriate content, just as much work was required to set up policies and procedures for putting that content up on AJN *Network* so that the processes were in place to enable these functions to proceed smoothly and be as automated as possible. Significant time needed to be spent researching legal issues. As technology advances, laws regarding electronic information and communication are constantly being challenged and changed. We sought legal counsel on many issues and needed to have several formal agreements constructed. Our user agreement covers responsibilities of users, particularly in regard to copyright issues. Agreements were also required for forum moderators and contracts were drawn up for producers and distributors of CAI programs. Forging frontiers with new technology requires walking a fine line that will protect the company and the users from potential risks while making information available in a timely electronic format.

Education and Training

Launching AJN *Network* required a significant education effort directed toward AJN Company staff and other companies and individuals involved with the project as well as the actual users.

Company Training

Although AJN employees work on a sophisticated cross-platform local area network, staff needed education about the technology and demonstrations of AJN *Network* in order to understand the project and to encourage their participation. The project coordinator acted as the change agent in both formal and informal meetings with staff. Strong support from administrative staff assisted this process. Each employee has access to AJN *Network* from their desktop. In addition, a computer workstation was placed in the employee cafeteria so staff can "surf" various sites on the Internet with sophisticated software like Mosaic. Exposure to a variety of resources and content will stimulate AJN employees in all departments to generate ideas on how the resources of the company can be transformed into electronic products for nurses throughout the world.

Site Training

The project coordinator conducted site training in North Carolina, Nevada, and Wisconsin. The educational process began with initial phone conversations between the project coordinator and the contact people in each state. A few pockets of resistance were encountered due to fear of the technology and a real lack of access to computer hardware. A hardware survey revealed that most hospitals had one computer with a modem, which was usually in the library or medical records department. A few had Internet access, but not modem access. Very few of the rural nurses had computers with modems in their homes.

Most training sessions were held in large university settings that could provide access to multiple workstations with modems. Classes were planned for a full day of lecture, demonstration, and hands-on experience. Although the majority of attendees were nurses, some training sites sent librarians from AHECs and rural hospitals who would act as trainers and technical support for the nurses. Many of the nurses traveled hours and sometimes overnight to the training sessions. Although some may have come out of curiosity, the overwhelming impression of the project coordinator was that these nurses came because of their sense of accountability to the profession and their peers, and a real desire to stay current with the technological trends in nursing.

Some of the nurses who attended the train-the-trainer sessions did not understand the concept of communicating and/or retrieving information with a computer and a modem. Often they confused this use of technology with two-way television, Internet access, or wide area networks. Some nurses had never seen a CAI program. The project coordinator had to begin with some basics before she could even demonstrate AJN *Network*. By midday many of the participants were overwhelmed with new information. However, the hands-on experience during the second half of the class succeeded in helping them overcome their fears and reservations.

During the afternoon, as planned in advance, the system operator was monitoring the servers. When the project coordinator requested a chat, he responded immediately with words of welcome and comments about their geographic area, current successes (or failures) of regional sports teams, and requests to send the project coordinator back with local products like Point beer. This humanizing element cannot be underestimated in helping people feel comfortable with the technology. The system operator also used this opportunity to make them aware of the 800 number voice helpline that they could call to request someone to "talk" them through any problems they might encounter after training.

At the conclusion of training, some nurses who had previously given away their computers to other departments because of lack of knowledge and resources, went back to their rural hospitals to reclaim them. It was a study in nursing empowerment!

Future Plans

Technological advances and experimentation with the existing network will direct the growth of AJN *Network*. Future plans center around the development of timely content that will be accessed in as user-friendly an environment as we can make it. We are committed to making this network available to as many nurses as possible regardless of computer platform. We intend to continue to make AJN *Network* available on commonly used systems with minimal requirements, but we will constantly incorporate new technology, such as digitized audio and video, so it can be available to users as they upgrade their hardware.

Content Expansion

Content will be determined by the AJN *Network* development team, the advisory committee, and user feedback. We will continually examine resources on the Internet, push the capabilities of our software, and keep seeking new content and innovative ways to display and interact with that content and our users.

Internet Resources

Since AJN *Network* became an Internet node in September 1994, we have been exploring various sources of information on the Internet that might be of use to nurses. Advanced AJN "Netters" quickly began to participate in LISTSERVs and Usenet groups. We plan to echo information for nurses, give information and directions on how to access other valuable sources of electronic information, and filter, edit, and publish information gleaned from examining themes in messages and trends as they emerge in multiple Internet resource areas.

New Content

An idea to establish an area for reporting about conferences originated when the project coordinator attended the National Rural Health Conference. Every evening, she posted a message describing presentations and key issues that were discussed. This area instantly became a popular place on the *Network*. We saw this as another excellent way to provide timely information to those who cannot attend major nursing conferences. In the future we will assign reporters to a conference who will describe audience reactions to presentations, interview attendees, report on debates, and post election results. Abstracts of presentations can be available prior to the conference and users will be able to post messages to the presenters and perhaps engage in a synchronous "chat" with some of the presenters a few weeks after the conference has occurred. Software to allow online conference registration is available and can be added to the system in the future.

Other plans currently under discussion include:

- Recruiting nationally and internationally known nursing experts to conduct online discussions on hot issues of the day using the "chat" feature;
- Conducting online focus groups to generate ideas for new products and to discuss improvement of existing products used by nurses;
- Developing games with an educational focus, perhaps similar to Trivial Pursuit, that would be ongoing, with questions contributed by users and recognition given to winners;
- Expanding use of the survey feature of our software by encouraging researchers to post surveys and questionnaires.

We will constantly be alert to the suggestions of our users, and we encourage the imagination and creativity of all associated with the *Network* to generate new ideas.

Once the grant is over, revenue will be generated to continue the development and operation of AJN *Network* through a subscription fee and online advertising. In addition, software is already available to set up a "shopping mall" online. This area will be used initially to market AJN Company products and will later expand to other advertisers.

Another plan to generate revenue is to offer space on our system to others. Small nursing organizations, for example, that do not have the personnel or resources to set up and provide technical support for their own system, can contract with AJN Company to provide those services.

Design

Our goal to make AJN *Network* as user friendly as possible will culminate in a metaphor or motif of a virtual nursing center. Content will be reorganized around this theme with forums dedicated to clinical specialties on their appropriate "floors" or "units" like medical, surgical, pediatrics, and maternity. CE articles will be found in the library, journal club discussions will take place in the conference room, and the newsstand in the nursing center lobby will have racks displaying the current news of the day. This approach will help nurses to navigate the system with familiar graphics and terminology. Because our system operator is collaborating with the developers of Res Nova to incorporate Mosaic software on our system, we will parallel develop Internet and dial-up versions of our motif.

The AJN Company is an environment rich in the many resources that are needed to develop an electronic information source for nurses. Guided by an eminently qualified advisory committee, and in response to regular surveys, AJN *Network* will continue to add new resources and endeavor to meet the information needs of nurses throughout the world. AJN *Network* has the potential to be the primary online resource for nurses practicing in any setting with patients. It should become an integral part of every basic nursing curriculum. As the role of nurses changes and their practice settings move out of organized hospital environments, this will be an invaluable tool for practicing nurses. Tools must be developed to match the capabilities of the new technologies and the needs of those who will use them. The AJN *Network* is being designed to meet that need.

Questions

1. When and how did the AJN *Network* first develop?
2. What aspects of rural nursing were identified as needing support? Consider both the literature search and the needs assessment in your response.
3. Briefly describe the project objectives and the project implementation process.
4. What does the *Network* include as content? What plans are suggested for content expansion?
5. How is AJN addressing user support and process issues? Consider the education and training components included as part of the grant.
6. Sketch your own view of the "virtual nursing center" concept.

References

Anderson, J., & Kimber, K. (1991). Meeting the continuing education needs of nurses in rural settings. *The Journal of Continuing Education in Nursing, 22,* 29–34.

Bigbee, J.L. (1993). The uniqueness of rural nursing. *Nursing Clinics of North America, 28,* 131–144.

Bushy, A. (1990). Rural determinants in family health: Considerations for community nurses. *Family and Community Health, 12,* 29–38.

Carwein, V.L., Sabo, C.E., & Berry, D.E. (1993). HIV infection in traditional rural communities. *Nursing Clinics of North America, 28,* 231–239.

Muus, K.J., Stratton, T.D., Dunkin, J.W., & Juhl, N. (1993). Retaining registered nurses in rural community hospitals. *JONA, 23,* 38–43.

Parker, M., Quinn, J., Viehl, M., Mckinley, A., Polich, C., Detzner, D., Hartwell, S. & Korn, K. (1991). Case management in rural areas: Definition, clients, financing, staffing, and service delivery issues. In A. Bushy (Ed.) *Rural nursing, vol. 2* (pp. 29–40). Newbury Park, CA: Sage Publications.

Turner, T.A., & Gunn, I.P. (1991). Issues in rural health nursing. In A. Bushy (Ed.) *Rural nursing, vol. 2* (pp. 105–127). Newbury Park, CA: Sage Publications.

Unit 3
Transforming Health Care

Unit Introduction

Information technology affects health care on many levels and in many ways. Decision support systems, case management guidelines, and outcomes evaluation—all will change the care patients receive. Primary care stands to benefit from wide area networking and community-based resource centers.

First, Marley and Farber review four clinical decision support systems (CDSS), two from the 1970s and two now on the market. They then move on to discuss the development of wide area clinical networks, such as that being developed by the University of Iowa Hospital and Clinics.

Newberry offers the South Carolina model and its concept of a statewide system for primary health care. Networks and interactive long-distance computing give new meaning to the concepts of multidisciplinary terms and case management.

MacFadden describes a community center developed by a 500+ bed hospital. Located off-site, the center provides consumers access to a library, including software. Its free membership program offers discounted immunizations, hospital preregistration, and notice of health screenings.

Verona defines case management as a multidisciplinary care delivery method, founded on managed care. She describes the processes for developing guidelines, computerizing distribution and archival functions, and implementing pilots for analysis of the process and its outcomes.

Steinwachs discusses quality performance measurement and integrating outcomes measures into management information systems. To link issues in managed care and acute care, he proposes focusing on (1) high-volume and/or high-cost procedures to determine what factors contribute to better and worse outcomes, and (2) high-cost and/or high-prevalence conditions contributing substantially to healthcare costs and/or disability.

6
How Health Systems Affect Care

AMELIA LEE MARLEY AND MARTIN FARBER

Introduction

Mission statements formulated by both nonprofit and for-profit healthcare organizations across the United States announce their intention to provide high-quality healthcare services through the efficient use of resources. Hence, it is not surprising that a recent survey of 51 member companies of the Center for Healthcare Information Management cited cost reduction and demonstration of quality outcomes as the two leading reasons healthcare organizations buy information technology (Shortliffe, 1987).

Cost reduction and quality improvement are rather obvious fundamental goals inherent in technology decisions or, for that matter, any other healthcare decision. To date, however, proof of the cause and effect relationship of the acquisition of technology on cost reduction or quality enhancement remains elusive. The human organism, a complex combination of interrelated biological systems, remains an enigma only partially understood. In the context of our health delivery system, replete with interrelated providers and systems of care, a picture of extreme complexity emerges, further confounding our ability to accurately identify or measure effects on healthcare consumers.

Approaches to Evaluation

Given these complexities, where do we begin in an evaluation of how computer systems have affected health care? Perhaps with recognition of how narrow any method we choose will be, and appreciation for that which we cannot directly measure or understand. That aside, this paper will present two approaches for evaluating the effect of computer systems on health care.

The first approach is to review clinical support systems and assess their effect on specific patient outcomes. Four specific clinical decision support systems will be described as well as assessment of their effect on the efficacy of treatment. These systems target quality as the primary objective, although cost inferences are easily made.

The second approach is to examine information networks that have provided for the timely distribution of clinical information to clinicians across large geographic areas. Given that the technologies to support this type of wide area networking have very recently been available, there has been little to no research on their long-term cost effectiveness. However, it is important to review the initiatives in this arena as their impact will likely be very significant.

Clinical Decision Support Systems (CDSS)

What is a clinical decision support system (CDSS)? Various names have been used to denote the concept of a CDSS. Some examples are medical expert systems, medical artificial intelligence systems, and clinical database systems. No doubt, other names will appear as advances in software technology occur. For our purposes, CDSS is defined as a system that combines two or more data elements pertinent to a specific patient and leads the clinician towards a clinical decision specific to the individual patient case. Key distinguishing characteristics include direct clinician/system interaction and direct influence by the system of the clinical decision. Specific system "advice" may or may not be present. The important point is that the clinical decision is influenced vis-à-vis the clinicians' interaction with the system.

The field of CDSS began in the mid-1950s. Many of the initial projects explored the validity and reliability of prototype systems and sought to evaluate fundamental computer design issues. Recently, a small number of systems have been introduced into actual clinical use (Miller, 1986). Given the continued reliance on paper and the manual processes supporting the paper-based medical record, it is clear that the CDSS remain primarily in the domain of research initiatives. The move towards the computerized patient record (CPR) by the national Institute of Medicine (IOM) will perhaps lead to the ultimate CDSS. However, it is important to note that the actual implementation of a CPR remains more of a vision for the future than a fully developed tool ready for installation. Most computer systems in health care have been single departmental applications, such as laboratory systems or administrative systems such as a billing system (Dick & Steen, 1991).

In 1986, Blum summarized the then current state-of-the-art clinical information systems as follows:

We are now developing the second generation of medical information systems. Experience with these applications is broad; the knowledge of the technology is vast. . . .Yet, advancements are constrained by the fact that the field requires expertise in both computers and healthcare delivery, that the literature is diverse and difficult to evaluate, and that the technology is changing so rapidly that it is not always clear how past experience relates to new applications.

In 1994, one could well describe the state-of-the-art CDSS in similar terms. It is likely, however, that the remainder of this decade will yield relatively faster progress. The exponential rate of technology growth, the consolidation of healthcare delivery systems, and political momentum towards a CPR will hasten our progress.

Review of CDSS

Four specific applications will be presented in this section; two systems developed earlier in the evolution of CDSS, and two contemporary systems more recently developed.

The Regenstrief Medical Record System

Developed at the Indiana University School of Medicine, the Regenstrief Medical Record System consisted of an evolving set of computer programs that correlated pharmacy, radiology, and laboratory information. The computer generated clinical reminders to physicians based on protocols written by physicians. Based on these protocols, the Regenstrief Medical Record System searched for events specified and produced a printout of recommendations for a specific patient. The so-called surveillance report contained all the recommendations for a specific patient encounter (McDonald, 1976).

In 1976, McDonald studied the responses of nine physicians to complete surveillance reports generated by 390 protocols. Physicians responded to 51 percent of the 327 events when prompted by the surveillance report and 22 percent of 385 events when the computer suggestions were not available. Hence, the response rate by physicians to events was doubled when prompted by the computer. Presuming the protocols defined good care processes, the computer improved care (McDonald, 1976). Patient-specific clinical outcomes were not incorporated into the study. The process itself was evaluated but not the patient outcome. What was important about this study was its emphasis on the "role" of the computer as a tool to sort through amounts of data too voluminous for the clinician to manage without error. McDonald's 1976 study of the Regenstrief Medical Record System demonstrated that physicians responded to reminders and hence followed standardized protocols of care because the prompt led them to what they would have done anyway had they been able to correlate all relevant clinical data without the assistance of a computer (McDonald, 1976).

Diagnostic System Developed at the University of Leeds

Another broad category of the earlier CDSS systems were those developed to assist in the diagnosis of patients. To the extent there was a correlation between the diagnosis and patient-specific problems, the clinical decision itself was greatly influenced. In 1971, the Centre for Computer Studies at the University of Leeds conducted a study of 552 patients with acute abdominal pain. Diagnostic accuracy of the computer-aided system was found to be 91.5 percent compared to a diagnostic accuracy rate of 81.2 percent by the senior clinician. Even more dramatic was a drop in the rate of appendices that perforated before operation from 36 percent to 4 percent.

The study was a prospective controlled trial involving patients admitted to Leeds General Infirmary with acute abdominal pain. Details of the case were entered into the computer and a diagnosis was produced. The computer's "prediction" and the final clinical diagnosis were noted and filed for later analysis. The computer prediction was not discussed with the clinical team until the initial clinical diagnostic assessments were made. Although the computer-assisted diagnosis was unavailable to the clinician for making an initial diagnostic decision, the study did provide preoperative feedback to the clinician, which did have a positive influence on the accuracy of the ultimate diagnostic decision (de Dombal et al., 1974).

Two Contemporary Systems

Moving into the arena of more recently developed CDSS, we will now review two contemporary systems. These two systems are currently packaged under the product name OACIS and First Empower.

The Open Architecture Clinical Information System (OACIS) was built on the premise that "smart summarization" of relevant clinical data from heterogeneous sources results in greater predictability of outcomes than using the medical record alone, and thereby enhances the clinical decision process.

The system consists of two major components: the database or "service model" and the workstation, which is the point of clinical entry. The service model describes the organization, and structures data in the database in generic terms. This generic structure forms an underlying, cohesive infrastructure so that all data queries are met by special cases of fundamental capabilities rather than as individually programmed solutions. The workstation adheres to microsoft windows conventions and therefore navigation is "intuitive." Data are organized and presented from the highest level of summary to the lowest level of detail, branching by degree of granularity rather than by function.

Winston Churchill is quoted as saying "out of intense complexities, intense simplicities emerge." OACIS is a CDSS built on this philosophy. Although very little research has been concluded regarding the effect of this system on quality and costs, many experts predict substantial gains as this type of CDSS is implemented.

Another contemporary CDSS is First Empower. This system takes a more traditional approach to computerizing the medical record in that it has incorporated the basic look and feel of the paper-based chart. The tabular design of a manual record is incorporated into the screen displays. From a single workstation clinical data can be displayed across episodes of care. Multimedia formats including voice, images, and graphics are incorporated in the system.

At the center of First Empower is a clinical database fed either directly or by interfaces to ancillary departmental systems. Tabs indicate different topics "filed" in the chart. Examples include medication administration and laboratory and radiology reports. A patient encounter summary screen exists to provide an overview of the patient. Sections included in the detail behind the summary might be physician, allergy, diagnosis, and legal notices. First Empower, like most contemporary systems, is highly configurable to meet specific organizational needs.

Again, empirical research is currently unavailable regarding the effect of this system on health care. However, it has been well received by both the United States and international markets.

Wide-Area Clinical Networks

Recent advances in telecommunications and distributed information processing hold great promise for improving clinical information access by generalists and specialists. On a global level, it may well be that computer networks servicing large geographic areas will have the greatest affect on healthcare delivery in the future. For example, the University of Iowa Hospital and clinics will invest $7.3 million over the next three years to link rural healthcare providers throughout Iowa. The need to share medical data and imaging technology across the state between general practitioners and university-based specialists are the major drivers for the project (Dunbar, 1994).

It is interesting to note that whereas financial systems were the focus for development during the 1970s and 1980s, clinical requirements are largely driving the development of wide area networks. Without the support of an information infrastructure that provides clinical information across patient episodes, an integrated healthcare delivery system will be dysfunctional and potentially more costly than the traditional delivery systems (Bergman, 1994).

Summary

Although clinical decision support systems were conceived in the middle of the 20th century, their prevalence remains minimal as we head into the 21st century. Computer applications that met financial and administrative requirements took the lion's share of capital investment. Perhaps capitated payment will simplify administrative and billing requirements and allow us to focus on good clinical decision making based on the integration of accurate data that is readily available, and presented in a clinically relevant format. The computer can and should be a tool for the clinician to improve care and provide access to all within our community at affordable cost.

Questions

1. Identify two approaches to evaluating the effects of computer systems on health care.
2. Describe briefly the concept of clinical decision support systems (CDSS). Refer in your description to the systems reviewed: the Regenstrief Medical Record System, the diagnostic system developed at the University of Leeds, the Open Architecture Clinical Information System (OACIS), and First Empower.
3. What progress has occurred since the writing of this chapter. Consider both CDSS and wide area clinical networks? Cite examples. Are the hopes the authors expressed being realized?

References

Bergman, R. (1994). Healthcare in a wired world. *Hospitals and Health Networks,* 28–36.

Blum, B.I. (1986). *Clinical information systems* (p. 66). New York: Springer-Verlag.

Dick, R.S., & Steen, E.B. (1991). *The computer-based patient record.* Washington, DC: National Academy of Sciences.

de Dombal, F.T., Leaper, D.J., Horrocks, J.C., et al. (1974). Human and computer-aided diagnosis of abdominal pain: Further report with emphasis on performance of clinicians. *British Medical Journal, 1,* 376–380.

Dunbar, C. (1994). University of Iowa links rural providers. *Health Management Technology,* 20–24.

McDonald, C.J. (1976). Protocol-based computer reminders, the quality of care and the non-perfectability of man. *New England Journal of Medicine, 295*(24), 1351–1354.

Miller, P.L. (1986). The evaluation of artificial intelligence systems in medicine. *Computer Methods and Programs in Biomedicine, 22,* 5–11.

Shortliffe, E.H. (1987). Computer programs to support clinical decision making. *JAMA, 258*(1), 61–66.

7
Community Family Practice Systems

W. Marcus Newberry

Technology Changing Health Care

The rapid development and merging of telecommunication and information system technologies promise to improve the accuracy of our decision making. The collection, storage, manipulation, and reporting of data are functions of what is being heralded as a new information-based society. As these functions become ever more powerful, the means for information transport and exchange also gain power.

Electricity, from its discovery to the wiring of the rural farm, is a useful analogy in visualizing the time and technologies that will be required before the rewards of informatics are universally distributed. As with electricity, we will tread our way through the cost/benefit of application and deployment guided by the precept that benefits should be accessible to everyone.

The application and deployment of more powerful decision-making tools among health professionals will impact the process for the diagnosis and treatment of disease. Perhaps more importantly, it can reorient the health-care system. Increasingly, we realize that the existing system is marked by the preoccupation with and dedication of resources to the care of individual patients after they have become ill. The care of the sick individual cannot be extrapolated to the care of a sick public. Clearly, there is a point of diminishing returns for this concept. Thus, it is not difficult to forecast a phased transformation:

- Developing information technologies will change current methods for diagnosis and treatment.
- The "universal" information system will make possible sweeping changes, challenging us to define new health values and goals.
- These new values and goals will call for a recasting of the current health-care resource distribution curve.

These are confusing times for the public and their health care. Cost notwithstanding, people seem to want more personal control over their health. Also, it seems, that many people now recognize life style as the key to good health. Yet, if people continue to believe that modern medicine can fix anything, relinquishing our preoccupation with sick care and shifting to an emphasis on prevention will require a transition period of reconciliation and accommodation. An expanded and empowered primary healthcare system can be the meeting ground for the merger of old and new values, the evolution of new techniques for sick care, and the full realization of prevention.

Empowerment of the system is now possible through the application of telecommunication and open architecture information system technologies. Currently networks and interactive long-distance computing can give new meaning to the concepts of multidisciplinary teams and case management to achieve seamless life cycle health care. Although these are sick care activities, their focus upon *outcomes* can be an important step in bringing sick care into perspective.

Primary Health Care

How might primary health care be empowered on the scale required for change to be systematic? This, of course, introduces the practical problem of implementing technology.

The South Carolina Model

In South Carolina, there are current activities pointed in this direction that are calculated to develop a statewide system. This model incorporates primary healthcare delivery, primary healthcare education, social services, public education, and telecommunications. The design of the system emphasizes networked computer systems to achieve interaction and transmission of relational databases. The goal is to coordinate services to achieve optimum health status for individuals and the population.

South Carolina represents a geopolitical area with the potential and need to address the creation and development of the primary healthcare system through a public/private partnership. Such a partnership currently exists between the state health professional associations (including the hospital association), the state research universities, state government through its various agencies (budget and control board, departments of health and environmental control, mental health, social services, education, and educational television), and multiple commercial firms with telecommunication and information system capabilities.

The 28 independent telephone companies of South Carolina have formally associated to create a statewide information highway with more land-based fiber-optic capability per capita in place than any other state in the Union. This capability coupled with wireless communication has been solicited and offered as a backbone to create and implement a statewide open architecture information system to provide for

- Instantaneous and constant linkage between all components of the system,
- High-speed and high-capacity data transmission between all components of the system,
- Computer-aided decision making,
- Diagnostic and therapeutic support distributed throughout the system,
- Monitoring and analysis of health status, healthcare outcomes, quality assurance, and financial data important to the system, and
- Education support to the healthcare providers, students on site, patients, families of patients, and the public.

The Department of Family Medicine at the Medical University of South Carolina has utilized computers as a clinical and educational tool in the clinic and physician offices for 20 years. A cadre of family physicians has been trained in such an environment, and the department has accumulated computer experience and databases on 46,265 patients. The department functions as a resource base for a statewide family practice residency training system located in a total of seven sites, all linked to each other.

There are two active telemedicine links in South Carolina. One is between the University of South Carolina and the family medicine clinic in Winnsboro serving primarily for remote video consultation. Another is between the Medical University of South Carolina and Hampton County in the rural western part of the state. This link is broadbased within the community and across various units of the university. Students from the College of Medicine and resident physicians from the Department of Family Medicine rotate with students from the College of Nursing and College of Pharmacy.

The state is preparing to move toward capitated payment for Medicaid patients. The system, under development in Hampton County, will be evaluated for facilitating this task. Also, the Veterans Administration is viewing the system as a mechanism for providing care near the site of residence with data transmission to the VA hospitals.

Partnerships such as these promise what will ultimately become seamless life cycle health care for all citizens of South Carolina. Data collection and analysis will permit more effective life cycle healthcare planning for individuals and populations. Citizens will be more actively involved in managing their own health care. Patients and practitioners alike will have access to healthcare knowledge and educational resources. Widespread access to information will allow the coordinated delivery of a full continuum of healthcare services and appropriate utilization of healthcare resources. All these changes will ultimately improve outcomes, both for the individual patient and for the population at large.

One of the immediate benefits of networked healthcare practices is the capacity for cost savings related to the pooling of administrative and financial functions. This efficiency is expected to be complemented by increased productivity of the workforce, as it has in other industries that have implemented these technologies. It is important to remember that current practitioners need to achieve subsequent financial benefit to accept what may otherwise appear to be an interesting but expensive cost center.

The primary healthcare system will link practitioners of different professional disciplines in such ways as to allow working relationships not previously possible on a widespread basis. Close contact between physicians and physician's assistants is no longer limited by geography. Pharmacists can be linked directly to healthcare practices, thus allowing the benefit of point of origin input to drug utilization. Software to notify providers when drug prescriptions are not filled by patients offers new paradigms for therapeutic compliance that could result in savings of life and cost. Physician shopping by patients for controlled substances could be quickly detected. The College of Nursing at the Medical University of South Carolina will utilize the system to design and implement a new approach to the practice of wellness and illness prevention. There will be important linkages to social services and the school systems. Such will be the capability and reach of the primary healthcare system and the enhanced definition of multidisciplinary teams.

The primary healthcare system relates to specialty healthcare providers in new ways. The system would establish the perspective that health care is more information (data) based than procedure based and that it is far easier and less costly to transmit data than people. In that light, there can be more far-reaching assessments of the value added to health care by specialists. For example, it could be argued that the value added by medical oncologists is in confirming specific diagnoses and outlining and monitoring treatment programs. Much of this is possible through transmission of data and the utilization of the medical oncologist's expert opinion. The benefit to patients and families comes in cost savings, comfort, and convenience. It will be important that future healthcare providers be trained for the system that provides the value added benefits of case management over gatekeeping.

Patient access and input to their own health medical records are part of an educational process. Software can initiate notification of patients and providers for certain aspects of wellness care; enhanced patient education for specific illnesses and therapies will be more available. Ultimately, targeted educational programs for patients, families, and populations can be directed through television.

Home care can be refined through patient and family education coordinated with sophisticated monitoring systems and home visits by appropriate healthcare providers. Data can be transmitted to health professionals wherever they may be at any given time. This will improve coordination of hospital utilization and enhance the interface between hospital care and alternate care/care sites.

These rapidly developing and merging technologies, and the growing acceptance of their use, have made the concept of the primary healthcare system feasible. Many daunting tasks remain ahead. Among these are creating multidisciplinary healthcare teams, standard healthcare records, healthcare protocols, healthcare outcomes measurements, interactive multimedia for health professional education, and organized educational materials for patients and their families. As healthcare activities join with the advancing telecommunication and information system technologies, health professionals will interact in new and productive ways. The interaction of healthcare professionals with those responsible for developing these technologies will be fertile beyond our current imaginings.

History teaches us that, although specific details cannot be accurately predicted, once progress has been set into motion, we cannot stop or control it entirely. The primary healthcare system described here may never evolve, but it is possible. Within the foreseeable future, it may be surpassed in some form.

The values and goals upon which this concept are based may be longer lasting. The concept envisions a system that, compared to the system of today, is

- More consumer driven,
- More accountable for results with online data, and
- More recognized for constant improvement with online data analysis.

Such a system will foster widespread and effective healthcare delivery research and provide expanded and enhanced education for students, providers, and consumers.

This new world, whatever form it takes, should be exciting!

Questions

1. Discuss how information technology will enable us to move from the present "sick care" model to a "life cycle" model for health care.
2. Describe the activities in South Carolina designed to advance primary health care.
3. Describe how the system that will result will differ from today's system.

Bibliography

Glowniak, J.V., & Bushway, M.K. (1994). Computer networks as a medical resource: Accessing and using the Internet. *JAMA, 271*, 1934–1939.
Lincoln, T.L. (1994). Traveling the new information highway. *JAMA, 271*, 1955–1956.

8
Resource and Community Education Center

Laura A. MacFadden

As the healthcare system undergoes change, the needs of the consumer are also changing. Education, wellness, and prevention are key areas in which hospitals and healthcare corporations should focus in order to provide quality services to the consumer.

These three areas can be enhanced by information technology, making it easier for both the provider and the consumer to gather the most up-to-date educational information.

The best way to empower and enable consumers of health care services is to freely give them access to information that will help them make good choices. (Kernaghan & Giloth, 1991)

Establishing the Center

Bayfront Medical Center is a private, not-for-profit 518-bed hospital in downtown St. Petersburg, Florida, with centers of excellence in cancer care, cardiac care, neurosciences, rehabilitation, trauma, and women's services.

In fall 1993, Bayfront recognized that consumers needed more information and education on prevention, treatment, and diagnosis of many types of illnesses (Proposal for Bayfront Life Services, p. 176). The hospital opened the Community Resource Center to fill this need.

A prime mission of the Resource Center is the consumer health and information library. At the library, consumers can read about conditions such as Alzheimer's disease and AIDS, and check out the latest treatments in areas such as radiation therapy or nutrition. In all there are more than 50 health topics covered at the library.

Consumers usually want information in layman's terms. With that in mind, Bayfront Medical Center believed that consumers might find a standard medical reference too intimidating. But if consumers prefer traditional medical texts, these are available at the Resource Center as well.

In addition, Bayfront felt that people did not want to visit a hospital setting for education or information. For the most part, consumers visit hospitals only when they need care or when their friends or relatives are there receiving treatment.

By choosing an off-site location, the hospital ameliorated the fear and intimidation of a hospital setting. Another benefit of the off-site location is that people can research information at their convenience, when they want to know, and not have to wait until their next visit to the doctor.

Space was leased in a downtown building; with funding provided by the hospital auxiliary for building renovations and state-of-the-art technology, the Resource Center opened to the public.

Serving the Public

The Resource Center is a free service that provides information through a wellness and health-related lending library of books, periodicals, pamphlets, and videos. There is also a community room designed for a variety of meetings, programs, health screenings, and physician lectures. The Resource Center health library is open 8:30 a.m. to 5:30 p.m., Monday through Friday. The community room is open in the evenings and Saturdays as needed for educational programs. Staffing consists of a coordinator who manages and markets the facility, an administrative assistant who handles scheduling, reservations, and membership data, and volunteers who update the clipping files of current health-related articles and assist with mailings and various other support functions.

Prior to opening the center, the hospital's information services department developed a team to review the latest software on the market that would provide quality information to the consumer on the latest healthcare trends, treatments, and methods of diagnosis. After evaluation of many different products, two were selected, both in CD-ROM versions and Windows-based applications.

Resources Available

The two products online at the Resource Center are MEDLINE and the Mayo Clinic Family Health Book.

MEDLINE is produced by the National Library of Medicine and is a computerized index of more than 3500 medical journals published throughout the world. This database provides access to the latest medical information and is a highly valuable research tool for patient care and education. CD-ROM technology has made it possible to store the entire MEDLINE database on compact disks, allowing consumers to retrieve information at their convenience at a computer terminal located in the Resource Center (Facts about the MedLine Database on CD-ROM). MEDLINE was selected by the hospital's information systems department because this software is widely accepted by the healthcare industry as the standard for medical information.

The Mayo Clinic Family Health Book, distributed by Sony Electronic Publishing, makes the book of the same title come to life by adding sound and animation to the medical reference document (Trivette, 1993). The software is very user-friendly, inexpensive to purchase, and easy to understand. It relays a lot of information through pictures and graphics. For these reasons, this software is available at the Resource Center and is used extensively by the public.

Center Membership

The information technology at the Resource Center not only provides the consumer access to a variety of healthcare information in both layman language and medical terminology, it also allows the staff to deliver a membership program to the community.

The Raiser's Edge by Blackbaud is a software package the staff uses at the Resource Center to deliver a membership program to the community. Easy to operate and understand, the software allows employees to produce many different forms, including letters, labels, and reports. The system offers multi-user capabilities through local area network (LAN) technology, providing speed and flexibility.

The Resource Center's Membership Program is easy to handle using this software program. Membership is free and provides many attractive benefits to the consumer. Among the benefits of memberships are discounts on immunizations, preregistration into the hospital admitting system, and advance notice of health screenings.

Biographical information on each member is entered into The Raiser's Edge program using a LAN workstation at the Resource Center. This same information is entered into the hospital's patient registration and accounting system, using a different personal computer workstation located at the Resource Center.

After all the data entry is complete, the member's name and membership number are sent to the printer, where a preprinted, laminated membership card is produced. To date, there are 1400 members of the Resource Center. More members are being recruited. And because of the information technology used at the Resource Center these consumers already have been preregistered and loaded into the hospital's patient database system, without duplication.

The information technology utilized at the Resource Center enables the staff to provide quality health-related information and services to the consumer. Without this technology, the staff would find it extremely difficult to provide services to the nearly 1000 consumers that are served each month. Information technology will allow the Resource Center to expand and grow in the services that it provides to the community.

Looking Ahead

Information technology changes rapidly. New products and services become available every day. Using information technology will give the Resource Center an advantage and make it easier for consumers to gather health-related information.

Potential New Services

One option being considered is to connect the two existing software programs to a telephone modem service. Having modem access to both MEDLINE and the Mayo Clinic Family Health Book would make information gathering easier. Consumers could get health and wellness information using personal computers without ever leaving their desks or homes. Additionally, more health-related information could be put onto computers, such as material from current books and pamphlets. Then the most current and up-to-date information would be easily available.

Another option is to develop a bulletin board service, if a healthcare bulletin board does not exist in the local area. This simple networking application would fill a need for people interested in communicating about diet, nutrition, prevention, and general overall healthy lifestyles.

Yet a third option is to provide online physician referral services. The Resource Center staff could make appointments for consumers calling for referrals, facilitating the process for both the consumers and for staff in physician offices.

The hospital is now investigating the possibility of using the Resource Center membership of 1400 to test new patient registration technology. Each member would receive a photo identification card including machine readable barcoded biographical and insurance information. Resource Center members arriving at any hospital facility would present their membership cards; the card would be scanned into the registration system for verification with the patient and correction if needed. Consequently, the registration system would contain accurate and current information, and the photographs would facilitate positive identification. Photos would be taken at Center membership meetings or when members presented themselves for service at the hospital.

Patient Education

Hospitals and healthcare corporations need to continue to educate the consumer to make decisions about treatment and prevention. Information technology is a definite asset in providing health-related information to patients and consumers. When the right technology and systems are used, the consumer can gain quick and easy access to the most current and relevant information available, thus empowering the consumer to make informed choices concerning health issues.

Questions

1. Describe the Community Resource Center developed by Bayfront Medical Center. Is the concept generalizable to other settings? What advantages might it offer?
2. Comment on the plans for new service offerings at the Resource Center. How would you suggest "growing" the Center?

References

Facts about the MedLine Database on CD-ROM. Marketing Brochure: CD PLUS Technologies, New York.

Kernaghan, S.G., & Giloth, B.E. (1991). *Consumer health information: Managing hospital-based centers.* Chicago: Hospital Research and Educational Trust.

Proposal for Bayfront Life Services, Inc.: Blackbaud, Charleston, SC, 1993.

Trivette, D.B. (1993). Five home medical packages keep you informed. In *Mayo Clinic family health book.* Monterey, CA: Sony Electronic Publishing.

9
Case Management Guidelines

ARLENE J. VERONA

Healthcare management, or the management of patient care, has long been discussed both within and outside of the healthcare industry. Organizations responsible for health care continuously remodel the care delivery process, seeking optimal health for the populations they serve while attempting to match and optimize resource costs to payments received. External forces have had a significant impact on the healthcare industry by raising quality of care issues, including access, as well as applying reimbursement modifications in attempts to curtail high healthcare costs.

We have come full circle in relation to healthcare services payment. Historically, the patient had full financial responsibility for his health care; this also provided individuality in his care choices. Then third-party payment removed the financial burden from the patient and his family while maintaining individuality of care choice; Medicare and Medicaid programs covered those not covered by third-party insurers. More recently, diagnostic-related groups (DRGs), prospective payment, and capitation have become the payment sources for managed care. Although they ensure payment, they limit time and resource payment for specific populations and diagnoses. They also limit individual choice. In essence, managed care integrates healthcare financing with the provision of care. Enrolled patients have limited access to the services and care providers of their choice (Iglehart, 1992). The patient who chooses to invoke individual choice assumes full financial responsibility. Managed care plans aggregate efficient provider groups to deliver specific services for a limited cost per enrollee (Eggert et al., 1991).

The foundation for case management currently rests in managed care, a result of national healthcare reform (Packard, 1993). Case management is seen as a means of containing increasing healthcare costs while ensuring citizens equal access to health care (Iglehart, 1992). A fundamental principle of managed care is that all healthcare-related choices made by clients, clinicians, and administrators have a price. The more one exercises freedom of choice, the greater the personal cost (Packard, 1993). Managed care shifts the financial burden of resource use from insurers to the patient and the provider (Berenson, 1991). Managed care systems use market forces of supply and demand to reward and encourage healthcare efficiency. Those providers identified as practicing efficiently will gain more patients through the managed care selection process (Hoy et al., 1991).

The term case management is used in several different contexts. It can refer to a type of patient care delivery model, differentiating the case management process of care from a primary care process. In this context, case management as a process is used to distinguish among providers and their responsibilities in the provision of care. Or case management can denote a defined set of activities performed within a professional organizational setting, for example, the clinical management of patients with specific clinical diagnoses. It can be used to discuss separate services provided by private practitioners, as is seen in requirements for independent case manager's approval prior to the rendering of services, and with third-party payors. It can refer to a model for professional practice, based on a scientific body of knowledge, which is multidisciplinary in nature and based on collaboration of healthcare providers (physicians, nurses, therapists, etc.).

For the purposes of this discussion, case management is defined as a multidisciplinary care delivery method, the goal of which is to achieve for an individual client, and the homogenous population of which that client is a part, an effective cost/quality ratio (Olivas et al., 1989). This is accomplished through effective and appropriate resource use standardization, collaborative team practice across disciplines, coordinated care continuity across an episode, and cost minimization.

Basic to this model is multidisciplinary collaboration. Case management integrates the various care standards practiced by the professional disciplines into one consolidated standard, or guideline. This integration is a necessary step to ensure care coordination and standardization across the disciplines by case type and to facilitate effective communication between disciplines. Coordination of care is strengthened by the consequential sequencing of each guideline and the addition of a temporal dimension to the integrated standard. Fragmentation of care is minimized when coordination of efforts of all responsible disciplines occurs. Pivotal to this process are revisions to exclude unnecessary activities and assure completion of the critical events. When goals are defined for each event in the standard's sequence, progress towards anticipated outcomes can be measured.

The case management process has been used for over 20 years as a method for rationally allocating healthcare resources across a variety of settings (Kovner et al., 1993). The New England Medical Center pioneered the adaptation of this concept—previously limited to social service activities with welfare clientele—to an inpatient acute care setting, with the nurse direct care provider described as "case manager" (DeZell, Comeau, & Zander, 1988). Their success with nursing case management is well described in professional nursing literature and has promoted the paradigm shift from nursing coordination of care to nursing management of care, primarily in the inpatient care setting.

Elements of Managed Care

The effectiveness of case management depends on the development and utilization of guidelines, which are synonymous with the terms *standards of care, clinical paths, protocols,* and *pathways.* The length and breadth of individual guidelines vary, and their purpose is threefold:

- To standardize the plan of care for a patient population,
- To provide a process standard for care for a specific patient, and
- To allow concurrent and retrospective comparisons of that patient's care with other patients assessed as having similar health concerns.

Retrospectively, trends or variances from anticipated paths within patient populations can pinpoint structural, procedural, or outcome-related modifications for optimizing quality or cost parameters.

Case management guidelines in use today are organization specific; most are discipline specific. Their overall structures are similar, following the process of assessment, plan development, plan implementation, and evaluation. Generic and applicable to any patient with a similar diagnosis, a guideline specifies time parameters for activities and identifies expected outcomes for each activity, category of activities, and for the guideline as a whole. The structure and terminology of guidelines vary within and across organizations, due to differences in how individuals and organizations use terminology.

Guideline development processes vary. Commonly, guideline development begins when a multidisciplinary work group forms to define a sequence of events patients have followed to optimize recovery and to achieve or maintain their health status. Organizational and professional standards, chart audits, literature reviews, and other documentation provide information sources for identifying and sequencing events. Further information is drawn from financial analysis, by case type, including ancillary service use, length of stay, and cost per case. Information from literature reviews and comparable organizations can be used to benchmark current practices and to challenge current organizational practices. Once events are identified, anticipated outcomes or goals for each event are delineated, the resources necessary for assuring event completion are named, and time frames for completion are approximated. Events may also be prioritized and identified as either critical elements or supportive elements. Nonessential events that utilize significant resources, contribute to the cost and length of stay, and do not assist in outcome attainment are identified and removed.

Costs are calculated for the guideline as drafted; these costs are compared to model payments from different payors. If these costs exceed the total payments anticipated, the guideline may be redesigned. The costs, as finalized, are factored into the negotiation of managed care contracts. Supportive information, such as research study results, may be imbedded into the guideline to assist practitioners in making care decisions.

Upon completion of the development process, the guideline is reviewed for accuracy and is moved through an agreed-upon approval process. Once approved, the guideline is available for use.

The essential items of the guideline, therefore, are the following:

- Events, sequenced in order of occurrence (dependencies of each event on other events are highlighted),
- Expected outcomes tied to each event or related series of events,
- Time frames for the occurrence of events, which ultimately provide an overall time frame for completion of the guideline, and
- Resources identified as necessary for completion of events.

For ease of use, the events deemed critical may serve as the *critical path*, rather than the entire document.

Evaluation of the guideline as it is used with actual patients is a necessary and critical step. Through ongoing analysis of variances and subsequent modification, the guideline becomes a useful tool. Events deemed critical should be evaluated over time to validate their importance in achieving desired outcomes. Guideline utilization does not then become a form of cookbook medicine, standardizing the care of patients without further thought; rather it provides a qualitative and quantitative measure against which patient care can be evaluated by both providers and reviewers. Guidelines do not replace professional judgment, but rather represent a recommended pathway for the expected course, facilitating concurrent variance monitoring against the standard. The responsibility for the proper care of each patient continues to remain with the practitioner.

A given guideline reflects the needs of a particular patient population, usually defined by a single clinical diagnosis. In reality, however, patients often enter care with multiple problems or develop additional problems during the care process. As a result, multiple guidelines must be used concurrently. In such cases, there must be a mechanism to resolve conflicts and redundancies among guidelines.

Organizations vary in their philosophy and vision of case management. Some organizations have promoted nursing personnel as case managers as well as care providers; others have utilized quality assurance or utilization review personnel, not actively involved in patient care, to case manage specific patient groups. Regardless of background, the case manager is responsible for monitoring the patient's course against the plan of care, documenting any variations, and providing feedback to the caregiver team.

There are three points in the continuum of care at which case management most typically begins:

- Admission to a hospital,
- Initial outpatient visit for a problem, and
- Enrollment in a managed care plan.

In all cases, there is an event that triggers the assessment or intake process. As a result of this process, client needs are identified; a diagnosis or wellness plan is determined. The assessed patient care needs initiate the selection of a guideline or multiple guidelines, which in turn identify the critical and supportive events to be accomplished and specific outcomes to be achieved. The composite set of guidelines becomes the plan of care specific to the individual patient. As each guideline event occurs, one of several possibilities results:

- The event occurs within the anticipated time frame and the expected outcome is met (no variation),
- The event occurs outside of the time frame but the expected outcome is met (variation to time frame),
- The event occurs within the stated time frame but the expected outcome is not met (variation from goal),
- The event occurs outside of the stated time frame and the expected outcome is not met (variation of time frame and outcome), or
- The event does not occur (event variance).

Should any of these variations occur, the patient care course continues, but the variations must be reviewed to determine causative factors and their impact on the overall expected outcome of the composite guideline. These variances are communicated within the caregiver team and with the patient as appropriate. They are also documented, with explanation, for subsequent analyses of aggregate performance of both the caregivers and the guidelines.

Initially, guideline development tends to focus on two areas:

- High-cost, high-volume patient populations, which have the greatest impact on the bottom line, and
- More homogeneous clinical situations, such as surgical procedures, which are more straightforward and thus analyzed more easily and with less risk.

Once organizations gain experience with guideline activities, they generally commit additional resources to further the case management and guideline development process.

Computers and Case Management

Computerization of the case management process is essential. From a clinical perspective, information systems facilitate efficient guideline development. By making data available, they minimize the time required for guideline development. Historical cases can be aggregated to define current care trends and costs; this analysis can help prioritize guidelines for development. Electronic transmission can expedite the review of draft versions, speed the distribution of approved new and revised guidelines, and notify practitioners of obsolete guidelines, efficiently removing them from use.

For purposes of record and research, obsolete guidelines should be archived and maintained in databases. Computer libraries of current and obsolete guidelines should be established, including initial implementation, revision, and withdrawal dates, and names of the personnel participating in the development and approval process.

Computerized libraries of current guidelines assist in the selection and assignment of guidelines for specific patients based on their needs. As a patient-specific plan of care is built, all contradictory or redundant events, sequences, and expected outcomes are electronically brought to the practitioner's attention. Upon resolution of any conflicts, notations of the decisions made and the persons responsible for them are electronically attached to the approved patient specific plan of care for audit purposes.

Once the patient-specific plan of care is developed, the computer can help the practitioner track the patient's course of care against the plan. The practitioner can view the plan as needed, either in detail (full narrative of the event, the time sequence, and the expected outcome) or in outline form. The events are documented using either of these two views. Documentation of this tracking process has two results:

- The course of patient-specific care is documented for purpose of the record, and
- The variations from the plan are recorded for analysis.

Computerizing the record of variances makes possible efficient retrospective review, evaluation, and revision of the guidelines. It also allows systematic feedback to caregivers of their aggregate performance against the guidelines. An automated case management system of this type has been piloted at the Lakeland Regional Medical Center.

The electronic collection of patient-specific information against standards would support the analyst dimension of case management. Information systems can provide efficient and effective data generation, data reduction, and variance reporting for analysis if the information input is organized according to the data's relationships. Effective analysis will be the product of data readily sorted and reported. The computerization of guidelines and concomitant documentation must follow a consistent structure and content to accomplish this important effort. The guideline structure should be based on logical data flows, to expedite retrieval of information needed. The structure provides the framework for the content. The content must follow agreed upon clinical practice and medical terminology within the healthcare community, to facilitate the actual practitioner's understanding and use. Content must be constructed using the same text statements, to minimize contradiction of terms.

When organizations utilize the same guideline structure and content, information analysis will be possible across organizations, permitting variance review to have a significantly wider consequence than in one organization and for one specific group of clients representing a clinical population. This expanded analysis capability would make available community norms against which current practice would be compared on an ongoing basis, and facilitate expedient revision to support optimal practice for the patient populations. Longitudinal studies, based on a clinical population's information collected over specific covered lives' segments, would provide significant information to ascertain benefits of health regimes and practices. Clinical research would be advanced by the availability of computerized volumes of clinical data based on guidelines, making clinical research results more readily available to practitioners.

Computerization of the information would expedite plan of care review, through demonstration of variance occurrence regularity outside of the preestablished standards on a patient-specific basis. When computerization of population information is available, the software should also signal the impending need for guideline revision because of trends occurring in variance to preestablished standards. These trends would result in a shift in outcome achievement, or a suboptimal resource utilization in either dollars or time.

Process of Implementation

Implementation of the process initially should be experimental or pilot in nature, selecting a few significant patient populations and interested organizational experts as participants in the design and implementation process. Realistic time frames for process initiation should be delineated and adhered to. At agreed upon time periods, the process and its outcomes should be measured relative to the anticipated outcomes to understand the significance of the change and its impact on the realization of the stated goals.

Determination of the patient populations to be initially involved in case management activities falls naturally from the organizational analysis. Using high cost/high volume and current payment levels by case type as the primary selection indicators, a reasonable number of patient populations and provider involvement should be determined. Minimal pilots should be implemented initially, in order to assure that the necessary organizational process changes can be accomplished and supported.

Selection and empowerment of the players are critical to the experiment. Clinical experts from all disciplines relative to the patient populations selected should be supplemented by financial, managerial, and analytical experts in the organization. The latter will provide information and evaluation assistance to the clinical team. The experimental team should be charged with the responsibility for guideline development and utilization within their patient population, and for providing ongoing communication within the organization regarding the pilot's status.

Patient involvement in the guideline development process should be considered by the team, as quality ultimately is meeting or exceeding the customers' needs (Marszalik-Gaucher & Coffey, 1990). The initial decisions regarding patient involvement should be reviewed after substantial data are present, to ascertain whether the involvement level is appropriate.

The guideline development process begins within the pilot team by reviewing the current practice as well as review of current standards, policies, and procedures. The guideline approval process should extend beyond the pilot team, to initiate organizational participation and assure a complete and critical view of the guidelines prior to use. During the period of guideline development and approval, the organization should review and revise policies, procedures, and forms to facilitate the pilot implementation and improve work efficiencies. Educational sessions for those staff impacted and for staff not involved in the pilot should focus on the rationale and process for the pilot study, the anticipated outcomes, and the pilot study time frames. Documentation policy reviews are useful prior to the pilot's onset, to assure that documentation practices utilized in the pilot will result in adequate information for guideline analysis and patient record requirements. Both variance reporting records and exception-based charting have been demonstrated to improve efficiency in manual and computerized modes.

The pilot area's involvement is determined through the aggregation of the study patient population and the selection of the pilot team members. Regardless of the number of pilot team members, all staff in the area should be involved in all activities designed for purposes of education and guideline review, as well as organizational review, revision, and implementation of policies, procedures, and practices. Staff involvement is essential in the early pilot phase and throughout the pilot study as the patient population served enlarges.

According to the agreed upon time frame, the initial guideline usage should begin on a minimum number of patients, upon the patient triggering the healthcare need (e.g., admission to the patient care unit in the inpatient setting). The pilot team should be charged with the responsibility of caring for the first patient groups, providing the authors of the guideline the opportunity to first utilize and assess its appropriateness. Patient involvement in this stage is highly desirable; understanding client expectations and requirements concurrently with actual guideline use will provide important commentary and potential variations. The plan of care for the first patients should be readily modified if event sequence or event outcomes do not represent the true clinical patient picture or client expectations. The guideline development team should meet frequently during the first patients' course, to identify impediments and to celebrate successful phase completion of each patient's care.

Within a predefined time frame or upon a preselected number of patients completing the guideline utilization, the pilot team should complete the first formal analysis. The information collected on initial patients should be reviewed to identify each individual patient's variations from the guideline, and the patterns and percentages of those variations occurring across the initial study population. The event variances should be studied to understand the rationale for their occurrence and their impact in achievement of the outcomes. Positive and negative variances should be analyzed. Variance analysis should include

- Classification of the causative agent,
- Patient/family compliance,
- Current health status of the patient,
- Identity of the caregiver, and
- Organizational structures or processes.

Patient and team satisfaction levels should be measured as a part of the quality outcome achievement determination.

The formal analysis process should also examine the following:

- Actual costs on a per patient basis,
- Aggregate costs for the composite patients utilizing the same guideline,
- Actual versus anticipated costs per case type,
- Comparisons of aggregate costs per case type against the prestudy actual costs, and
- Length of stay for inpatients
    by individual patient
    by case type
compared against anticipated and prestudy actual length of stay by case type.

The team should use the resulting qualitative and quantitative data to determine the initial achievements recognized through the case management process.

When this analysis identifies impediments or indicates that anticipated outcomes were not achieved, the guideline and the processes of care should be revised. In this process, the team should consider revisions to event timing and sequencing; event removal, addition, or reiteration; and outcome modification. Organizational processes and structures should be assessed to determine whether they are capable of change. If they are, then the necessary revisions should be identified and implemented in an expedient manner. If such change is not possible or cannot be accomplished in an efficient manner, guideline modification should be accomplished to assure event completion within the current structure and process. Once the revision is complete, guideline approval and implementation should occur; the original guideline should be archived.

Summary

Managed care is expected to become the dominant means of financial payment for health care. As a result, there will be diminished opportunities for cost shifting, the process of improving charge to cost ratios on a payor-specific basis. Pioneers implementing case management will see more significant financial savings and thus revenue improvement than will those who delay implementation. As early leaders become more cost efficient, they will succeed in bidding on and obtaining the managed care patient populations because of their documented cost and quality. Others, in order to maintain or gain patients, may have to bid lower than their real costs, anticipating to make up needed revenues on other patient populations. This will suffice for the short term only, as managed care dominance increases.

Health care must continue to improve, both in quality and in cost. Healthcare delivery processes must continue to be revised or redesigned to meet this requirement. Internal and external forces will continue to drive this improvement process. Case management is not new; the process of case management in a multidisciplinary environment is a challenge that has long been discussed. Managed care simplifies the expectations of payment for care. Care standardization has always been the individual practitioner's practice; the use of documented guidelines will assist in standardizing multidisciplinary health professionals' practice, improving communication, and optimizing client outcomes. Information systems must be made available to facilitate the case management process, to utilize practitioner resources for efficient and effective patient care, and to provide significant information to aid in care improvement.

Questions

1. Describe the role of case management in managed care, with specific reference to multidisciplinary care delivery.
2. Define the elements of a case management guideline.
3. Briefly outline the guideline development process.
4. Explain the role of information systems in case management and in the guideline development process.

References

Berenson, R.A. (1991). A physician's view of managed care. *Health Affairs, 10,* 37–47.

DeZell, A., Comeau, E., & Zander, K. (1988). Nursing case management: Managed care via the nursing case management model. In: F. Shaffer (Ed.), *Patients and purse strings, II* (pp. 249–264). New York: National League for Nursing.

Eggert, G.M., Zimmer, J.G., Hall, W.J., & Friedman, B. (1991). Case management: A randomized controlled study comparing a neighborhood team and a centralized individual model. *Health Services Research, 26,* 471–507.

Hoy, E.W., Curtis, R.E., & Rice, T. (1991). Change and growth in managed care. *Health Affairs, 10*(4), 18–36.

Iglehart, J.K. (1992). The American health care system—managed care. *New England Journal of Medicine, 327,* 742–747.

Kovner, C.T., Hendrickson, G., Knickman, J.R., & Finkler, S.A. (1993). Changing the delivery of nursing care. *Journal of Nursing Administration, 23*(11), 24–34.

Marszalik-Gaucher, E., & Coffey, R.J. (1990). *Transforming healthcare organizations.* San Francisco: Jossey-Bass.

Olivas, G.S., et al. (1989). Case management: a bottom-line care delivery model, part I: The concept. *Journal of Nursing Administration, 19*(11), 16–20.

Packard, N. (1993). The price of choice: Managed care in America. *Nursing Administration Quarterly, 17*(3), 8–15.

Select Bibliography

Babington, L. (1993). Cautionary notes on innovation in nursing practice. *Nursing Administration Quarterly, 17*(3), 22–26.

Cesta, T.G. (1993). The link between continuous quality improvement and case management. *Journal of Nursing Administration, 23*(6), 55–61.

Katzenbach, J.R., & Smith, D.K. (1993). *The wisdom of teams.* Boston: Harvard Business School Press.

Migchelbrink, D., Anderson, D., Schultz, P., & St Charles, C. (1993). Population-based managed care: One hospital's experience. *Nursing Administration Quarterly, 17*(3), 45–53.

Nolin, C., & Clougherty, L. (1994). Will critical paths keep you out of trouble? *Inside Case Management, 1*(6), 4–5.

O'Connor, P. (1984). Healthcare financing policy: Impact on nursing. *Nursing Administration Quarterly, 8,* 10–20.

Tahan, H. (1993). The nurse case manager in acute care settings. *Journal of Nursing Administration, 23*(10), 53–61.

Zaltman K., Duncan, R., & Holbeck, J. (1983). *Innovation and organizations.* New York: Wiley.

10
Patient Outcomes of Health Care: Integrating Outcomes Data into Management Information Systems

Donald M. Steinwachs

Introduction

Healthcare managers are being challenged by a rapidly changing environment driven principally by cost and competitive pressures. Financial and clinical managers are being asked to respond to the perceived needs of stakeholders in the healthcare system. Payors, both private and public, are looking for value; consumers want freedom of choice and lower out-of-pocket costs; insurers want to avoid risk and make a profit (or net revenue); and providers want to protect their incomes and the values of the systems of care they have built. In an environment of conflicting goals and expectations, information that links cost and quality of services has assumed a central role. Those managers who understand the cost and quality performance of their healthcare products and services will have the opportunity to lead a healthcare system that is undergoing dynamic and fundamental changes.

In the following sections, the role of patient outcomes data in quality performance measurement will be discussed. This will lead into an examination of issues that will have to be addressed if patient outcomes-based measures of quality performance are to be integrated into management information systems. The final section will discuss the potential for using patient outcomes information to improve cost and quality performance in health care.

Quality Performance

The measurement of quality performance is based on a well-developed paradigm that healthcare *structure* (personnel, technology, and facilities) underpins the *process* of care (diagnosis, treatment and management of disease and injury) that contributes to the health *outcomes* experienced by patients (Donabedian, 1993; Brook & Lohr, 1987). Historically, quality performance measurement has placed greater emphasis on structural and process characteristics than on the range of health outcomes experienced by patients. This is changing; health status outcome measures are emerging as the foundation for quality performance indices of the future. The rationale is simple. Healthcare services should lead to health status outcomes that patients value and payors think are worth purchasing, within resource and technology constraints. Patients value their functional capacity (i.e., are able to do what they want to do and are not limited by poor health) and most payors also value functional status (i.e., people are able to be productive).

Patient Outcomes Measurement: State of the Technology

The measurement of patient outcomes is being broadly conceptualized to include:

- Disease status, including current status and end results of the disease process (e.g., mental and physical impairments);
- Health status as indicated by functional capacity, including physical, mental, and social; and
- Satisfaction with healthcare services and satisfaction with health status outcomes, sometimes referred to as quality of life.

The importance of recognizing these three dimensions can be seen in some of the recent research supported by the Agency for Health Care Policy and Research (AHCPR) as part of their Patient Outcomes Research Teams (PORT). In the PORT on cataract surgery, patient satisfaction with vision is more highly correlated with visual functioning ($r = 0.34$) than with visual acuity ($r = 0.03$) (Steinberg et al., 1994). Thus, what the patient values is not significantly related to the clinical measurement (Snelling visual acuity) that is traditionally recorded in the medical record and has been used to measure outcomes. Furthermore, one might guess that most payors would also give greater importance to changes in functional capacity (e.g., ability to read, drive a car) than changes in the ability to read a Snelling eye chart. Other studies of patient outcomes are reinforcing these findings (Steinwachs, Wu, & Skinner, 1994).

As a result, there is a growing interest in the routine application of health status instruments that are valid, reliable, and sensitive to the type of healthcare services being examined. In most cases, these instruments are designed to be either self-administered or completed by an interviewer.

Two categories of health status measures meet these criteria. One category includes numerous condition-specific measures, such as the one cited above that was developed to measure visually related functioning, the VF-

14 (Steinberg et al., 1994). These measures tend to be brief, sensitive, and specific. Their major limitation is that they are applicable only to one set of conditions and cannot be used across a range of patients with different health problems.

The other category is referred to as generic health status measures because they can be applied to any person, independent of the condition or diagnosis they have. These measures include the Short-Form 36 or SF-36 (Ware & Sherbourne, 1992), the Sickness Impact Profile or SIP (Bergner et al., 1981), and the Quality of Well Being Scale or QWB (Kaplan & Anderson, 1988). The SF-36 has the advantage of brevity measuring eight dimensions of functioning whereas the longer SIP has the advantage of somewhat greater sensitivity and measures 12 dimensions of functioning, plus has a summary total score. The QWB is comparable in length to the SIP and has the advantage of producing a single summary score based on utility weights, ranging from zero equals death to one equals the highest level of functioning.

Research comparing condition-specific to generic measures of outcome has found little difference in explanatory power. The general conclusion is that generic measures perform as well as condition-specific measures in explaining functional outcomes, while having the advantage of being universally applicable. The advantage seen by many in disease-specific measures relates to the clinical relevance and interpretability of the information.

A reasonable conclusion is that we have the technology to measure clinical and functional health status, plus satisfaction (Rubin & Wu, 1991). There are costs associated with the capture of these data, their analysis, and their interpretation (Steinwachs et al., 1994). In return for the investment, new insights into treatment effectiveness is gained, and information that can help guide decisions regarding how to better match treatments to patients (Wennberg et al., 1987). Furthermore, the full range of information is likely to be critical to answering the managed care issues of tomorrow, what services should be approved, for which patient, and under what circumstances to control costs, assure good outcomes, and minimize disenrollment due to dissatisfaction.

Analyzing Patient Outcomes

A conceptual model for analyzing patient outcomes is emerging from research and quality improvement studies. The basic elements are depicted in Figure 10-1. There is a set of information sought at baseline that is intended to reflect the patient's characteristics and status before treatment. This includes sociodemographic characteristics, diagnosis, severity, extent of comorbidities, disease status (if different than the measure of severity), generic health status, and satisfaction. Other items that have been found

Time - - - - -> - - - - -> - - - - -> - - - - -> - - - - -> - - - - ->		
Baseline	**Intervening Care**	**Outcomes⁺**
Sociodemographic		
Diagnosis Severity Comorbid conditions		Severity Comorbid
Treatment	Change in Tx	Treatment
Clinical status Health status Satisfaction		Clinical status Health status Satisfaction
Patient knowledge* Self-management capacity* Provider characteristics* Managed care features* Social support*		Knowledge* Self-management* Changes* Changes* Changes*

*These categories of information may be optional, depending on the nature of the condition being examined, and the types of management issues that are being addressed.

⁺Outcomes may be measured at one or multiple time intervals after the baseline; there are no accepted guidelines for timing of outcome measurements, nor whether or not timing should vary across different conditions and treatments.

FIGURE 10-1. Conceptual model for analysis of patient outcomes related to a specific diagnosis.

useful may vary by condition, including knowledge of the condition, self-management capacity, and extent of social support.

At one or more specific time intervals after the baseline assessment, most of these same items of information need to be obtained. In addition, information is required on changes in treatment, if any, during the follow-up interval.

The analysis usually involves the application of multivariate statistical models in which baseline disease severity, comorbid conditions, health status, and intervening treatment is used to predict outcomes, including disease status, health status, and satisfaction at follow-up. Models with high predictive power over time and across variations in treatment and patient characteristics will provide more valid and useful information for management. If there is little or no variation in treatment, including variation associated with the extent of patient adherence to treatment, it is more difficult to know if the model is valid. Specifically, variability in treatment provides a test of the model's capacity to discriminate between outcomes associated with better or worse treatment (e.g., as defined by adherence to treatment guidelines).

Where alternative appropriate treatments for a condition exist, it is desirable that there be variability in the sociodemographic, social support, and self-management capacity characteristics of patients who receive each treatment. Here, the statistical model should provide information regarding whether or not there are differences in outcomes for similar patients who get alternative treatments, as well as for dissimilar patients who get the same treatment.

The paradigm is built on the opportunity to exploit random and systematic variations in health care to gain information on patient, provider, and treatment characteristics related to patient outcomes; specifically, variability is desirable among:

- Patients and their characteristics,
- Provider decision making regarding treatment, and
- Patient adherence to treatment.

Observing this natural variability provides a basis for statistically assessing the effectiveness of treatment(s) in terms of disease status, health status, and satisfaction outcomes. To achieve this objective involves choosing diseases for which clinically meaningful variations are likely to exist and choosing samples of patients that cut across diverse populations being served by different providers and healthcare organizations. The Institute of Medicine has suggested criteria for choosing specific diseases for effectiveness evaluation; these criteria are very useful (Institute of Medicine, 1990).

Integrating Patient Outcomes into the Management Information System

The healthcare management information system (MIS) is usually structured to capture information at the time of patient enrollment or registration and at the time services are received. This potentially provides two of three key elements for analyzing patient outcomes, namely, the baseline characteristics of the patient, the patient's condition (e.g., diagnosis), and treatment prescribed and/or received, plus intervening treatment. However, baseline need not always be measured at the time of a visit or hospital admission.

For chronic conditions it may be preferable to measure baseline independent of services to assess average status and not status at the time medical care is sought, which is probably worse than average if care was sought in response to symptoms or complications.

Most clinical information systems (CIS) capture similar information to MIS, with the important addition of clinical status measures at the time of diagnosis and at the time of follow-up care, if any is received. In both MIS and CIS, some information on treatment may be absent if the patient has received services from other providers, or other systems of care, including services obtained through out-of-pocket payment.

The critical third element missing from MIS and CIS is the routine capture of outcomes information on all patients, whether or not they return for follow-up care. In general, outcomes should be measured at the same time interval from baseline for all patients, otherwise patients will be at different points in the natural history of the disease (injury). This can be done by sending patients questionnaires by mail, or by interviewing patients by telephone or in-person at a fixed interval after baseline. As the domestic information highway is extended into people's homes, this may provide a new modality for capturing outcomes information. Patient questionnaires/interviews can be an expensive process to do well, but statistical calculations can be used to determine the minimum sample size needed to examine the outcomes being evaluated. Also, healthcare organizations may want to come together to pool data on patients, further reducing sample size requirements and increasing variability in the overall patient group. One example of this is the Consortium on Outcomes Management formed by the Managed Health Care Association (MHCA). Sixteen managed care organizations are participating with 11 employers to examine patient outcomes for common and expensive conditions (Steinwachs et al., 1994).

The links between MIS, CIS, medical record, and the development of patient outcomes database are summarized in Table 10-1. It is evident that this is not a simple extension of MIS, but it is a linked parallel system that augments traditional MIS and CIS to provide the information needed to understand cost and quality performance. In general, a combination of data sources is required that can make maximum use of MIS and CIS. In addition, there needs to be patient questionnaires at baseline and follow-up. There are pros and cons for including a physician data form or questionnaire. The cons include the difficulty of gaining physician cooperation and the cost of the physician's time for completing questionnaires. The pros include the physician's capacity to provide reliable diagnostic, severity, comorbidity, and treatment information at the time the patient is being seen. How these are weighed in a final decision may vary by type of disease and treatment and by how the information is expected to be used (e.g., physician questionnaires may be more important if the purpose is to use the information to change physician practices).

TABLE 10-1. Data Sources for Patient Outcomes Analysis

Data Elements	Data Sources
Sociodemographic	MIS, CIS, PQ*
Diagnosis	MIS, CIS*, PDF, PQ
Severity	CIS*, PDF, PQ (?)
Comorbid conditions	MIS, CIS*, PDF, PQ*
Treatment	MIS, CIS*, PDF, PQ (adherence*)
Clinical status	CIS*, PDF, PQ (follow-up*)
Health status	PQ*
Satisfaction	PQ*
Patient knowledge	PQ*
Self-management capacity	PQ*, PDF
Provider characteristics	MIS, ADS, PDF*
Managed care features	MIS, ADS*
Social support	PQ*

Potential data sources include management information systems (MIS), clinical information systems (CIS) or medical records, physician (provider) data form (PDF), patient questionnaire (PQ), or other administrative data sources (ADS).
*Preferred source(s) considering cost, difficulty, and validity in the author's opinion.

What Management Questions Will Patient Outcomes Data Answer?

From what has been discussed, it should be clear that patient outcomes analyses are designed to answer important clinical management questions (i.e., what types of patients benefit from which treatments and under what circumstances). These analyses also can address management concerns involving the structure of insurance benefit coverage, allocation of resources, design of system service capacity, and the management of cost and quality. There are relatively few concrete examples to cite, but one could anticipate several areas in which patient outcomes information might influence management decision making:

- When more expensive treatments, including specialty services, show little or no patient outcomes benefit over less costly treatment, the less costly treatment would be encouraged through staffing and resource allocation decisions.
- When patient outcomes do not meet payor (e.g., employer) expectations (e.g., return to work is delayed), management may seek to invest more resources toward improving specific patient outcomes.
- As new and expensive technologies are introduced into practice, outcomes information could provide a means to assess additional benefits and to identify types of patients who do not benefit and should not be referred.

- As high-cost providers, including teaching hospitals, seek to market their services to managed care organizations, outcomes information becomes critical in documenting the value of services to the purchaser.

These are some of the management targets for patient outcomes information, in addition to the more frequently cited applications in quality monitoring and quality improvement.

Value Performance

One definition of value is that it is equal to the ratio of cost to patient outcomes, adjusting for factors affecting the patient's prognosis that are outside of the control of the provider or healthcare organization. Examples of this measure can be seen in some of the cost-effectiveness assessments of technologies that extend life. Here it is possible to calculate cost per additional year of life, or preferably quality adjusted year of life.

Using this definition of value, greater value can be achieved by reducing costs, improving outcomes, or doing both. More complicated to evaluate are scenarios in which value is improved by reducing both cost and outcomes, but cost is decreased more substantially than outcomes, thus increasing overall value. In a competitive marketplace, the payors are searching for value and so are patients, although their view of cost is what comes out-of-pocket and not the total cost of care. Using the patient outcomes methodology shown in Figure 10-1 and adding in costs of care, value can be calculated. Further analysis can reveal sources of variation in value and suggest characteristics of patients, treatments, and providers associated with lower or higher value.

One application of value measurement is in assessing the impact of quality improvement. Quality improvement efforts all too often lack critical information regarding the full range of outcomes experienced by patients. To the extent this is applicable, they may miss opportunities. In the current efforts of the MHCA Consortium on Outcomes Management, the baseline data suggest that there is significant under-treatment of severe adult asthma based on existing treatment guidelines (Steinwachs et al., 1995), in part due to providers not prescribing corticosteriods (76 percent reported having corticosteroid inhalers) and in part due to patients not taking corticosteroid regularly (54 percent of those with inhalers reported using them less often than daily). Some of these individuals have been hospitalized in the previous two years for asthma; 34 percent of severe asthmatics who are working reported missing one or more work days in the previous four weeks due to asthma; and 44 percent reported canceling usual activities in the past four weeks due to asthma. In analyzing the outcomes information at follow-up, it will be possible to assess the extent to which prescribing and adherence to corticosteroid therapy is predictive of lower hospitalizations, fewer lost work days, and fewer days where usual activities are canceled. Using this information, it will become possible to calculate the value of corticosteroid treatment in terms of medical care service costs and functional status outcomes.

In terms of other outcome measures, only a third of the patients report "excellent" levels of satisfaction with their specific aspects of their care, and only half report having the knowledge and information they need to self-manage their chronic condition (e.g., prevent attacks and anticipate attacks and adjust medication). As one-year follow-up data become available, it will be possible to assess the relative contribution of each of these indicators of quality on outcomes. Using this information should assist managers and clinicians in making choices regarding which aspects of care improvement should be given highest priority.

Summary

The emerging technology of patient outcomes management was characterized by Paul Ellwood (1988) as leading to "... a national data base containing information and analysis on clinical, financial, and health outcomes that estimate as best we can the relation between medical interventions and health outcomes, ... (providing) an opportunity for each decision-maker to have access to the analyses that are relevant to the choices they must make." We remain a long way from this goal, but that is clearly the direction in which we need to move. The challenges are numerous, and include what do we measure, on whom, and when do we measure outcomes of health care? Once measured, how do we interpret the results in ways that can lead to better health care in the future? In summary, I would like to share one statement of caution and one strategy for meeting this challenge.

The caution about which I remind myself each time I begin an analysis of outcomes is—under circumstances of no care or inadequate care, some few patients experience good outcomes, whereas under the best of medical care available, some patients experience poor outcomes—biomedical and health services research continues to search for the answers as to why and mechanisms to intervene and improve outcomes. There are many reasons for variability in outcomes, ranging from treatments that are not uniformly efficacious to the unexplained recuperative powers of the human body.

There are two strategies that appear to be promising in the development of outcomes information. One strategy is to focus attention on high-volume and/or high-cost procedures to understand what factors contribute to better and worse outcomes. The AHCPR PORT studies have emphasized high-volume and high-cost care relevant for the Medicare and Medicaid programs (e.g., cataract surgery). This strategy places a focus on value issues, assures adequate numbers of cases for study, and attracts interest from all stakeholders in the healthcare enterprise. The principal limitation to this strategy is that it generally does not focus on those at risk, but only those who seek and receive a specific diagnostic procedure or treatment. Hospitals and providers who do focus on procedures and acute/intensive care can use this strategy on their patients.

The second strategy is to focus on high-cost and/or highly prevalent conditions (diagnoses) that contribute substantially to healthcare costs and/or disability (e.g., loss days of work or limitations in usual activities). These conditions are frequently chronic or recurrent and might best be studied by sampling individuals with the condition and tracking them at periodic intervals independent of the care they are receiving (e.g., adult asthma). This strategy can be applied in insured/enrolled populations and can be used to probe into how well patient care is managed over time.

Taken together, these two strategies begin to link the issues facing managed care and acute care institutions. Managed care has to develop long-term strategies to assure good outcomes and efficiency in an enrolled population. Acute care institutions need to provide high-quality intensive services that lead to high value for the purchasers (including managed care) and good outcomes for the patients. For managed care, outcomes management is looking for better ways to reduce the use of acute care institutions, but when they are needed, to assure the choice of institutions is associated with high value.

The immediate challenge is to move a patient outcomes assessment research and evaluation technology into application in healthcare provider institutions. This is feasible to do, but it does require an investment. Based on the MHCA experience, there are efficiencies to be gained by forming consortiums to pool resources to adapt measurement, analysis, and interpretation technologies to their needs. In addition, there are advantages to pooling data across organizations; it increases variability within the sample and provides comparisons to judge relative performance.

References

Bergner, M., Bobbitt, R.A., Carter, W.B., & Gilson, B.S. (1981). The sickness impact profile: Development and final revision of a health status measure. *Medical Care, 19,* 787–805.

Brook, R.H., & Lohr, K.N. (1987). Monitoring quality of care in the Medicare program. *JAMA, 258*(21), 3138–3141.

Donabedian, A. (1993). The role of outcomes in quality assessment and assurance (see comments). *Quality Review Bulletin, 19*(3), 78.

Ellwood, P.M. (1988). Shattuck lecture—outcomes management. A technology of patient experience. *New England Journal of Medicine,* 318(23), 1549–1556.

Institute of Medicine. (1990). *Clinical practice guidelines: Directions for a new program.* M. Field & K. Lohr (Eds.). National Academy of Science Press.

Kaplan, R.M., & Anderson, J.P. (1988). The quality of well-being scale: Rationale for a single quality of life index. In: S.R. Walker & R.M. Rosser (Eds.), *Quality of life assessment and application* (pp. 51–78). Lancaster, England: MTP Press.

Rubin, H.R., & Wu, A.W. (1991). Patient satisfaction: Its importance and how to measure it. In: G. Gitnick (Ed.), *The business of medicine: A physician's guide.* New York: Elsevier Science Publishing Company.

Steinberg, E.P., Tielsch, J.M., Schein, O.D., Javitt, J.C., Sharkey, P., Cassard, S.D., Legro, M.W., Diener-West, M., Bass, E.B., Damiano, A.M., Steinwachs, D.M., & Sommer, A. (1994). The VF-14—an index of functional impairment in cataract patients. *Archives of Ophthalmology, 112,* 630–638.

Steinwachs, D.M., Wu, A.W., & Skinner, E.A. (1994). How will outcomes management work? *Health Affairs,* 153–162.

Steinwachs, D.M., Wu, A.W., Skinner, E.A., & Campbell, D. (1995). *Asthma patient outcomes study: Baseline survey.* Report prepared for Managed Health Care Association Outcomes Management System Project Consortium, Health Services Research and Development Center, Johns Hopkins University.

Ware, J.E., & Sherbourne, C.D. (1992). The MOS 36-item short form health survey (SF-36): I. Conceptual framework and item selection. *Medical Care, 20,* 473–483.

Wennberg, J.E., Roos, N.R., Sola, L., Schori, A., & Jaffe, R. (1987). Use of claims data systems to evaluate health care outcomes: Mortality and reoperation following prostatectomy. *JAMA, 257*(7), 933–936.

Section 2
Planning and Managing the Move

Unit 4
Charting the Course

Unit Introduction

Like any move, the move into the information age requires planning. Fortunately, formal models and proven methodologies can facilitate information systems planning and link it to business strategies. Information architecture can provide a strategic advantage in health care, and the chief information officer position can offer critical leadership.

Focusing on the evolution of integrated delivery networks (IDNs), Helppie and Stretch describe a formal planning process that can be institutionalized and tied to the evolution of enterprise business strategy and plans.

Gabler links information delivery architecture to strategic advantage for health care. Modular, open architecture makes possible flow-oriented, multisystem design, and can give management the ability to manage costs and outcomes, respond quickly, and offer strategic value.

Penrod sees strategic planning as proactive and integral to strategic management. Planning models vary and must be tailored to the healthcare institution. Penrod proposes a six-step model and discusses evaluation.

Hersher updates her profile of the chief information officer (CIO), highlighting leadership and the new organizational view mandated by evolving integrated delivery networks. The CIO fills multiple functions, including those of change agent, information architect, and standard setter.

11
Information Systems Strategic Planning: A Healthcare Enterprise Approach

RICHARD D. HELPPIE AND TERRANCE T. STRETCH

This chapter outlines a number of the major changes affecting the health-care industry, emphasizing those with substantial implications for information systems (IS). It then describes the benefits and challenges associated with adopting a formal IS strategic planning program within the healthcare enterprise, describes a proven process for developing IS strategic plans and of institutionalizing IS planning as a process, tied intimately with the evolution of enterprise business strategy and plans, rather than an episodic and isolated determination of computer technology needs.

Changes in Health Care

Even while the federal healthcare reform wars have been waged in Washington, the healthcare delivery system in the United States, driven by market forces and fear of the politicians, is evolving from a fragmented industry composed of thousands of individual providers, various financial risk-accepting entities, and numerous corporate and individual purchasers to a consolidated industry featuring regional integrated delivery networks (IDNs). These changes affect the management and the information systems of every participant in the healthcare delivery system. Tomorrow's IDNs will evolve from many roots—health plans, insurance firms, hospital systems, physician groups, new investors, and perhaps other sources. Regardless of an IDN's origin, all players in the healthcare industry must, at a minimum, adopt new strategies. Many must take on entirely new corporate identities and vision. Whether one's core business strategy is to become the central force in forming and operating an IDN or to participate as a member in some other enterprise's network, the changes in the healthcare environment emphatically dictate strong IS.

Even more than previously, the creation and evolution of those systems depend, now and increasingly in the future, upon an equally strong process of strategic information systems planning as healthcare enterprises and their software vendors struggle to move through this period of tumultuous

121

change. IS have become an integral component of enterprise business strategy, shifting in the executives' view from their previous overhead/pacing factor, inhibitor (and sometimes preventer) of strategy execution to capital resource allocation choice/enabler, extender (and sometimes creator) of strategy execution.

Some discussion will illustrate this profound shift and, hopefully, provide incentive for an enhanced approach to strategic IS planning.

In a world of fragmented, reimbursement-funded healthcare providers, the various providers had little concern for the scheduling of activity, leveraging of resources, and approval of claims at any of the other providers. Consequently, IS were largely devoted to postevent tabulation of activity within a specific provider. The transfer of information was from an individual provider to third-party payors. IS planning was often devoted to capacity and volume estimations, rather than functional expansion or the creation of capabilities to better manage enterprise resources.

In a world of integrated delivery networks where all providers share economic risk, it becomes vitally important that patient care is managed throughout the healthcare enterprise. Scheduling of activity, utilization of resources, and the approval of care at other providers now affect the revenue, profitability, and the very survival of the healthcare enterprise. Indeed, the manner and method of providing care at a specific site, for a specific malady, by a specific caregiver have now become subject to prospective and in-process management rather than post-event tabulation. The need for the transfer of information among providers has therefore risen exponentially.

The paradigm shift from care as a source of revenue to care as an expense drives the shift in enterprise management and information requirements. A system designed to document that services were provided to an individual and then request money from one or more payors is simply inadequate for managing the obligation to provide services to a set population for a fixed amount of money. Regardless of whether the buyer is a purchasing alliance, employer coalition, or some other entity, providers will compete for patients, premiums, and populations on the basis of cost and quality. Provider networks that can demonstrate quality outcomes at reasonable costs will win new business in the competitive environment. Aggressive marketing, sales, and costing systems are needed to successfully compete on the basis of price and delivery.

The traditional approach to IS planning looks backward, noting deficiencies, and documenting requirements. It cannot possibly be expected to meet the needs of a future healthcare delivery enterprise. Concurrent with the definition of organizational identity and enterprise vision, the IS vision must be defined via a process that might be characterized as intercepting the future. This process consists of describing an IS that will support the current and future enterprise vision and identity, and constructing a preliminary design using a combination of proven, advanced, and anticipated information management technologies. The delivery network will be composed of owned, leased, and contracted facilities and providers. The healthcare enterprise will not be defined by bricks and mortar, but by IS, culture, and contracts. The most important characteristics of the IDNs strategic IS plan and of its systems will be adaptability and openness.

The need to manage across an entire continuum of care in a financial risk environment, using both semipermanent and temporarily aligned service entities, requires IS that can quickly connect and disconnect merged, affiliated, or contracted entities. In this regard, the era of monolithic databases for all applications gives way to specific repositories. Likewise, traditional construction of indexes and numbering schemes to identify and track patients and subscribers is outmoded and must be replaced with network-resident modules (agents) that identify individuals based on algorithms that use the natural information found in the computer systems of all entities.

Health care will be purchased on the basis of cost and quality by large, organized buyers. Whatever form these new, organized buyers ultimately take, the demands for information management will veer markedly from historical requirements. At the time of this writing, quality measures still presume the presence of an acute or chronic condition that requires intervention. The healthcare delivery system swings into action when a patient requests intervention, and the IS are accordingly designed for this reactive environment. Observers have opined that quality is spelled c-o-s-t because the measurements to evaluate the effectiveness of care are inconclusive at best. At worst they do nothing for the portions of the population who do not seek medical intervention.

In the new healthcare world order, purchasers will demand that provider networks prove the wellness of their covered population and demonstrate improvements in health status. Thus, the IDN competes to become the low-cost producer by ensuring that its population avoids high-cost services. The IS designed for this purpose must include a widely accepted means of measuring health status. Such a means of measurement must be understood by the average citizen, the provider of health care, and the ultimate purchaser. The means of health measurement must also statistically prove that the higher the measure of health status, the fewer the number of interventions for acute conditions. The health delivery system now becomes more active, verifying the health status of a covered population on a routine basis so that early, less costly interventions and prevention programs can be administered. The IS now moves from a passive recipient of events to an active manager of wellness for the patient population.

The consolidation of the healthcare system and the changing incentives have spurred dramatic changes in the business relationships of physicians. The formation of physician–hospital organizations, physician organizations, and other such entities have provided a transition vehicle for the rising influence of primary care physicians. When the need for a medical inter-vention arises, jointly developed care protocol and productivity standards guide the delivery of physician and caregiver services. Healthcare delivery networks must construct sophisticated clinical IS handling capabilities to ensure that protocols and standards are communicated and adopted. Ad-ditionally, all practices are measured for outcome effectiveness and impact on health status.

Successful healthcare delivery systems have a financial risk-accepting component within their network. Successful healthcare delivery networks will construct managed care applications that use the same clinical data as the care-supporting IS to identify patient populations, control costs, and market themselves as the quality leader.

Successful healthcare delivery networks will have robust IS that com-municate among entities within the health system, across dispersed geog-raphies, and with income sources, including insurers and employers. These IS will be developed as networks owned by a health provider system. Sim-ilar to electronic mail networks and automated teller machines (ATMs), these organization-specific networks will eventually link to the networks of other organizations.

Throughout the development of an IDN, it will be necessary to make concurrent investments in IS to manage the remainder of the pre-reform system as well as support the strategic needs of the post-reform system and the transition between them.

The purchase of IS in a hospital-centric, fee-for-service environment was often accomplished by compiling lengthy feature/function lists. These lists were typically limited to the needs of individual departments, which were incorporated into requests for proposals to software vendors. The software vendor then answered the specific queries and was led through a process that was limited to satisfying the needs of the requesting departments. The construction of an IDN means that the transfer and use of information among all the departments and across the IDN's operating entities now has a greater importance than the departmental feature/function of the past. The procurement process must be based on overall data and communica-tions architectures adopted by the IDN. Selection of vendor partners must demonstrate how they will assist in managing the network, rather than pro-viding a few specific features. A partnership orientation must supplant the traditional vendor–customer relationship to ensure success for the evolving IDN.

If times are difficult today for the healthcare providers, their software vendors have no easier lot. The success of packaged software depends on a large market of homogenous customers with common and stable infor-mation requirements. However, just the opposite is the forecast: the implo-sion of a large market to a small number of quite diverse IDNs with dif-ferent and very volatile business and information requirements occasioned by their different origins, composition, and regional economic characteristics. As a result, healthcare enterprises will need to take an ever greater role in systems integration and may, in fact, have to examine the continued viability of their reluctance to develop custom software when their business requirements are truly unique.

The purchasing aspect of healthcare IS planning should not be taken lightly. Successful IDNs will continue to require IS proficiencies and project management skills within their work forces. However, the concurrent trend to limit permanent employees will require them to purchase more products, advice, and services. More work, requiring greater expertise, with fewer employees means that partnerships will be the rule of the day.

Obtaining value from information technology, niche products, tools, techniques, architecture, and services requires IS planning that includes the sponsorship and involvement of senior executives and technical staff at each step in the process. Achieving the IDN's goals for clinical effectiveness, market share, and financial performance will require a truly strategic view of IS–and a correspondingly strategic approach to planning for those IS.

The Benefits of IS Strategic Planning

Virtually all traditional hospital enterprises have adopted a formal planning process for their overall business planning and most have also initiated more or less formal planning activities for their IS activities. Other members of the healthcare industry, especially smaller, entrepreneurial enterprises, have made less progress in this regard.

In the interest of affirming the righteousness of those converted, and perhaps of swaying the minds of those as yet unpersuaded, we suggest a number of benefits of a formal practice of IS planning. We believe the benefits can be addressed in two categories: those benefits to overall enterprise management and those of specific benefit to IS management.

Benefits to Enterprise Management

The following are the major benefits to the healthcare enterprise as a whole from a successfully implemented process of IS planning:

- Consensus within the enterprise of the role of information systems in achieving enterprise strategy—not only supporting its execution, but of creating opportunities to extend it;
- Focus of investments in IS on areas of greatest impact and highest payoff;
- Placement of board and executive management decisions regarding IS investments on a proper business footing, comparable to other capital resource allocation decisions;
- Comprehensive, multiyear view of the funding requirements for IS; and

- Effective management framework for directing the implementation of the IS strategic plan.

Role of IS

The planning process forces a dialogue within the senior ranks of the enterprise of what they want from information technology. This dialogue will align expectations, opportunities, resources, organization, participation in executive management activities, funding, and accountability. For example, adopting a position that information and information technology constitute a strategic resource, comparable to human, facilities, and capital resources (see Figure 11-1), will determine the type of leadership for the function, the level of participation of that leader in the general business decision-making process, the operational and capital budgeting approaches, and the level of accountability.

High Payoff Investments

The planning process allows the enterprise to concentrate its limited resources on efforts with the greatest overall impact by concentrating on those that have the best demonstrated business case. Under such an approach, IS investments that create competitive advantage will rise to the top over departmental or administrative investments. It also focuses implementation planning on sequencing projects. If, as has been often the case in the past, IS has been an inhibitor—or even a preventer—of the execution of enterprise strategy, it must now take up a much stronger and active role, as an implementor, an enabler, and, on occasion, a creator of strategic opportunities for differentiation of the healthcare enterprise and the creation of competitive advantage. Clinical applications, such as telemedicine, extend the reach of the enterprise to new geographic markets; automated clinical

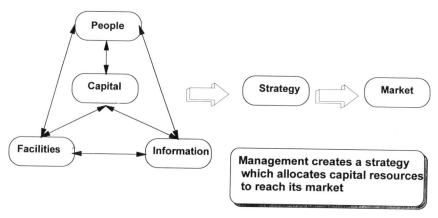

FIGURE 11-1. Information is a strategic enterprise resource.

protocols demonstrably enhance both the quality and cost of patient care. Integrated supplier/enterprise approaches to materials management bring just-in-time inventory management to health care. Distance learning permits medical schools to extend their geographic reach for continuing medical education, extending their links to physicians, nurses, and other practitioners and enhancing the bonds with these core delivery system constituencies. The availability of core molecular biology equipment, software, and data permits research centers to attract, retain, and support the work of researchers in an era of dwindling grant funds.

IS Decisions on a Business Footing

Carrying this same argument forward, this business/payoff approach permits IS management to present its proposals for use of enterprise capital on an even footing with other competing proposals for investment in human or facilities resources.

Funding Framework

The IS planning process will identify IS operational and capital efforts. The business case presentation of the plan makes explicit the multiyear financial implications of alternative investments and allows enterprise management to consider the lifecycle costs and benefits of the initiatives. Even when the defined benefits of proposed IS initiatives are not easily quantified, a complete analysis of costs permits selection of the most appropriate funding means, including cash from operations, grants, special fund-raising, leasing, or other debt financing approaches.

Effective Implementation Management Framework

The planning process should result in a portfolio of projects to be executed, moving the IS environment from one projected stage to the next. In addition, the process should have established a governance process for IS that can be used during execution to monitor progress, make appropriate midcourse corrections, and hold both IS and user participants accountable for their performance against the plan.

Benefits to IS Management

The following are the major benefits that can accrue to the healthcare enterprise's IS management as a whole from a successfully implemented process of strategic IS planning:

- Congruence of IS goals with enterprise goals;
- Comprehensive IS architecture for IS—data, applications, technology, and management;

- Substantial work products for accelerating and parallelizing the early phases of the implementation of the IS strategic plan;
- Preservation, when appropriate, of existing IS investments and project initiatives;
- Clear definition of the funding, benefits, success, and accountability; and
- Effective management framework for directing the implementation and enhancement of the strategic plan.

Congruence of Goals

If conducted successfully, the IS planning process will ensure that the goals and priorities of the IS function are clearly understood by everyone within the enterprise. IS will be focusing its energies where they can have the greatest impact and, to a great degree, IS can avoid the mismatch between expectations, resources, and delivery that plagues many IS environments.

Comprehensive IS Architecture

The historical reliance of healthcare enterprises on prepackaged departmental software solutions—comprehensive healthcare information systems (HIS); departmental applications such as laboratory, radiology, pharmacy; and specialty segment applications such as durable medical equipment (DME), home health, reference laboratory—is at risk during the period when the industry, the technology, and the vendors are evolving. In more stable times, a single provider could successfully adopt a primary HIS, select other packages, and construct point–point interfaces between them. In an IDN environment with both fee for services and managed care components, the combinations of applications, the technical complexity of interfaces, and the selection process will call into question the old approach. There are too many participants, too many legacy environments, and dramatically changing business rules and requirements. The creation of the formal architecture will provide a beacon illuminating the make–buy–integrate decisions that will be necessary during implementation.

Although the notion of a formal architecture is familiar to most enterprises, the changing nature of the healthcare environment will require new emphasis on two other areas as well. The importance of a formal data architecture will increase dramatically as the number of packaged software products increases. The enterprise or the IDN must implement a data warehouse to collate information in an easily accessed form from many applications so that the semantic (meaning) differences between data in various applications becomes as apparent as their syntactic (format) differences. Secondly, the need for a formal communications architecture will increase and become an independent component of the strategy as the geographic dispersion of processing and data continues.

Although new architectural elements will arise, some of the old favorites will remain and take on added importance and complexity. Security, reliability, resilience, backup, and recovery are still essential—even more so when managing distributed resources over a wide area. Password protection for access to application functions and data will not be sufficient when unencrypted packets are passed on connectionless networks, available for examination by any attached device. An uninterruptible power supply (UPS) in the computer room is helpful for an orderly shutdown of certain elements of the environment, but will likely not support continued operation unless the local area network/wide area network (LAN/WAN) distribution electronics are also protected by UPS. Time to restoration of business operations will become the measure of contingency management plans, eliminating/reducing time in diagnosis, procurement, configuration, and installation of replacement components.

Accelerated Implementation

Those opposed to conducting formalized IS planning often do so under the banner that planning merely delays implementation. Quite the contrary, a comprehensive plan can accelerate implementation by prioritizing those products with value to multiple implementation projects and permitting many projects to be conducted in parallel with solid coordination. A well-defined understanding of the enterprise's business environment will jumpstart the requirements analysis in every application effort. An enterprise data model and definition of key business process information requirements will frame database, application, and technology analyses.

Principal IS Strategic Planning Challenges

On its face, IS planning would appear to present its greatest challenges in the technical arena. Although the technical complexities of today's environment are challenging, we suggest that they pale in comparison to the enterprise, political/behavioral, cultural, and management/financial challenges for HIS. One could write at length on each of the issues. Table 11-1 presents a summary of key planning challenges encountered over the years. The point is not discouragement, but forewarning. It is *people* who create, adopt, implement—and sometimes thwart—plans. Carefully addressing the issues in the planning process will increase the chances for successful implementation. Perhaps the most important issue, though, in thinking about IS planning at the enterprise level is to ensure the proper blend of talents. IS planning and development without the active sponsorship and direction of executive management will always be expensive, time consuming, and of low value. IS planning, development, and deployment without the proper technical expertise will always be expensive, time consuming, and prone to failure.

TABLE 11-1. Challenges in the IS Planning Process.

IS Planning Challenges	Challenge Area				
	Enterprise	Technical	Political/ Behavior	Cultural	Mgt./ Financial
General uncertainty in enterprise business environment	✔				
Potential acquisition, divestiture, reorganization, alliance entry/exit	✔				
Lack of an enterprise business plan and strategy	✔				
Lack of clarity within the enterprise as to business plan and strategy	✔				
Shifting, conflicting busness, IS priorities within the enterprise	✔				
IS management inclusion in business, strategic discussions, decisions	✔			✔	
Executive sponsorship for planning, implementation	✔		✔		✔
Tactical/overhead view of IS vs. strategic resource view		✔			
Islands of automation environment		✔	✔		
Balancing enterprise standards with unique user needs		✔	✔		
Balancing enterprise priorities with business unit/departmental priorities		✔	✔		
Legacy transition—data, applications, technology, IS management		✔			
Obtaining executive agreement on strategic role of IS	✔		✔		
Agreeing on IS priorities and prioritization process	✔		✔		
Business unit/departmental *territoriality* re IS resources			✔		
Climate of trust (it's OK to be a second priority if there is confidence that the secondary items *will* be addressed			✔	✔	
Balancing the delivery, timing, and pace of implementation			✔		✔
Balancing directly-user-beneficial with infrastructure projects			✔		✔
Antiplanning bias in the enterprise or the IS function				✔	
Balancing business unit/departmental autonomy with need for enterprise-level solutions			✔	✔	✔
Centralization/decentralization polarization				✔	
Sacred Cows—enterprise or IS			✔	✔	
Excessive resistance to change				✔	
Too-easy concession to implementation obstacles				✔	
Matching financial resources with expectations	✔				✔

TABLE 11-1. *Continued*

IS Planning Challenges	Challenge Area				
	Enterprise	Technical	Political/ Behavior	Cultural	Mgt./ Financial
Balancing multiyear funding commitments with annual budgetary pressures					✔
Balancing capital and operational budgeting and funding					✔
Ensuring a *Get it Done!* mentality (an excuse is *not* as good as a result)				✔	✔
Effective management oversight and control					✔
Validation and risk assessment/ mitigation throughout implementation					✔

The Process of IS Strategic Planning

We present here a three-phase methodology for the conduct of IS strategic planning that we believe offers healthcare enterprises a proven approach to successful planning—and the means to ensure both a successful implementation and institutionalization of the planning process itself. The three phases are depicted in Figure 11-2 and are described below.

Phase I: Define Business Context, Direction, IS Vision

The purpose of the first phase of the IS strategic planning process is twofold: (1) to ensure a formal definition of the current and intended business environment, and (2) to define an IS vision for the enterprise that will guide the development of the IS strategy.

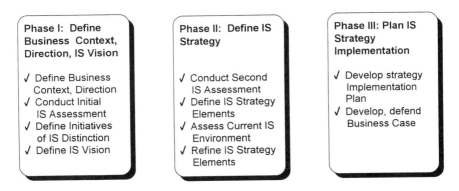

FIGURE 11-2. A three-phase approach to strategic IS planning.

Phase I comprises seven basic tasks:

- Conduct executive and planning team education. Facilitate a one-day briefing session on issues affecting the healthcare industry in general, the enterprise's segment(s) in particular, and the planning process in which they are about to participate.
- Define, document the scope of the planning effort. Establish the fence-posts: what enterprise business units, departments, applications, technology, and IS management issues are open to study or fixed for purposes of the plan.
- Develop an enterprise portfolio. Document and agree on a description of the key business characteristics of the enterprise including mission, critical success factors, key strategies, competitive strengths, weaknesses, opportunities, threats, marketplace environment (customers, suppliers, alliance partners, competitors), high-level structural analyses (legal, organizational, geographic, process, data).
- Develop a high-level IS overview. Compile basic information about the current IS environment—data, applications, technology (platforms and communications), management. Compare/contrast the current environment with the information developed in the enterprise profile.
- Define IS initiatives of distinction. Identify opportunities for the IS function to assist in the execution of enterprise strategy or even to create strategic opportunities for the enterprise.
- Define the enterprise IS vision. Conduct a one-day workshop to define the broad outlines of the role and mission of IS within the enterprise, the major IS contributions and goals to be achieved over the planning horizon, the general magnitude of investment, and operational dollars involved in achieving them.
- Define the enterprise data/application portfolio. Within the context of the IS vision, define the independent variable of the IS strategy, a statement of what data are essential to the enterprise and how those data will be created, maintained, transmitted, and displayed.

Several comments are in order regarding phase I. The educational workshop session is intended to create a common framework for the conduct of the IS planning process. Although many in the enterprise's senior management will be acutely aware of the major changes sweeping the healthcare industry and the implications of these changes for their enterprise, others on the planning team may not have been similarly exposed to the issues. Further, senior management participation in and contribution to the workshop establishes their level of interest and commitment to the planning process.

The scope definition task is as important in terms of what is ruled out as what is ruled in to the planning process. If management has made a determination that it is not willing to move from a particular technology platform or not willing/able to invest more than a certain amount of cash per year in implementing the plan, it is important to identify those constraints as soon as possible to prevent unproductive analysis and the useless raising of expectations.

The enterprise profile becomes the agreed framework and criterion against which IS initiatives, investments, and results will be developed and evaluated in the remainder of the planning effort. It is not a substitute for an overall enterprise business plan and strategy, but rather an extraction of selected information from such a plan to assist in the IS planning effort. That said, the enterprise profile can well serve other purposes in the enterprise—for example, as a tool in the enterprise business plan/strategy process; a basis for business process reengineering and quality improvement programs; a training and communications aid for staff and alliance partners. As will be seen below, the approach calls for an assessment of the current IS environment in terms of its ability to contribute to the accomplishment of the strategy. In phase I, the purpose of considering the current environment is to gain an appreciation of the relative coverage of the current IS environment with respect to the areas of the enterprise identified as strategic in the enterprise profile. A common result of this task is the recognition that a very circumscribed focus of IS relative to the overall needs of the enterprise has developed over time—and a recognition of the need for a much expanded vision of the role of IS.

The IS initiatives of distinction task focuses on identifying specific opportunities for IS to contribute to the achievement of enterprise strategy. It concentrates on distinguishing *strategic* IS applications (those that directly affect enterprise competitiveness—for example, telemedicine, physician office linkage and support, effective cost accounting in a managed care setting—where time-to-market, differentiation, and acceptance of reasonable cost/risk penalties dominate) from *tactical* IS applications (those associated with business activities that, although necessary, do not affect enterprise competitiveness—most accounting and administrative applications, plant operations and other back-of-house operations, for which cost reduction, efficiency, low risk are the watchwords).

Figures 11-3 and 11-4 present the strategic–tactical initiative distinction graphically, drawing on a technique developed in consumer research to profile customer key buying factors in terms of potential product/service characteristics. In this application of the technique, we have indicated four primary axes, each ranging from none to high: performance, risk acceptance, reliability, low cost.

The IS vision accomplishes two goals: (1) it frames the discussion of IS strategy in phase II; (2) more importantly, it is the first point of commitment for senior management. Their participation in its creation and visible support for it are essential to the development of consensus and commitment over the planning process, especially at the time of setting final priorities and allocating funds to individual initiatives.

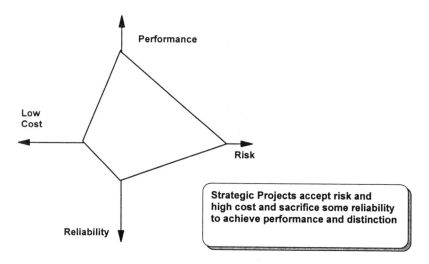

FIGURE 11-3. Characteristics of *strategic* IS initiatives.

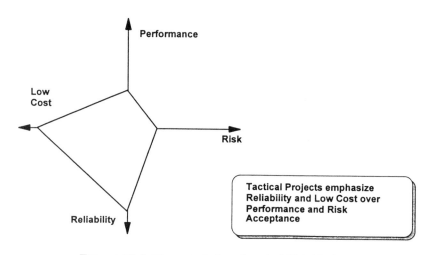

FIGURE 11-4. Characteristics of *tactical* IS initiatives.

Phase II: Define IS Strategy

Phase II comprises four basic tasks, though some degree of iteration may be required to bring the strategy to closure. The strategy addresses the question *where do we want to be?* and cannot be addressed completely without an understanding of *where are we?*

- Document current IS environment. Create a fact book about the current IS environment, an inventory, and summary of what is in place and underway and of how well it matches the needs of the enterprise.
- Define the IS strategy elements. Project the policy and implementation framework for IS forward over the planning horizon in terms of data, applications, technology (platforms and communications), and management of the IS function.
- Assess the current IS environment. Determine how well the current IS environment fits the initial strategy, where there are existing investments that can be incorporated into the strategy, where there are missing elements of the strategy.
- Refine the IS strategy elements. Refine the statements of strategy based on what has been learned in the assessment process.

Here, too, several explanatory comments seem in order. As noted earlier, the truly independent variables in the IS strategy are data and applications. Together, they define the charter for IS: support the creation, maintenance, distribution, and access to information essential to achieving enterprise strategy. Once there is agreement on core strategies in these areas, one can move on to address the other strategy elements. Technology choices, for example, are shaped by these initial decisions. If a major application strategy is to acquire and integrate vendor-supplied applications for core business activities, then until the vendor community moves forward substantially from its 1994 position, a fully open, distributed, client–server technology platform may not be possible due to a lack of packages that operate in such a technical environment. Similarly, decisions about applications and technology will shape strategic decisions about the organization, location, and size of the IS function.

Today's healthcare environment is simply no longer campus based. Geographic dispersion will become even greater as the industry continues to consolidate, align, and extend its activities from diagnosis and treatment to prevention and maintenance. As a result, the careful planning of an enterprise communications network is an essential—and distinct—portion of the IS strategy formulation. To use a biological illustration, we have fully entered the era of the *exo-computer,* a technology environment in which the network serves as the skeleton of the computing environment and to which various computing organs, servers and clients, are attached. Data transfer and high-bandwidth requirements at the individual desktop, as well as the increased need for individual users to access data from many sources, will no longer permit a view of the network as either twin-ax wires extending from the mainframe to the terminals or as a collection of EtherNet LAN's with an SNA Gateway. High-capacity, reliable, secure networks, centrally managed and interconnected throughout the enterprise, the IDN, and the industry will require careful planning, especially at this time of rapid change in the industry and in networking technology.

Phase III: Plan IS Strategy Implementation

Phase III of the planning process comprises five principal tasks:

- Define a portfolio of IS strategy implementation projects. Define discrete projects to effect the IS strategy elements, addressing purpose, benefits, deliverables, risks, and principal tasks.
- Develop schedule and budget estimates for each project. Create a schedule and project budget for each project in the implementation portfolio.
- Develop the overall IS strategy implementation plan and management framework. Develop an overall implementation schedule and project management framework suitable to ensuring effective monitoring and communications of implementation progress, accomplishments, problems.
- Document the business case for the IS strategy. Ensure an adequate understanding of and balance among the benefits and costs of each project and of the overall portfolio.
- Present the IS strategy and implementation plan to senior management for formal approval. Conduct a briefing session for senior management on the results of the planning process and secure approval for implementation.

Finally, a few supplemental thoughts on phase III. First, phase III returns to the business focus of phase I: the IS strategy takes its meaning and derives its value from making explicit, meaningful contributions to enterprise strategy formulation and execution. The frame of the implementation plan and business case is a capital authorization request, different in kind but not in nature from any other funding request.

The business case may not, however, be as straightforward as a clearly understood, traditional return-on-investment analysis. In fact, to the very extent that the IS strategic plan succeeds in focusing on strategic initiatives, it may be that much more difficult to quantify all of the anticipated benefits. A tactical IS effort, because it is working on the margin of the way things are, is more susceptible to this sort of financial analysis. Strategic initiatives can, however, be subjected to a formal and rigorous assessment of their direct contribution to enterprise goals and then measured in execution to ensure delivery or be abandoned if they are not succeeding.

The final presentation to senior management has a symbolic value as well as a practical benefit of achieving a formal approval of the plan. By once again visibly endorsing the process and the product of the planning effort, management sends a message throughout the organization of its views on the role and significance of IS to the enterprise and sets the stage for continued involvement in the oversight of the implementation effort.

Institutionalizing the Process of IS Planning

Information systems strategic planning is a process, not an event. The Joint Commission on Accreditation of Healthcare Organizations (JCAHO) can mandate the preparation of IS plans. It cannot, however, mandate their effective use. That has to come from within the enterprise. We believe there are three principal considerations in institutionalizing the IS strategic planning process:

- Capture the imagination and commitment of senior management as to the potential of the IS function to create and sustain competitive advantage.
- Transform the planning process, the IS strategic plan itself, and the management of the implementation from its traditional passive, instantly-out-of-date paper document focus to an active, always current, always done electronic database focus to which senior management has ready access for IS and other purposes.
- Create and shape desired behaviors during the initial planning cycles regarding enterprise perspective, prioritization, resource allocation, and project management.

For many of the current generation of clinical care chief executives and their boards of directors, information systems have been inextricably bound up with patient accounting, patient management, and reimbursement reporting. Many senior medical researchers and educators grew up in an era in which the role of the computer was ancillary to their core intellectual and laboratory work. They understood full well that no patient or physician ever chose a hospital because of its outstanding billing system. Nor did any prospective research or teaching faculty member select a medical school on the basis of its word processing and electronic mail facilities.

Automated care protocol planning and monitoring, robotic medicine, teleradiology, videoconferencing, computerized gene sequencers, computerized brain imaging, problem-based/lifelong learning/systemic educational approaches have radically changed the role of the computer in today's leading healthcare enterprises.

As in all other industries, the administrative, *overhead* era of computing is over. In a very real sense, the ability of senior healthcare IS executives to help their organizations make the transition to a competitive, *capital* computing era will be a major factor in the long-term success of their enterprises. Doing so will require that the IS executives capture the imagination and commitment of senior management by clearly demonstrating the linkage between enterprise success and information technology. Actually delivering on the projects outlined in the initial plan and a continuing dialogue with senior management on the IS role will keep the fires stoked.

How many times does one hear an executive say, "Well, we did a five-year IS plan in 1984, and another in 1989. I guess it's time to do another now in 1994"? Such an episodic view will not suffice for general business planning—nor, in today's fast-moving healthcare business and technology climate, will it work for IS planning. However, for many organizations, the effort associated with prior planning efforts is a major deterrent to creating an ongoing process of IS planning. Paper work products and the lack of linkage with the actual management of plan implementation render the plan obsolete the moment it is created. Something else is needed: automated tools.

Such tools should support, first, the *creation* of the IS plan—enterprise profile, IS vision statement, IS current environment assessment, strategy element definition, implementation project profiles, implementation plan, and business case. Second, project management facilities linked to the planning database should provide senior management, user, and IS technical management tailored views of the status of implementation. Third, by supporting construction of the plan in a structured framework, and facilitating easy updating of the enterprise knowledge base throughout the implementation process, the automated tools will permit the enterprise to maintain the freshness of the plan, without the administrative headaches associated with paper-based methods and work products.

The essence of the IS planning process is as much or more about consensus development, prioritization, and development of an enterprise perspective than about specific information technology issues. Unless the process of managing these behavioral and cultural issues is mastered, there is simply no way to force a continuing climate of planning for information systems. It is just too much work. In the early cycles of the planning process, however, those leading the effort can dramatically enhance the odds of successfully institutionalizing an IS planning climate by implementing planning *project behaviors* that they ultimately want to survive as ongoing *enterprise mechanisms* for the implementation of the plan and the continuing planning process. Put differently, whereas the IS management strategy element is the final segment of the IS strategy to be formally created, leaders of effective planning projects usually have created the key elements early in the effort—placing it carefully in their desk drawers and pulling out each page when it is time for the planning team to discover it!

Conclusion

A common objection to planning is that there is no point in planning, because there are always going to be unexpected situations that arise. True enough. However, the failure to plan guarantees that every situation will be unexpected! Information technology is too integral to healthcare enterprise success to bet on a perfect record of IS responses to the waves of unexpected situations that will occur without an effective IS strategic plan and a planning climate!

Questions

1. Discuss the development of integrated delivery networks (IDNs) within the context of the changing healthcare system.
2. Describe the benefits of IS strategic planning, with attention to enterprise management and IS management.
3. Outline the three phases of the planning process: vision, strategy, and implementation.
4. Describe how to ensure that IS strategic planning is "a process, not an event."
5. Explain the importance of automated tools, project behaviors, and enterprise mechanisms to successful planning.

Bibliography

Brooks, F.P. (1975). *The mythical man-month: Essays on software engineering.* Reading, MA: Addison-Wesley Publishing Company.

French, J.A. (1990). *The business knowledge investment: Building architected information.* Englewood Cliffs, NJ: Prentice-Hall, Inc.

Martin, J. (1982). *Strategic data planning methodologies.* Englewood Cliffs, NJ: Prentice-Hall, Inc.

Martin, J. (1989). *Information engineering, book I: Introduction.* Englewood Cliffs, NJ: Prentice-Hall, Inc.

Martin, J. (1990). *Information engineering, book II: Planning and analysis.* Englewood Cliffs, NJ: Prentice-Hall, Inc.

Murray, C., & Cos, C.B. (1989). *Apollo: The race to the moon.* New York: Simon and Schuster.

Rockart, J.F., & Bullen, C.V. (Eds.) (1986). *The rise of managerial computing: The best of the center for information systems research* (Sloan School of Management, MIT). Homewood, IL: Dow-Jones-Irwin.

Spewak, S.H. (1993). *Enterprise architecture planning: Developing a blueprint for data, applications and technology.* Wellesley, MA: QED Publishing Group.

Strassmann, P.A. (1985). *Information payoff: The transformation of work in the electronic age.* New York: The Free Press.

Tichy, N.M. (1983). *Managing strategic change: Technical, political and cultural dynamics.* New York: John Wiley & Sons, Inc.

Zachman, J. (1987). A framework for information systems architecture. *IBM Systems Journal, 26*(3).

12
Information Systems: A Competitive Advantage for Managing Health Care

JAMES M. GABLER

The term "competitive advantage" is often used to describe business initiatives in health care and elsewhere. Yet only history can judge whether in fact an initiative did make a difference. Time must pass before the competitive impact of a particular product or service can be appropriately evaluated. Moreover, an apparent competitive advantage is difficult to sustain because it is limited by *time* until a competitor matches or exceeds the advantage. Regaining the advantage may be even more difficult.

Competitive Advantage in an Information Society

Information is as critical a resource as are people and money. Today more people work with information than produce manufactured goods, making our postindustrial society an information society (Naisbitt, 1982). White collar work is almost all information intensive, using the brain rather than muscles. It is interesting to observe that information about an industry creates its own value. For example, the net-asset values of *TV Guide* and the *Official Airline Guide* are greater than those of the top four TV networks combined and the top 10 airlines combined, respectively (Williamson, 1993). Consumers are willing to pay for information that enables them to better access the industry itself. And so, like money, information even has a time value.

Timely information often creates a competitive advantage. The retailing and textile industries have sophisticated processes that capture daily purchasing patterns and turn that information into marketing advantages, for example, rapidly altering distribution and production plans to take immediate advantage of actual sales patterns. These loosely integrated networks tie together separate, independent businesses to reduce information float that can often return more benefits than reducing monetary float.

Sustaining a competitive advantage in an information-oriented society requires a strategic, communication-based information architecture that can quickly adjust its content and presentation as customers change. The architecture for information delivery must be in place before any product or service can consistently utilize timely information. The availability of an information delivery vehicle is more critical to establishing and sustaining a competitive advantage than are the key information components required for specific products or services delivered by the vehicle.

This advantage is further enhanced for the early investors because market saturation and/or costs can limit or prevent competitors duplicating the delivery vehicles. For example, when banking was deregulated, most banks focused on new products and services; but only a few banks developed networks of automated teller machines (ATMs). Today, a *few* ATM networks dominate as national delivery vehicles across the banking industry. Typically, there will be more than one delivery vehicle in an industry, but competitive saturation eventually limits the total to a few (three to five on a nationwide basis).

As an information-intensive industry begins to fully recognize their value, information delivery vehicles become a requirement for participation because all "players" share the few surviving national delivery vehicles. This, however, significantly shifts the competitive paradigm from delivering information to optimizing the use of the information delivery vehicles. Much proprietary information (e.g., airfares) must now be shared on the delivery vehicles (e.g., airline reservation systems) to maximize customer exposure, requiring new strategies for competitive advantage (e.g., target marketing). The most successful organizations in this more visible information environment will be those that are "smarter" at using the information delivery vehicle(s) (Hopper, 1990) *and* the additional information available on the shared delivery vehicles. This shift is not a creative advance, but a fundamental redefinition of the industry requiring new innovative approaches. Past history and experience are less reliable in this new shared visible information environment (and may even inhibit it).

Clearly, information-intense industries are discovering the enhanced value of nationwide shared information delivery vehicles. In the early stages, there is a competitive edge in owning the delivery vehicles, which may continue over time as the vehicles consolidate into a few national networks. However, the real competitive advantage lies in the use of these vehicles. This second stage of information delivery vehicles is much larger, but is more dispersed, has more competitors, and is constantly changing under increasingly competitive pressures. The most successful organizations will be those that recognize the long-term competitive advantage lies in the use of these vehicles and prepares their information infrastructure to take advantage of this new environment.

The Airline Industry Example

The airlines offer striking examples of information as competitive advantage (Keen, 1986). When airlines were deregulated, most airlines competed for market share through fare wars; only a few airlines invested heavily in reservation systems. Today those *few* systems dominate the industry as national and international delivery vehicles.

In 1984, Delta Airlines admitted it suffered for failing to invest early in reservation systems. American Airlines generates more income by selling its reservation system to travel agents than by flying passengers.

Timely information served as a basis for offering new services and extending established ones. Through its frequent-flyer program, American Airlines captured not only market share but also information on the flying public, which they combined with hotel and car rental information. The resulting service differentiation and target marketing improved customer ties while generating additional revenue through custom-tailored travel packages.

The loosely integrated, strategically interconnected design of American's travel agency services gave competitive information advantages over other airlines' reservation and frequent-flyer information systems. The same was equally true for United Airlines.

Now that reservation systems are recognized as necessary to compete in the transportation industry, all airlines own or use a reservation system. In fact, the demise of People's Express (Freedman, 1989) is directly attributable to their lack of a reservation system, making them vulnerable to the seat inventory capability of competitors' reservation systems (e.g., match fares but with a limited number of seats) and handicapped by the lack of adequate customer service tools (e.g., know before going to the airport that a flight was full). It is clear that timely integrated information can optimize existing resources and enhance services.

Competitive Advantage of Information in Health Care

In health care, information systems can provide a competitive advantage for management if the systems are implemented as modular parts of an information communication architecture rather than strictly as support for specific functions, such as billing, registration, cost accounting, and lab. Given the pressures of competition and limited resources, healthcare providers must be able to add, drop, or change information system components as quickly as they can adjust programs and services provided to patients. Whereas investing in a monolithic system tends to limit options, investing in a communication architecture can protect against being locked in to one vendor—frustrated by competing priorities and incompatible alternatives.

In fact, the specialization and diversity within health care requires an interconnectivity foundation to effectively address both financial and quality of care issues. If a care provider is integrated by an information delivery vehicle that funnels information through the organization, extending that structure to key relationships outside the organization can be relatively simple with existing technology if an open architecture design is used.

It is flexibility that allows open architecture to be used within a facility, across an enterprise, throughout an integrated delivery system, and to integrate a community health information network (CHIN). Supporting these networks within networks increases the options for modularity, which in turn increases the flexibility for rapidly adjusting the business and its information infrastructure to quickly meet competitive pressures.

Thus, this modular integration model supports multiple opportunities for business relationships and joint ventures inside and outside an organization—opportunities limited or excluded by centralized storage models that depend heavily on ownership and/or direct control. The critical difference is the design, not the technology.

The Role of Information Professionals

With their ongoing contact with all departments in the organization, information professionals are positioned to develop a unique perspective on how all the pieces fit together. This perspective should be utilized to make money for the organization, not just save money. It should add value, not just reduce costs. Executive management should view information system expenditures as an investment, and the information professionals should justify this perspective with verifiable results. This requires that executive management and the organization as a whole develop an information perspective and a strategic communication vision.

Information systems are most effective when their top manager becomes an active participant on the executive management team. That team can then pursue opportunities to use information to gain a competitive edge. Because any contact with the healthcare buying public is an opportunity to capture strategic information, it is imperative that the information linkage (the delivery vehicle) be considered from the origination of every program or service offered by an organization. Information-oriented leadership must find opportunities and turn them into competitive advantages by preparing a strategic information infrastructure, recognizing industry trends, and seizing opportunities when they arise.

To create a competitive advantage, executive management must value the capture of information and its flow through the organization. Otherwise, the information resource will eventually be utilized by their competitors (and their successors).

All managers must recognize that information integrity originates at the information source and degenerates as manual handling increases prior to its capture in an information system. If the personnel capturing the information can make immediate use of both the collected and other related information, they will be better motivated to ensure its quality and timeliness. If the information is perceived as benefiting only upper management, it will be less reliable, regardless of any management edicts.

This updated form of the original GIGO principle (garbage in, garbage out) has implications that can be effectively and efficiently addressed by an appropriate information architecture. Disruptions in the information chain, like the food chain, tend to have a much larger overall impact than would initially appear at the point of disruption.

The Information Architecture

According to Porter (1985), "Interrelationships among business units are the principal means by which a diversified firm creates value, and thus provide the underpinnings for corporate strategy." In health care, competitive advantage must come from diverse and specialized areas in the form of better, faster, more productive information solutions and enhanced interrelationships among the entities. The ability to capture and subsequently provide meaningful information within and across these entities can bring added value to healthcare services. Because functions within health care are highly specialized, and because medical technology and knowledge are expanding rapidly, the healthcare industry must have a new information delivery architecture to manage costs and outcome quality.

Design Approaches

This new architecture represents the most recent generation in information designs, moving beyond the process-oriented designs of the 1970s and the database-oriented designs of the 1980s, as shown in Figures 12-1 and 12-2.

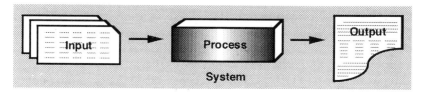

FIGURE 12-1. Process-oriented designs.

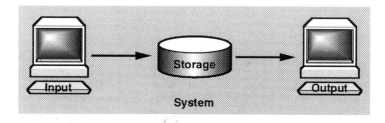

FIGURE 12-2. Database-oriented designs.

The systems of the 1990s will be flow oriented, characterized by data movement and multisystem designs, as shown in Figure 12-3. The capture process must be moved to the source at which data are generated, to eliminate errors associated with manual data capture and its subsequent entry. As in earlier systems, output can be used in various ways, but flow designs use subsets of the output from one system as input to another system.

For example, systems A and B in Figure 12-3 could be lab and pharmacy, which provide a subset of clinical information (charge events) to patient accounting represented by system C. System D could be the general ledger that receives journal entries as a subset of the patient accounting information in system C. This model could similarly be extended right to include a separate cost accounting system or left to include the registration system.

Connectivity issues are being addressed with proven tools such as local area networks (LANs) and standards for moving summarized data. However, if flow designs are overlaid with single database concepts, the resulting architecture will limit the potential for modularity. Information flow creates different architectural and control issues, but the flow-oriented designs can be much more responsive to the capture, accuracy, control, usage, and relevance of information from a functional perspective (i.e., more people oriented). The technology is available, but more than technical expertise is needed. An information architect is critically necessary.

Due to prevalent database orientations, many available systems still tend to combine multiple functions in a single database. Although separation may not seem easy or natural due to familiarity with combined designs, functional system separation can often be better addressed with commercially available information systems. These separate functional systems can then be architecturally combined, recombined, or replaced as desired. The integration of these modular systems occurs on the network (the information delivery vehicle) rather than on a single database; this modular inte-

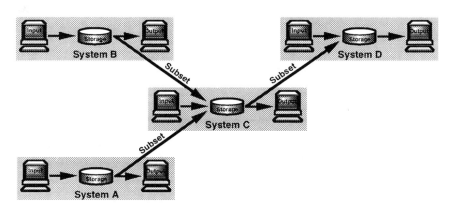

FIGURE 12-3. Flow-oriented designs.

gration is the most distinguishing characteristic of flow-oriented designs. Other characteristics are as follows.

Single Entry

Information can be entered once and reused without reentry when appropriate subsets of information are moved between systems. The flow of these subsets may be immediate; but if immediacy is not necessary, periodic batch flows remain simpler and more reliable. A single official source for each information item and a cohesive flow design can ensure that information is reconcilable (i.e., balances between systems).

Operational Accountability

Information can be captured at the source as part of the system tool used to perform detailed tasks (i.e., developed from the line workers' viewpoint). Job performance accountability can also help ensure detailed accuracy, allowing accurate information subsets to be quickly extracted as a by-product.

Functional Modularity

Each system module can focus on a functional work unit's similar usage patterns and performance criteria. The resulting modules generally reflect the structure of the organizational entities. This direct relationship to function allows management to determine a system's value to the organization relative to costs and priorities. Accountability is also clear.

Open Architecture

This design can accommodate modular, incremental changes resulting from growth and replacement. Because few limits are placed on hardware or software options, functional areas have freedom in system selection and require very few productivity compromises. The open design allows each module to simply "plug in" to the modular architecture, with standards such as HL7, ASTM, ANSI X.12, ACR/NEMA, MEDIX, etc., facilitating and accelerating the process. Furthermore, this approach allows off-the-shelf, turnkey systems that minimize development time, learning curves, and costs.

Information Architect

Flow designs require a new and critical role. An information architect, rather than a technician, is needed to define the scope and boundaries of each functional system and to maintain the integrated modular structure. By defining an official source for each information item, the architect can more easily control the synchronization and reconciliation of information flows. By minimizing the subsets of information to be transferred, duplicate information can be more easily managed. Synchronization is more easily maintained when two-way transfers are avoided. Communications must also be standardized. Information flows must be logically defined and monitored to ensure information integrity between systems. The architect must also ensure that the information is suitable for the receiving system and must control architectural cohesiveness through authority over system connectivity and flows.

Benefits

To justify an architectural design change of this magnitude, there must be significant benefits over existing designs. Clearly, such benefits do exist and have in fact been demonstrated in many installations of modular integrated systems utilizing LAN technology. These benefits include the following.

Operational Productivity

Because functions are separated by systems, there is a clear accountability for the productivity of each system. Likewise, the relationship between functional areas can be clearly defined, allowing productivity issues to be more quickly isolated for improvement.

Understandable Systems

Open architecture of the type described here focuses on the functional roles of individual systems rather than the technical details (e.g., one does not need to understand copier technology to understand the role and value of a copier). It is easier to identify and quantify the role and value of a single functional system than to determine the role and the value of one function of a large, multifunction system. This enables management with technical appreciation to understand and manage a modular architecture without detail technical expertise.

Organizational Adaptability

This modular architectural structure is readily adaptable to organizational requirements. Its decentralized technical structure can support either centralized or decentralized controls, whereas a centralized technical structure is not amenable to decentralized control.

Management Control

This structure offers management a high degree of control. In response to changing business priorities and resources, management can more quickly adjust *timing* because modular components can be added, replaced, or deleted relatively independently of the rest of the architecture. Management can control *costs* based on the relative value of the system to the organization, ensuring that value exceeds cost as business sense requires. Because the value of an operational and/or strategic impact can be subjective and hard to quantify, it is upper management's responsibility to determine the relative value of each area for system-wide priorities. Middle and lower management must then sell their information system's value in terms of upper management's criteria rather than from their own point of view.

With a modular architecture, management can control the *benefits realization* process. Measurable commitments should be made by the functional area's managers during the approval process (e.g., workload levels, personnel allocations, expenses, etc.). Line managers should then be held accountable for the delivery of those commitments, which are also more easily measured in a modular flow design. Management can also focus on the productivity issues enhanced by each information system.

System statistics can be used to measure productivity and pinpoint areas of greatest gain. Detailed analysis of these statistics can optimize resources; with an objective and highly precise tool for evaluation, creative managers can discover new efficiencies.

For example, some hospitals have reduced their length of stay by changing the dates when hip replacements are performed relative to the start of physical therapy. Meaningful information capture and feedback facilitate this type of analysis.

Decreased Risk

Because of its lower initial and incremental costs, this modular architecture involves less risk. Risk is further decreased by narrowing the focus for each system, or individual target area, and providing a single focus for accountability, functionality, costs, and benefits. This architecture also allows the use of turnkey systems, which can eliminate system development costs and time, thus placing the focus on implementation and production.

Workgroup Commitment

A workgroup that relatively freely chooses its own productivity tools (system) experiences pride of ownership. Control of its own tools makes the department logically accountable for its own job performance. This accountability reflects a recognized role for the functional area within the organization, increasing commitment to the overall organization.

This clarity of role, in turn, generates a synergistic environment and encourages the mutual resolution of problems. Areas with their own resources are more likely to collaborate with one another in resolving working level problems.

Economies

Multiple, smaller systems generally have both lower initial and incremental costs and a lower total cost than do the typical single, large systems in the marketplace. Additional economies accrue over time as a result of continued vendor competition because the organization is not "locked in" to one vendor. This generally yields continuing economies up to twice that of typical large-volume pruchasing discounts. Further economies result from the continued focus on workgroup usage and productivity rather than on technical development, maintenance, and enhancement.

Natural Redundancy

By design, this architecture has no single point of total failure. A single system failure primarily affects only that functional area. Other areas may lose access to the failed system, but can continue to serve their own areas. Additional and/or special hardware is not generally required, but management can selectively apply fail-safe technology to areas where it is determined that a functional role is sufficiently critical to justify the additional expense.

Strategic Structure

Because network adjustments can be made quickly and relatively easily, the organization can more quickly take advantage of opportunities that arise—provided that the information linkage was part of the initial foundation in the decision/planning process. With the growing focus on quality of care, the ability to address clinical issues is increasingly critical. This modular architecture empowers management to control the technology rather than vice versa while strategically positioning the organization.

Strategic Value

Sustaining quality customer service is the competitive edge in any business, and especially in health care. Internally, this means efficiently providing the best patient care; externally, it means maintaining and expanding the customer base served. Maintaining a competitive edge in the 1990s will require the strategic architecture described above. With this structure in place, management can manage costs by

- Relating the value for functionality to specific expenses, and
- Increasing accountability for productivity.

Healthcare providers can strengthen their customer relationships by linking patients, physicians, and payors. With easier access and added value, utilization patterns can be encouraged by ease of use rather than forced by ownership, control, etc.

   Timing is paramount and flexibility is critical, but this strategic modular architecture can be created with limited financial resources. Overall costs can be reduced if all planning strategically includes linkages to the information architecture from inception rather than added as an afterthought. Although there are always constraints on the resources available, an information perspective must guide the decision process.

Information systems should be measured by their effectiveness in meeting business objectives, not by their utilization of sophisticated technology. With a strategic information vision and the architecture described above, healthcare institutions can take the major step toward creating and sustaining a competitive advantage.

Questions

1. How does an information perspective affect management decisions?
2. How can patient demographics be used for target marketing?
3. How can information systems encourage physician usage? What role does timeliness of information play in encouraging this physician usage? In what ways can services be most easily accessed inside and outside the facility?
4. How can timely information be used to enhance patient and visitor contact?
5. Contrast the two stages of information delivery vehicles in terms of the types of competitive advantages that can be obtained in each.
6. How does the communication architecture allow true clinical care applications to be more economical and justifiable?
7. Contrast the three design approaches described in this chapter. (Hint: Categorize a familiar system and note strengths/deficiencies.)

References

Freedman, D. (1989). Canceled flights. *CIO 2*(7), 48–54.

Hopper, M. (1990). Rattling SABRE—New ways to compete on information. *Harvard Business Review, 90*(3), 118–125.

Keen, P. (1986). *Competing in time.* Cambridge, MA: Ballinger Publishing.

Naisbitt, J. (1982). *Megatrends.* New York: Warner Books.

Porter, M. (1985). *Competitive advantage.* New York: Free Press.

Williamson, M. (1993). Finding the business future. *CIO 6*(21), 58–59.

Bibliography

Freedman, D. (1989). The myth of strategic I.S. *CIO 4*(18), 42–48.

Gabler, J. (1993, March). Shared information boosts competition in healthcare networks. *Computers in Healthcare,* pp. 20–26.

Gabler, J., & Lopez, M. (1994, May). Open systems architecture: How to make it work. *Healthcare Informatics,* pp. 64–70.

Porter, M. (1980). *Competitive strategy.* New York: Free Press.

13
Methods and Models for Planning Strategically

JAMES I. PENROD

Strategic planning began to be embraced by corporate leaders in the mid-1960s as "the one best way" to devise and implement strategies that would enhance the competition of each business unit. True to the mold of scientific management, this one best way involved separating thinking from doing and spawned the growth of corporate strategic planners (Mintzberg, 1994). Too often, however, this model of strategic planning has failed to connect the thinking and doing within the healthcare organization. Implementational discipline has not matched the planning effort. Even worse, many corporate planners do not even have a good process. It has been treated as an executive adventure—something the intuitive generalist knows must be done—but without a system, it becomes a weekend or short term experience, perhaps aided by third-party consultants (Bean, 1993). Unfortunately, strategic planning for information and communication systems has been and continues to be an area often guilty of these practices.

What then is needed as a remedy for a malady that has reached epidemic proportions in the United States? First, there must be a clear differentiation between strategic planning and long range planning. Many times long range planning has been repackaged and sold as being strategic. Second, a strategic planning model or applied planning technology needs to be employed. Finally, the model should promote a methodology that is strategic, proactive, teamwork based, and that leverages the mission and goals of the healthcare enterprise (Bean, 1993).

Strategic Planning Defined

Long-range planning optimizes for tomorrow the trends of today. In contrast, strategic planning exploits the opportunities of tomorrow while minimizing the negative aspects of inevitable or unexpected challenges. Strategic planning goes hand in hand with strategic management and is the activity through which major strategic decisions are confronted, decisions that (Shirley, 1982):

- Define the institution's relationship to its environment,
- Generally take the whole organization as the unit of analysis,
- Depend on inputs from a variety of functional areas, and
- Provide direction for and constraints on administrative and operational activities throughout the entire institution.

Strategic planning differs from long-range planning in that its focus on issues makes strategic planning more appropriate for politicized circumstances. Typically, strategic planning summons forth an idealized vision of the organization, whereas long-range planning does linear extrapolations of the present. Strategic planning identifies decisions and actions relating to a range of possible futures identified through environmental assessments, whereas long-range planning tends to get locked into a single stream of decisions and actions leading to a most likely future (Bryson, 1988b).

As defined by Bean (1993), strategic planning is "the process of determining the long term vision and goals of an enterprise and how to fulfill them."

Strategic planning can result in many benefits:

- A clear and inspiring strategic vision,
- Increased external support,
- Increased certainty in the lives of organizational members,
- A context for resource allocation and reallocation,
- An improved image for the organization, and
- Enhanced expertise and teamwork in the organization.

Strategic Planning Models

Healthcare organizations vary immensely in size, complexity, governance structure, and decision paths; their leaders differ in management style. Accordingly, planners must analyze their organization and tailor a strategic planning process to fit (Keller, 1983).

One of the most important parts of this is in understanding the different aspects of strategy:

- *Strategy is a plan*—a consciously intended course of action to deal with a situation. As plan, strategy deals with how leaders try to establish direction for organizations.
- *Strategy is a ploy*—a specific maneuver intended to outwit a competitor. As ploy, strategy moves into the realm of competition, where threats, feints, and other maneuvers are employed to gain advantage.
- *Strategy is a pattern*—a pattern in a stream of actions. As pattern, strategy focuses on actions, noting that the concept is empty if it does not take behavior into account.

- *Strategy is a position*—a means of locating an organization in an environment. As position, strategy looks at how organizations find their positions and protect them in order to met competion, avoid it, or subvert it.
- *Strategy is a perspective*—its content consisting of not just position, but of an ingrained way of perceiving the world. As perspective, strategy raises questions about intention and behavior in a collective context.

Although in some ways these definitions may compete, in more important ways they complement. No single definition takes precedence over the others; each adds important elements encouraging the organization to address fundamental questions.

The first steps an institution should take in choosing a model are to analyze what has led to the adoption of a planning process and to examine its institutional history, including:

- Style and context of the organization,
- Relative power of external and internal forces shaping decision making,
- Nature and success of planning in the past,
- Biases and prejudices against planning and their relative strength, and
- Supporters and detractors of planning and their power to obstruct the process.

The resulting insights should be reflected in the charge to plan and the model itself. The model must adapt to accommodate these insights in order for the planning process to become integrated in the decision making and governance of the institution (Norris & Poulton, 1987).

In selecting a planning model, certain elements must be considered. According to Moynihan (1988), planning for information and communication systems should:

- Be ongoing, regardless of the level of technology used;
- Be eclectic;
- Be broad but bounded in scope;
- Be driven by institutional problems and opportunities, not by technical developments;
- Involve a formal process, have the support of senior management, use up-to-date planning methods, and result in documented output;
- Involve senior managers, major users, and information systems staff;
- Include a review of the mission and organization of the information and communication systems function;
- Involve the identification of potentially important technology developments;
- Address the information and communication systems organization's technical and managerial competence;
- Formalize an organizational architecture that addresses patient care, medical system, hospital, and departmental levels;
- Result in an organization-wide technical architecture and vendor policy;

- Formulate an organization-wide application system architecture;
- Develop an organization-wide tool architecture; and
- Yield an organization-wide architecture for voice, data, and image networks.

Initiating a strategic planning process for information and communication systems is not a trivial undertaking. It cannot produce positive results overnight, but takes time to evolve and to be assimilated into the organizational culture. However, certain factors will lead to success if the institution seeks persistently and patiently to ensure their presence:

- *Have a vision of the future.* Define an infrastructure architecture that can continually evolve to support the mission and goals of the Healthcare enterprise.
- *Fit the process to the institution.* Placing a focus on institutional priorities, active mechanisms for broad based participation, and a process that culminates in policy, procedures, information flow, and decision making is critical.
- *Select a model and use it.* Adaptation of a model will develop communication and feedback channels that work and link planning to managing in information and communication systems.
- *Evaluate the process and the outcomes.* Seek answers to assesssment questions from the institution served rather than from the information and communication system unit.
- *Make good impressions.* Act in ways you wish to be remembered later.
- *Listen with respect and be open to influence.* Look for and listen to ways that ideas can lead to better meeting institutional needs.
- *Find a balance for governance and decision making.* Top management support is necessary but does not by itself ensure successful planning. Good plans must address the expectations of the participants in the process and help fulfill their decision-making needs.
- *Avoid simple thinking.* Use teams, task forces, and client groups in analyzing challenges and seeking input for decisions.
- *Resist the bureaucratic frame or linear strategies.* Build information and communication systems that support networked organizations and help break down existing bureaucratic barriers.
- *Emphasize strong values.* The articulation of shared values engenders trust from others, and trust induces an increased openness to influence.
- *Focus on strengths.* Do not ignore weaknesses, but build from strengths and opportunities.
- *Encourage leadership by others.* Shared leadership provides multiple avenues for sensing environmental change, recognizing problems, and improving organization wide performance.
- *Check your performance.* Seek unbiased assessment of individual as well as unit performance.

- *Know when to change the process.* If the process is to work, it must adjust to environmental changes. Strangely enough, formal models with good feedback loops do this better than personality driven *ad hoc* models (Penrod, 1993).

A Proposed Model

The elements of the planning model described below are primarily taken from the work of Robert Shirley and John Bryson and reflect well the concepts of William Bean's leveraged strategic planning technology. Shirley's work has evolved from classical business-oriented strategic planning models and focuses on higher education. Bryson's model was developed for use in public and nonprofit organizations. Merging these methodologies and tailoring the model for particular circumstances allow for adaptation to most healthcare settings; the author of this article has in fact utilized the model in an academic health center.

Figure 13-1 depicts the planning model that has been postulated. The figure shows the interrelationship between the various steps and illustrates potential feedback loops used in modifying ongoing cycles. The advice that follows draws upon Shirley and Bryson and the experience of this author. The steps below reflect their recommendations for the strategic planning process; tailoring the process to the specific environment remains critical in any adoption of these recommendations.

Step 1: Establish Planning Parameters

Document and clarify the initial agreement, including purpose; steps; form and timing of reports; role, functions, and membership of the coordinating committee and of the team to write and implement the plan; commitment of resources in support of planning; and specific documents or requirements to be incorporated into the process (Bryson, 1988a,b).

Step 2: Assess the Environment

In an external environmental analysis, identify and assess major forces in the economic, social, technological, political/legal, demographic, and competitive areas presenting specific opportunities, threats, and constraints. In an internal environmental assessment, identify organizational strengths and weaknesses, using the elements of a simple systems model. This latter assessment should focus on outputs and include a stakeholder analysis.

Step 3: Determine Values

Systematically identify the values of primary stakeholders or constituencies and integrate those findings into the process. This requires a sensitivity to

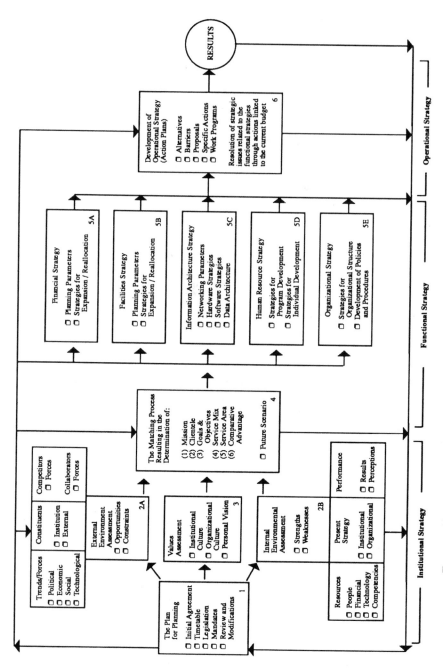

FIGURE 13-1. A strategic planning model for information resources in healthcare facilities.

institutional cultures and should result in a vision statement that articulates a philosophy for managing the organization. It may be helpful to have managers within the organization develop vision statements for their individual units (Block, 1990).

Step 4: Specify Areas for Strategic Decisions

Develop a guideline for the future. Address the decision areas below, acknowledging interactions and interdependencies and revising across all areas before making final determinations.

Organizational Mission and Purpose

In an extended mission statement, describe:

- Fundamental purposes of the organization;
- Characteristics that distinguish the organization from other units;
- Obligations assumed by the organization with respect to its clientele;
- Types of units and nature and role of support services offered by the organization;
- Relative emphasis on areas such as patient care, education, research, and administration; computing, voice, video, and data networks; centralized and distributed facilities; institutional and external services;
- Major stakeholders to be served;
- Style of governance and decision making structures that the organization employs;
- Philosophy of the organization related to effective/efficient use of resources, including human resources.

Clientele to Be Served

Identify the audience of clientele being targeted. Define organizational stakeholders in sufficient depth to set expectations and to evaluate whether they are being met.

Goals and Outcomes

Develop goals that state the desired outcomes and accomplishments. Develop a futures scenario to use as the vision of success. Establish goals with five to ten year horizons; identify time bounded, measurable, behaviorally oriented objectives related to the accomplishment of specific goals, and linked to a budget cycle.

Service Mix

To define service mix, develop a mechanism for reviewing organizational units and support services offered during the time covered by the strategic plan. This may involve considering whether an information resources management approach or a chief information officer function is viable within the institutional culture. Also develop a means for establishing priorities among the service mix and a process outlining how new services will evolve.

Geographic Service Area

Identify the primary service area of the information and communication organization. If responsibility and resources for computing and communications are assigned to different segments of the institution, clarify organizational guidelines for the respective service mix and service areas (Heterick, 1988).

Comparative Advantage

Identify features that differentiate the information and communication systems unit from other institutional units and from the information and communication organizations of competing hospitals and clinics.

Step 5: Form Functional Strategies

Develop strategies that address fundamental policy questions affecting the information and communication system mandates, mission, services, clients, financing, management, and structural design. Because strategic decisions almost invariably involve conflict, pose the issue as a question that the organization can address, list the factors that make it strategic, and state the consequences of failure to address the issue.

Group strategic issues by area, including financial, facilities, architecture (network, hardware, software, data design), human resource development, and organization. Formulate strategies, establishing time lines and operational parameters and linking the strategies to a broad-based, multiyear budget.

Step 6: Develop Action Plans

Develop operational strategies to deal with issues identified. These action plans may be within organizational units or other hospital units; they may span part or all of the information and communication system organization or of the entire institution. Regardless of where they are to be carried out, relate action plans directly to functional parameters (financial, facilities, architecture, etc.) to ensure appropriate trade-offs, integrated action plans, and respected institutional bounds.

Evaluate the Planning Process

Formal and informal processes should measure effectiveness (doing the right things) and efficiency (doing things right). Regular reviews by management should determine whether the process produces decisions and which parts of the process work.

Because determining strategy requires a blend of rational and economic analysis, political maneuvering, and psychological interplay, the process must be highly tolerant of controversy (Keller, 1983). The key is to identify those components of the process that need not be participatory and can be centrally directed, while subtly but firmly providing direction to those areas where participation and consensus are critical. The planning structure must achieve a balance between top-down and bottom-up planning. Moreover, it should (Shirley, 1987):

- Evidence top management support,
- Involve appropriate constituents meaningfully and in an ongoing way,
- Concentrate on substance rather than on form and paperwork,
- Provide for continuity of involvement by key individuals and from one cycle to the next,
- Employ the appropriate quality and quantity of data and analysis in decision making, and
- Work to culminate deliberation with decision making.

Methods of Evaluation

As those ultimately responsible, senior management should evaluate the decisions emerging from the information and communication system planning process. Questions of interest to senior management, which might be answered in an executive summary of the annual report (Below, Morrisey, & Acomb, 1987) include the following:

- How is the information and communication system performing in relation to the milestones outlined in the strategic plan?
- What are the key information and communication system budget items for the organization and the institution over the planning period?
- What are the critical strategic issues that will affect (1) the hospital's performance, and (2) the performance of the information and communication system organization? Why?
- Why are the strategies identified in the plan appropriate to the institution?
- What are the critical success factors necessary for successful implementation of the plan?

Evaluation tasks vary in difficulty. The evaluation of decisions probably requires the most judgment. However, perceptions of decisional results can be collected and quantified in fairly straightforward ways. The evaluation of data and process is usually easier and may be accomplished through the accumulation of periodic analyses throughout the planning cycle. Appropriately written action plans and behavioral objectives provide a strong platform for analysis (Shirley, 1982).

Hospitals or medical centers belonging to larger systems may be assigned specific criteria and report formats by their system planning office. When possible, criteria for the system and the institution should be meshed so unnecessary duplication is avoided. It may prove useful to enlist a consultant who can bring an unbiased perspective and lend credibility to the evaluation effort.

Summary

Information and communication systems are being increasingly used in patient care, research, education, and management, at every level of the institution and in every medical discipline. The importance of strategic planning for resources in these areas and the preponderance of poor practice gave rise to this attempt to develop a generic guide to strategic thought and action. Clearly, those who become planners must be careful in adapting strategic planning concepts. Every situation is different, and planning can be effective only if tailored to a specific situation. To be successful, a strategic planning process must fit the environment of the organization and institution where it is implemented. Above all, planning requires political astuteness, a solid understanding of the culture of the place and time, and a resolve and methodology to implement what has been planned.

When successful, strategic planning and management becomes far more than the *strategic programming* generally practiced. It enables institutional and information and communication system leaders to understand the difference between planning and strategic thinking, so they can focus on what managers learn from all sources and then synthesize that learning into a vision of the direction that should be pursued by the organization and supported by the electronic infrastructure (Mintzberg, 1994).

Questions

1. Why has strategic planning as practiced since the 1960s failed so often?
2. How does strategic planning differ from long-range planning?
3. What are the critical success factors for information and communication systems strategic planning and management?
4. Who in your healthcare organization would be involved in review ("buy off") at the institutional strategy level? At the functional strategy level? At the operational strategy level?

5. Briefly outline an evaluation process for an information and communication system unit. Who in the unit would be responsible for each element of the process?

References

Bean, W.C. (1993). *Strategic planning that makes things happen.* Amherst, MA: Human Resource Development Press.

Below, P.L., Morrisey, G.L., & Acomb, B.L. (1987). *The executive guide to strategic planning.* San Francisco: Jossey-Bass.

Block, P. (1990). *The empowered manager.* 2nd ed. San Francisco: Jossey-Bass.

Bryson, J.M. (1988a). A strategic planning process for public and non-profit organizations. *Long Range Planning, 21,* 78.

Bryson, J.M. (1988b). *Strategic planning for public and non-profit organizations.* San Francisco: Jossey-Bass.

Heterick, R.C. (1988). *An information systems strategy.* CAUSE Professional Paper, 9-10. Boulder, CO: CAUSE.

Keller, G. (1983). *Academic strategy: The management revolution in American higher education* (p. 164). Baltimore: Johns Hopkins University Press.

Mintzberg, H. (1994). The fall and rise of strategic planning. *Harvard Business Review* January–February, 107–114.

Mintzberg, H. & Quinn, J.B. (1992). *The strategy process: Concepts and contexts.* Englewood Cliffs, NJ: Prentice-Hall, pp. 12–19.

Moynihan, J. (1988). Propositions for building an effective process. *Journal of Information Systems Management, 5,* 61–64.

Norris, D.M., & Poulton, L. (1987). *A guide for new planners.* Ann Arbor, MI: Society for College and University Planning, 16-7.

Penrod, J.I. (1993). Reflections on IT planning. *EDUCOM Review, 28*(2), 22–28.

Shirley, R.C. (1982). Limiting the scope of strategy: A decision based approach. *Academy of Management Review, 2,* 262–268.

Shirley, R.C. (1987). *Evaluating institutional planning,* 16-8. Evaluating Administrative Services and Programs: New Directions for Institutional Research (No. 56). San Francisco: Jossey-Bass.

Bibliography

Freund, Y.P. (1988). Planner's guide: Critical success factors. *Planning Review, 16,* 20.

Langly, A. (1988). The roles of formal strategic planning. *Long Range Planning, 21,* 47–48.

Lelong, D., & Shirley, R.C. (1984). Planning: Identifying the focal points for action. *Planning for Higher Education, 12,* 4.

Kaufman, R.A. (1991). *Strategic planning plus.* USA: Scott Foresman.

Krallinger, J.C. & Hellebust, K.G. (1993). *Strategic planning workbook.* New York: John Wiley and Sons.

Shirley, R.C. (1988). Strategic planning: An overview. *Successful strategic planning: Case studies, new directions for higher education, 64,* 11–12.

Wallace, R.E. (1986). Why strategic planning? *Journal of Information Systems Management, 3,* 51.

Wallace, R.E. (1989). *Information systems planning for competitive advantage.* Wellesley, MA: QED Information Sciences.

14
The Chief Information Officer: Past, Present, and Future

BETSY S. HERSHER

The need for senior global executives in response to the sudden shifts and challenges within the healthcare industry has touched every function in the hospital and in the emerging integrated health networks.

The Chief Information Officer

The role of the chief information officer (CIO) in the healthcare enterprise has evolved as a result of the 1982 TEFRA regulations and reporting requirements and other historical developments, as shown in Figure 14-1. As hospitals fought to remain viable and competitive, they began to view information as a key corporate resource—a drastic change from their previously rather *laissez faire* attitude.

Medicine was advancing rapidly, but traditional healthcare information systems were not supporting that growth. For a systems industry that was started in 1967, the progress made by 1982 was not sufficient to put information directly into the hands of the users, particularly clinical users.

Data processing directors found it difficult to meet these new needs. The reporting structure in which they were placed was not supportive of relationships with key users, and the level of their positions within the organization did not provide the power or authority to effect change. Many data processing directors were technical by training and territorial and controlling in approach.

Defining the CIO Role

Today, the CIO role has evolved to the point in healthcare that leadership is the key trait being sought. This leadership has many dimensions within the dynamic healthcare environment (Figure 14-2).

Aspects of the CIO role have changed dramatically as healthcare has responded to the challenges facing the industry. Rapidly evolving technology supports the linkages and interfaces needed to develop integrated

Bank Processing
Shared Services (Outsourcing)

1967–1979
- Self Development
- Packaged Software

1979–1985
- Age of Enlightenment
- TEFRA/Diagnostic Related Groupings (DRGs)
- Information Systems Come out of the Basement
- Clinical Systems
- Departmental Systems
- Decentralization
- Minis and PCs Explode
- Emerging CIO Role
- Emergence of the Computer Savvy Doc

1985–1991
- Role of the Healthcare Executive Changes to a Business Orientation
- Information Technology Savvy Managers Appear
- Interface and Integration Become Critical
- Decision Support and Cost Accounting Systems
- Nursing Informatics
- HL-7 and Open Systems Change Healthcare Information Systems

1991–Present
- Integration Engine
- Outsourcing
- Reengineering
- CIO Comes of Age
- Technology Catches Up
- Computerized Patient Record
- Information Resources and Technology Become Mission Critical

1994
- Chief Systems Officer

FIGURE 14-1. A brief history of information resources and technology in health care.

delivery systems (IDSs). This technology also supports the development of computerized patient records and clinic data repositories. The factors for the success of a CIO function have also changed (Figure 14-3).

The role of the CIO in healthcare and the required skill set have evolved rapidly in response to the acceptance and requirement for information as a key corporate resource, widespread decentralized computing power, and users who are quickly growing comfortable with technology (Figure 14-4).

Through this role of providing access to data, the CIO has become a change agent. No longer solely the implementor of systems, the CIO is the architect of the overall plan for systems integration and connectivity.

The Corporation/Integrated Health Network
- Is committed to information as a key corporate resource
- Views the CIO as a key senior executive

The CIO
- Reports to the highest level possible, either chairman, chief executive officer (CEO), or chief operating officer (COO)
- Is a provider of access to data/facilitator
- Has oversight of all the corporation's technology, hardware, and software
- Is the key contributor to the overall architecture plan for the organization
- Champions a strategic information plan that is synergistic with the corporate long range strategic plan
- Viewed as a resource to the integrated delivery system

FIGURE 14-2. The chief information officer (CIO) function: critical success factors.

Shoshana Zuboff, Associate Professor, Harvard Business School and author, *In the Age of the Smart Machine*

The CIO is an adaptation with a limited niche. I'd like to think that what we're going to evolve toward will look more like general managers. Organizations need general managers who understand the innovations that technology will enable. This is not a matter of saying that if we learn how to use the technology we don't need the CIO. Rather, technology has in it explosive implications about how we organize ourselves.

As long as we keep technology in a box, in a function, separated from other functions and concerns, its strategic benefits are not going to materialize in a way that is regular, sustainable and integrated into the real life of the business. I think part of the problem is the functionalization of domains including (that of) the CIO.

(Technology will be strategic) when people in the field know how to leverage information to create value and have the environment to be able to do so. I just don't think it's in the cards for most CIOs to understand how critical this is.

F. Warren McFarlan, Ross Graham Walker Professor of Business Administration, Harvard Business School

We will find many more CIOs with substantial general management experience as well as IT experience. It's going to be very hard for the CIO to be the best technologist in all details. When running a large operation, almost by definition (the CIO) must move away from the issues at the cutting edge. We're going to need (talented technologists) for as far as we can see into the future. But those people are going to have an entirely different set of skills and career paths than people actually responsible for making things happen inside the organization. Where will the CIOs of the future gain management experience? Out working where the real rubber meets the road in the company.

It may be in the factory, it may be the marketing organization not in staff jobs, but out where you bleed so that you get a much cleaner feeling as to exactly how technology impacts in an environment, where it doesn't work well, what the implications of that are.

FIGURE 14-3. On leadership: excerpts reprinted with permission from the *CIO Magazine* (January, 1991).

Chief Information Officer Skills in a Traditional Environment	Chief Information Officer Skills in an Integrated Health Network (IHN)
• Leadership/Leadership/Leadership • Business Orientation • Results/Action Orientation • Communicator • Flexible • Comfortable Sharing the Expert Role • Team Player • Change Agent/Provide Solutions • Strategist/Planner • Vision • Architect • Facilitator • Orchestrator • Negotiator • Coalition Builder • Catalyst • Manage the Technology • Management/Project Management Political Savvy • Risk Taker • Educator	• All the Skills Listed for the Traditional Chief Information Officer • Able to Deal with Dramatic Changes and Respond Quickly and Decisively • Confident/Mature Style, Comfortable Partnering, Sharing and Influencing • Entrepreneurial • Able to Deal with Formal and Informal Relationships while Building Consensus • Managing Relationship and Priorities/ Able to Balance a Broader Scope of Priorities • Keep Patient Focus and Business Imperatives at the Forefront • Able to Develop a Broad Network Strategy Supporting the Whole Enterprise • Ability to Deal Well with Community and In-House Physicians

FIGURE 14-4. CIO skill sets.

Source: Kevin A. Hahn, Vice President/Chief Information Officer, Froedtert Memorial Lutheran Hospital and Horizon Healthcare, Inc., and Betsy S. Hersher, President, Hersher Associates, Ltd., "Profiles and Challenges for Today's Integrated Health System CIO," presentation at Healthcare Information and Management Systems Society (HIMSS) February 1995.

The decreasing cost of technology and the increasing availability of powerful departmental tools dictate that someone must orchestrate the flow of information, foster the integration of systems, ensure the integrity of data, and monitor for redundancy. The CIO must have the vision to view these issues from a senior executive perspective, to match business and organizational needs to the appropriate information and technology platforms.

The emergence of clinical systems and sophisticated connectivity tools points to the role of architect/leader, not controller, of information resources. The successful CIO must be able to provide access to sound technical resources and to act as a consultant to sophisticated users in the organization.

As the party responsible for setting standards and procedures in support of the growth of technology and maximizing the benefits of the technology investment, the CIO must be able to deal with the abstract, be flexible, and monitor, but not necessarily directly manage, all the departmental resources and resources with the IDS. This involves dealing with many new issues today, among them the following: benefits realization, executive information requirements, clinical workstations and clinical repositories, the computerized patient record, data administration, reengineering, managed care issues, outsourcing, outcomes measurement, rapidly changing technology, and consolidation of services.

Successful Reporting Structures

In a single entity, the CIO needs to report to the highest executive level possible with the highest title appropriate for that organization and must sit on the senior executive council.

The role of the corporate CIO is evolving rapidly, as IDSs and various reporting structures become operative across the country. In the corporate setting, the CIO should be on the same level as the senior financial officer and all other senior officers.

Emerging enterprises and turf issues have resulted in a variety of gymnastics in defining reporting relationships. Ultimately, the most successful structure for an individual hospital's vice president of information systems (VPIS) in a merged entity is to report directly to a corporate CIO. Without this reporting structure, the value and survival of corporate CIOs are at risk. Moreover, the CIO needs access to the major information systems resources within the corporation. This does not mean that the director of laboratory computing in hospital A should report directly to the hospital VPIS or to the corporate CIO. It does mean that the VPIS at hospital A should report directly to the corporate CIO while acknowledging the chief executive officer of hospital A as his/her major client.

The organizational charts shown in Figures 14-5 and 14-6 represent a corporate CIO organization and the CIO reporting structure within the corporation.

Clinical Systems and the Role of the Physician

For years there has been a struggle between clinicians and the data processing director. When the data processing director was under the control of finance, the clinicians felt their needs were not being met. Minicomputers and excellent new departmental system vendors allowed clinical departments to begin their own computerization efforts. Once computerized, they did not want their systems under the control of the data processing director. Generally, they did their own thing, without consulting or getting help from information systems.

As the CIO concept has matured, many forces have contributed to the growing effort to work closely with physicians and satisfy their critical data needs. Reporting requirements and clinical and physician auditing have forced the industry to focus more attention on clinical systems. Administrators and physicians alike need quick access to data for reporting and

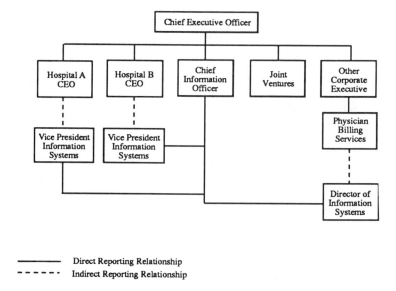

FIGURE 14-5. Corporate entity.

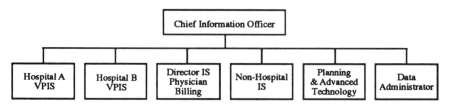

FIGURE 14-6. Corporate chief information officer organization.

decision support. Hence, CIOs and physicians are working together to provide timely, accurate information. The importance of clinical information has become mission critical. CIOs and clinicians are working closely in healthcare settings of all sizes and configurations to achieve the required access to data and develop clinical repositories and workstations. This cooperation and the resulting benefit to the healthcare enterprise have been influenced by the addition of a clinician to the CIO's team.

A New Organizational View

In an environment marked by the explosion of technology issues and of increased user demands, the senior information systems executive cannot do it all and must rely upon the support of others. The CIO needs to hire excellent people in specific areas of expertise to be able to manage strategically. A mark of an excellent CIO is the ability to share the expert role.

The organizational chart shown in Figure 14.7 is a composite of what is currently happening around the country and what the consultants and CIOs contributing their thoughts to the author of this chapter suggest will be future trends. These functions are described below.

Data Administration

This function addresses the overall planning, control, and management of data and databases as a corporate resource, with special attention to

- Support of the mission and business objectives of the organization;
- Development and administration of data policies, standards, and procedures to define ongoing projects and effectively utilize data;
- Coordination and development of the database and other data structures to minimize redundancy and maximize the realization of the data.

Client Services/User Support

There is an increased demand for responsiveness to the users. This function can encompass the following:

- Information center,
- Benefits realization,
- Education and training,
- Decision support systems,
- Office automation,
- System implementation and support,
- Help desk,
- User liaisons, and
- Clinical officer.

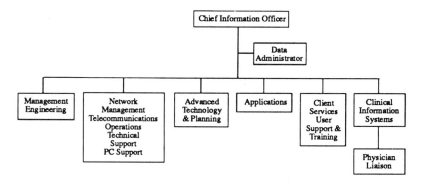

FIGURE 14-7. A new chief information officer organizational view.

Network and Technology Management

This function, and the individual meeting it, will fast fill one of the most critical roles in the CIO's organization. This will be the key technical guru who should be responsible for the following functions:

- Network management,
- Operations,
- Technical support,
- Telecommunications,
- Education, and
- Help desk.

This function will have a significant impact on a complex multisite organization and be responsible for the continuity between systems internally and effective communications between external sites.

Together with the data administrator, the network and technology manager will have a significant impact on the CIO's organization in the future. They hold the key to connectivity and data repositories, as they work together to address these questions:

- Who has the data?
- What are the data?
- What form are the data in?
- How are the data extracted for use?

Clinical Information Management

This function can encompass but not necessarily control systems in the following clinical areas:

- Laboratory,
- Radiology,
- Pathology,
- Pharmacy, and
- Nursing.

Clinical Officer

This role can report separately to the CIO or be included as part of clinical information management. The key success factor is that the individual filling this role assume a consultative attitude to departmental users. The role may be well served by a clinician, such as an in-house physician who is "computer savvy" and has excellent rapport with the rest of the clinicians and medical personnel. For the clinician to succeed in this role, the CEO, CIO, and clinical information manager need to share an exact understanding of the function and be clearly nonterritorial in their approach.

Advanced Technology/Planning/Research and Development

This function can keep up with regulatory issues and their impact on technology and healthcare trends as well as leading edge application development and emerging technology research. This is an excellent place to have the users explore some of their ideas. It is becoming commonplace to consider medical records as a critical department reporting to the CIO.

Future Requirements for the CIO

Among the skills CIOs need for continued growth are great flexibility and the executive ability to manage and support information flow without absolute control of decentralized systems. The CIO will need to have the strategic vision to set the overall architectural platform for the organization and function as a change agent and risk taker. Leadership, communication, and political skills will be paramount. The CIO must be able to ensure the continuity and integration of systems, thereby supporting the future growth of the enterprise without controlling all resources.

The CIO will need to be a great negotiator, building long-term business relationships. Business sense and the ability to communicate ideas and support solutions will be important for success. The CIO will have to be a survivor and be viewed as absolutely credible in order to set standards and procedures for the organization.

The successful CIO is viewed as a leader and resource for technology. A CIO must be very flexible and comfortable dealing in ambiguity and dramatic change, thereby allowing the CIO to respond quickly to initiatives and challenges that face the organization. A CIO must possess a global view of managing relationships and systems. Because there are often several CIOs involved in an integrated health network (IHN), a mature, credible leader is "comfortable" and manages by influence and facilitation rather than by control.

Partnering, using influencing skills without formal power, and creating comfortable formal and informal relationships in a variety of venues are not simple talents. It is a real asset to be able to balance the need for immediate action and decision making within a service and enabling environment. Balancing all this with the need for standardization of policies and accepted procedures across the IHN is a difficult task.

The CIO in an IHN serves many masters with complex problems. Developing a broad vision and network strategy, while at the same time juggling the needs of cooperation, specific entities, and departmental priorities, requires the skills of an excellent leader.

Consensus building for enterprise-wide decision making surfaces several talents that have not been synonymous with this role in the past: user education, marketing, and consensus building.

Questions

1. What is the role of a CIO in an integrated delivery system?
2. What are the benefits to the healthcare enterprise of a close CIO and clinician collaboration?

Unit 5
Addressing the Impact of Information Technology on Organizations and Ethics

Unit Introduction

Unit Introduction

The new capabilities provided by technology have profound effects. Organizations must recreate themselves, managing change and altering behaviors of their members. Professionals must reexamine their moral obligations in a healthcare environment where information is electronic.

In looking at the organization, Lorenzi and Riley describe its relationship with its informatics systems and the change process. Noting the variability of change, they review classic change theories that reveal underlying behavior issues, and present strategies for managing change.

As Havens explains, the information age places fundamental ethical principles into a new context and gives added dimension to such issues as confidentiality and privacy. As computerized knowledge systems evolve, moral obligations will continue to be inherent in the relationships among healthcare providers, organizations, and patients.

15
Health Informatics and Organizational Change

NANCY M. LORENZI AND ROBERT T. RILEY

It's exciting to think about a new vision particularly when you're the creator/driver of it. You see the need clearly. You feel the urgency in your stomach. You're motivated to change. You see the fire with your own eyes. You smell the smoke in your own nostrils. The tent is on fire. You have to change. Why are others in the organization so lackadaisical? Don't they smell the smoke? Don't they see the fire? Don't they feel the urgency to change?

(Belasco, 1990)

The healthcare profession as a whole is undergoing rapid changes with technology, politics, economics, and demographics all either forcing or enabling these changes. Change is a constant reality in both our personal and private lives. Our children grow up today taking for granted such things as powerful personal computers that we could not even envision at their ages. Our societies, our professions, and our daily work lives are changing. Moreover, this pace of change appears to be accelerating, not slowing down.

It is impossible to introduce a health informatics system into an organization without the people in that organization feeling the impact of change. Informatics is about change—the change of data into information with a possible evolution into knowledge. Data become information only after the data are processed (i.e., *changed*) in ways that make the data useful for decision making; those enhanced decision-making capabilities are inevitably going to affect the organization. Figure 15-1 shows this simple but critical circular relationship between the organization, its informatics systems, and the change process. The organization and its people influence, shape, and alter the nature and use of the informatics systems that, in turn, influence, shape, and alter the nature, operation, and culture of the organization that, in turn, etc.

Remember the saying, "Sometimes you get the bear; sometimes the bear gets you." The analogy in change processes is that if we do not manage our change processes, they will manage us—an undesirable alternative at best. The lower our feelings of control during the change process, the lower our "resiliency" (Conner, 1994) will be, our ability to bounce back from the

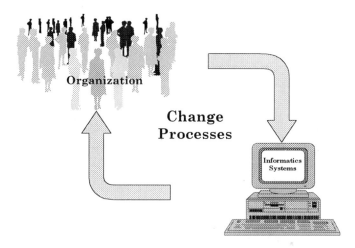

FIGURE 15-1. Circular change relationship between informatics systems and the organizations and their people. (Reprinted with permission from Lorezi et al., Transforming Health Care Through Information Case Studies. Springer-Verlag, New York, 1995.)

stresses of the change and to prepare for the inevitable next change in today's environment. When change processes are not managed well, the price is potentially high in terms of organizational stress. A Kepner Tregoe study conducted in a number of large United States companies found many of them suffering from "initiative overload" with high levels of cynicism among the employees. An article in *Management Review* ("Change for change's sake," 1994) described executives as seizing on one change initiative after another, desperately seeking a quick fix. These are the realistic outcomes of poorly managed change processes.

Change and Health Informatics: An Example

At a 1993 conference on the topics of informatics and change (*Draft Proceedings*, 1993), Dr. Bernard Horak, a healthcare consultant, presented an example of the implementation of a new information technology in a hospital he had studied. In this scenario, adapted by Lorenzi and Riley (1994), the perceived role of the nurses as the integrators of patient data/information was challenged when the physicians began doing direct order entry.

Scenario

When using a *manual system* on an inpatient unit, the nurse usually serves as an integrator and reviewer. The physician scribbles something down on a piece of paper, which is given to a nurse, unit clerk, or paraprofessional to do something with. A nurse typically "cleans it up" and transmits the information or order to pharmacy, radiology, laboratory, dietary, etc. Occasionally the lab or pharmacy will call the physician back. However, the nurse in general serves as the conduit for the transfer of information. When nurses fill this role, they learn a lot. Moreover, they have a total view of what is happening with the patient as they filter and organize information from various sources. This is a classic work flow design. What happens when a system is implemented that calls for the physician to enter orders directly into the system?

In one hospital, the nurses did not like this type of new system. The nurses believed that the system reduced their role in the overall care process. It took them out of the reviewer, case manager, and integrator roles that they were trained to do and that they had always done. The nurses said their two most important roles are (1) the nurse as integrator and (2) the nurse as reviewer, and this new system usurped both roles.

The nurses were very concerned. In the old system, the physicians were used to issuing vague or approximate orders. For example, the physicians would scribble "d.c." or "d/c" for discontinue. They would order "x-rays" and the nurses would figure out that a P.A. and lateral chest were wanted. If the physicians tried to enter their orders as they traditionally did, they would either get nothing back or something they didn't want. The physicians did not know how to order because they had not actually placed orders before. When the physician scribbled an order, the nurse knew the physician, knew exactly what was wanted, and would make it happen. With the new system, this was not possible.

There was a significant decrease of the role of the nurse as an integrator and reviewer of care. Physicians began to make mistakes that nurses had previously caught, such as ordering incorrect drugs or incorrect dosages. There was lower coordination between the nursing plans and the medical care plans. In their new role, nurses tended to show less initiative in making treatment suggestions. In summary, what was lost was the second overview review and analysis by a trained professional. The "second" person had lost the overview perspective. On the other hand, some positive things did occur. Relieved of the paperwork of ordering, nurses had two to three more hours per day to spend on hands-on patient care.

Using This Scenario

The remainder of this chapter presents both theoretical concepts and practical techniques for dealing with informatics change processes. We suggest that you try to relate each of the concepts or techniques back to this scenario, especially in terms of your current or potential role(s) in the areas of health informatics and management. What change forces were at work? What might have been done to prevent the friction that developed?

Types of Change

Changes within an organization can often be identified as one of four types with the definite possibility of overlap between two or more:

- Operational—changes in the way that the ongoing operations of the business are conducted, such as the automation of a particular area;
- Strategic—changes in the strategic business direction (e.g., moving from an inpatient to an outpatient focus);
- Cultural—changes in the basic organizational philosophies by which the business is conducted, for example, implementing a Continuous Quality Improvement (CQI) system; and
- Political—changes in staffing occurring primarily for political reasons of various types, such as occur at top patronage job levels in government agencies.

These four different types of change typically have their greatest impacts at different levels of the organization. For example, operational changes tend to have their greatest impacts at the lower levels of the organization, right on the firing line. Those at the upper levels may never notice changes that cause significant stress and turmoil to those attempting to implement the changes. On the other hand, the impact of political changes is typically felt most at the higher organizational levels. As the name implies, these changes are typically not made for results-oriented reasons but for reasons such as partisan politics or internal power struggles. When these changes occur in a relatively bureaucratic organization—as they often do—the bottom often hardly notices the changes at the top. Patients are seen and the floors are cleaned exactly the same as before. The key point is that performance was not the basis of the change; therefore, the performers are not affected that much.

Resistance to Change

It has been said that the only person who welcomes change is a wet baby! It seems to be part of the human makeup to be most comfortable with the status quo unless it is actually inflicting discomfort. Even then, people will often resist a *specific* change. This is probably the phenomenon of "the devil you know is better than the devil you don't know." It is a shock for inexperienced managers the first time they see subordinates resist even a change that they requested.

Resistance Against What?

There can be countless reasons for resistance to change in a given situation, and the term *resistance to change* is often used very broadly. One of the first aspects that must be analyzed in a given situation is the difference between

- Resistance to a particular *change,* and
- Resistance to the perceived *changer(s).*

In the first case, the resistance is actually directed against the changes in the system. In the second case. the resistance *occurs* because of negative feelings toward specific units, specific managers, or the organization in general. In this latter case, virtually any change would be resisted just because of who is advocating or requiring it. Both forces have to be dealt with, but it is critical that we identify the primary one.

When a new health informatics system is introduced, three factors are very important:

- What is the general organizational climate—positive or negative, cooperative or adversarial, etc.?
- What has been the quality of the *process* used to implement previous informatics systems?
- What has been the technical quality of the informatics systems previously implemented?

Even if we may be new to an organization, we inevitably inherit to some degree the organizational climate and history. Negative "baggage" of this type can be a frustrating burden that adds significantly to the challenge of successfully implementing a new system. On the other hand, the ability to meet this type of challenge is a differentiating factor for truly skilled implementers.

Intensity of Resistance

Resistance can vary from the trivial to the ferocious. Also, the very perception of resistance can vary widely from one observer to another. One might perceive an end user who asks many questions as being very interested and aggressively seeking knowledge. Another might see the same person as a troublemaker who should just "shut up and listen!"

We can safely assume that every significant health informatics implementation is going to encounter some resistance; however, the intensity can vary widely. In an organization with decent morale and a history of managing changes reasonably well, significant numbers of the people may be initially neutral toward a particular proposed systems change. However, there will still be a negative component to be managed. At the very least, this negative component must be prevented from growing. In other situations, the proportions of positive, negative, and neutral people may vary widely.

The Cast of Characters

For any given change, people can occupy a wide range of roles that will strongly influence their perceptions of the change and their reaction to it. As on the stage, some people may occasionally play more than one role. In other cases, the roles are unique. Unless we clearly identify both the players and their roles in any change situation, we risk making decisions and taking action based upon generalizations that are not true for some of the key players. The following categories provide one way of looking at the various roles involved in an overall change process.

- The *initiator* or instigator perceives the problem situation or opportunity and conceptualizes the change to be made in response.
- The *approver* or funder is the power figure who blesses and financially supports the proposed change.
- The *champion* or cheerleader is the visible, enthusiastic advocate for the change. The champion constantly tries to rally support for the change and maintain that support during periods of adversity.
- The *facilitator* attempts to assist in smoothing the organizational change process. The facilitator is sometimes involved from the beginning, and sometimes is only called in for disaster relief once the change process has gone awry.
- The *developer* or builder is responsible for the technical aspects of the change (e.g., developing the new informatics system). These aspects can range from the broad technical conceptualization to the narrowest of technical details.
- The *installer* is responsible for implementing the change, including the necessary training and support activities.
- The *doer* is the "changee"—the person who has to perform his or her work in the changed environment.
- The *obstructionist* is a guardian of the status quo and typically conducts guerrilla warfare against the change. If the obstructionist is also a doer, the reason may arise from a personal fear of the change. However, the obstructionism may also arise from forces such as political infighting (e.g., who gets the credit) or institutional conflicts (e.g., union resistance to a labor-saving system).
- The *customer* is the end beneficiary or victim of the change in terms of altered levels of service, cost, etc.
- The *observer* does not perceive that he or she will be immediately affected by this change but observes with interest. These observations often affect strongly how the observer will react if placed in the doer role in the future.
- The *ignorer* perceives that this change has no personal implications and is indifferent to it. In the broadest sense, this category also includes all those who are unaware of the change.

An overview term often applied to all these roles is *stakeholders*. With the exception of the ignorers, all the categories have some stake or interest in the quality of the change and the change implementation process. The roles are subject to change, especially during a change process that extends over some time. For example, an initial ignorer might hear rumblings of discontent within the system and change to an observer, at least until the feelings of angst subside.

For those implementing change, the following steps are critical:

1. Identify what roles they themselves are occupying in the process,
2. Identify what roles the others involved in the process are playing, being careful to recognize multiple roles,
3. Identify carefully which role is speaking whenever communicating with those playing multiple roles, and
4. Monitor throughout the process whether any roles are changing.

Magnitudes of Change

Change—like beauty—is in the eye of the beholder. A proposed change that virtually terrorizes one person may be a welcome alleviation of boredom to the person at the next station. Also, the types and magnitudes of reaction are often difficult for an "outsider" to predict. When working with change and change management, it often helps to have a simple way of classifying the types and sizes of change.

Microchanges and Megachanges

A practical model that we frequently use divides changes into *microchanges* and *megachanges,* with no great attempt at elaborate definitions. As a first approximation, the following scheme can be used to differentiate between the two:

- *Microchanges*—differences in degree,
- *Megachanges*—differences in kind.

Using an information system as an example, modifications, enhancements, improvements, and upgrades would typically be microchanges, whereas a new system or a very major revision of an existing one would be a megachange. This scheme works surprisingly well in communicating within organizations as long as we remember that one person's microchange is another person's megachange. Later in this chapter, we will present a more rigorous analysis of the magnitude of change that can be used if necessary.

Classic Change Theories

The rate of change in virtually all organizations is escalating, and healthcare organizations—after a slow start—are no exception. The phrase *change management* has become fairly common, appearing in management articles everywhere. What is change management? What is a "change agent" or a change management person? How does change management help people feel less threatened? How did it evolve, and why does everyone seem so fixated on it today?

Change management is the process by which an organization gets to its future state—its vision. Whereas traditional planning processes delineate the steps on the journey, change management attempts to facilitate that journey. Therefore, creating change starts with creating a vision for change and then empowering individuals to act as change agents to attain that vision. The empowered change management agents need plans that are (1) a total systems approach, (2) realistic, and (3) future oriented. Change management encompasses the effective strategies and programs to enable the champions to achieve the new vision. Today's change management strategies and techniques derive from the theoretical work of several pioneers in the change area.

Early Group Theories

In 1974, Watzlawick, Weakland, and Fisch published their now classic book, *Change: Principles of Problem Formation and Problem Resolution.* Theories about change had long existed. However, Watzlawick et al. (1974) found that most of the theories of change were philosophical and derived from the areas of mathematics and physics. Watzlawick and his coauthors selected two theories from the field of mathematical logic upon which to base their beliefs about change. They selected the theory of groups and the theory of logical types. Their goal of reviewing the theories of change was to explain the accelerated phenomenon of change that they were witnessing. Let's briefly look at the two theories that Watzlawick et al. reviewed to develop their change theory.

The more sophisticated implications of the *theory of groups* can be appreciated only by mathematicians or physicists. Its basic postulates concern the relationships between parts and wholes. According to the theory, a group has several properties, including members that are all alike in one common characteristic. These members can be numbers, objects, concepts, events, or whatever else one wants to draw together in such a group, as long as they have at least one common denominator. Another property of a group is the ability to combine the members of the group in a number of varying sequences and have the same combinations. The theory of groups gives a model for the types of change that transcend a given system.

The *theory of logical types* begins with the concept of collections of "things" that are united by a specific characteristic common to all of them. For example, mankind is the name for all individuals, but mankind is not a specific individual. Any attempt to change one in terms of the other does not work and leads to nonsense and confusion. For example, the economic behavior of the population of a large city cannot be understood in terms of the behavior of one person multiplied by four million. A population of four million people is not just quantitatively but also qualitatively different from an individual. Similarly, although the individual members of a species are usually endowed with very specific survival mechanisms, the entire species may race headlong toward extinction—and the human species is probably no exception.

The theory of groups gave Watzlawick's group the framework for thinking about the kind of change that can occur within a system that itself stays invariant. The theory of logical types is not concerned with what goes on inside a class, but gave the authors a framework for considering the relationship between member and class and the peculiar metamorphosis that are in the nature of shifts from one logical level to the next higher. From this, they concluded that there are two different types of change: one that occurs within a given system that itself remains unchanged, and one that occurrence changes the system itself. For example, a person having a nightmare can do many things in his dream—like fight, scream, jump off a cliff, etc. But no change from any one of these behaviors to another would terminate the nightmare. Watzlawick et al. concluded that this is a first-order change. The one way out of a dream involves a change from dreaming to waking. Waking is no longer a part of the dream, but a change to an altogether different state. This is their second-order change, as mentioned earlier.

- *First-order change* is a variation in the way processes and procedures have been done within a given system, leaving the system itself relatively unchanged. Some examples are creating new reports, creating new ways to collect the same data, refining existing processes and procedures, etc.
- *Second-order change* occurs when the system itself is changed. This type of change usually occurs as the result of a strategic change or a major crisis, such as a threat against system survival. Second-order change involves a redefinition or reconceptualization of the business of the organization and the way it is to be conducted. In the medical area, changing from a full paper medical record to a full electronic medical record would represent a second-order change, just as automated teller machines redefined the way that many banking functions are conducted worldwide.

These two orders of change represent extremes. First order involves doing better what we now do, whereas second order radically changes the core ways we conduct business or even the basic business itself.

There is a middle level that seems to be missing from these two extremes. Golembiewski, Billingsley, and Yeager (1976) added another level of change. They defined *middle-order change* as lying somewhere between the extremes of first- and second-order change. As defined by Golembiewski et al., middle-order change "represents a compromise; the magnitude of change is greater than first order change, yet it neither affects the critical success factors nor is strategic in nature." An example of a middle-order change might be the introduction of an electronic mail system into an organization. There is an organization-wide impact, but there is no reconceptualization of the basic business. E-mail is more of a tool for operational and communications efficiency.

Some personality types will welcome changes that they perceive will make their jobs easier whereas other personality types use their day-to-day work rituals to build their comfort zones. In the late 1960s, one unit in a medical center started to code all of their continuing medical education courses with ICD 9 codes. Even though these codes were never used and took a great deal of time to complete, the organization did not want to change the process as time passed because "we have always done it this way." The old process lasted through two directors. When a new director went to change the process, there was definite resistance to this change.

The five most important words to an individual involved in any change process are, "How will this affect me?" This is true regardless of the level or degree of change or the person's organizational position. The most traumatic changes are obviously in the second-order change category, but one person might perceive changes in the first or middle order as more traumatic than another person might perceive a second-order change. One of the challenges for the change manager is successfully managing these perceptions. How the change manager implements the process of change can have a decided effect on the resistance factors.

When the Watzlawick book was published, many people were unfamiliar with the applications of theories of change into contemporary society; thus, the book was a major contribution for alternative ways of looking at the changes that occur daily. Although Watzlawick et al. comprehensively presented the theories of change and offered their model of levels of change, they did not offer practical day-to-day strategies. We are interested in the effective strategies for managing change and have reviewed many social science theories to determine the psychology behind the change management concepts and strategies that are widely used today. We believe that today's successful change management strategies emanate from several theories in the areas of psychology and sociology. Small-group theories and field theories provide the antecedents of today's successful change management practices.

Small Group Theories

The *primary group* is one of the classical concepts of sociology, and many sociological theories focus on small-group analysis and the interaction process analysis. These theories outline and delineate small-group behavior. Small-group theories help us to understand not only how to make things more successful, but also how to analyze when things go wrong. For example, a practical application of small-group research was presented by Bales in the *Harvard Business Review* (1954). Bales, applying small-group principles to running a meeting, makes the following suggestions:

- If possible, restrict committees to seven members.
- Place all members so they can readily communicate with every other member.
- Avoid committees as small as two or three if a perceived power problem between members is likely to be critical.
- Select committee members who are likely to participate in varying amounts. A group with all highly active participants or all low participants will be difficult to manage.

We have all seen small-group behavior at work. For example, a job candidate is interviewed by a number of people. Information is then collected from the interviewers and is shared with a search committee. The search committee selects their top candidate, and that person is hired. If the person hired does not work out, a member of the search committee may very well say, "I knew that Mary would not work out, but I didn't say anything because everyone seemed to like her."

Many of the changes that new technology brings are discussed, reviewed, and debated by groups of people that usually fall within the small-group framework. If negative sentiments about a product or service are stated by a member of the group who is an opinion leader, the less-vocal people will often not challenge the dominant opinion. For example, a medium-sized organization was selecting a local area network (LAN) system. Although the senior leader wanted one system, some of the other people not only had suggestions, but documentation of the qualities of another system. During the meeting to decide which system to purchase, the senior leader stated his views first and quite strongly. A couple of the lower-level staff members started to confront the senior person; however, when there was no support from any of the other people present, they did not express their strong preferences for their system of choice. When the system finally arrived, the senior leader's initial enthusiasm had dwindled. He then confronted the technology people as to why they had not made him aware of the shortcomings of the system selected.

These examples illustrate a key change management requirement: to effectively manage change, it is imperative for change agents to understand how people behave in groups and especially in small groups.

Field Theory

Kurt Lewin and his students are credited with combining theories from psychology and sociology into the field theory in social psychology (Deutsch

& Krauss, 1965). Lewin focused his attention on motivation and the motivational concepts that underlie an individual's behavior. Lewin believed that there is tension within a person whenever a psychological need or an intention exists, and the tension is released only when the need or intention is fulfilled. The tension may be positive or negative. These positive and negative tension concepts were translated into a more refined understanding of conflict situations and, in turn, what Lewin called "force fields."

Lewin indicated that there are three fundamental types of conflict:

1. The individual stands midway between two positive goals of approximately equal strength. A classic metaphor is the donkey starving between two stacks of hay because of the inability to choose. In information technology, if there are two "good" systems to purchase or options to pursue, then we must be willing to choose.
2. The individuals find themselves between two approximately equal negative goals. This certainly has been a conflict within many organizations wishing to purchase or build a health informatics systems. A combination of the economics, the available technologies, the organizational issues, etc., may well mean that the organization's informatics needs cannot be satisfied with any of the available products—whether purchased or developed in house. Thus, the decision makers must make a choice of an information system that they know will not completely meet their needs. Their choice will probably be the lesser of two evils.
3. The individual is exposed to opposing positive and negative forces. This conflict is very common in healthcare organizations today, especially regarding health informatics. This conflict usually occurs between the systems users and the information technology people or the financial people.

People can easily be overwhelmed by change, especially within large organizations where they may believe they have little or no voice in or control over the changes they perceive are descending upon them. The typical response is fight or flight, not cooperation. Managers often interpret such human resistance to change as "stubbornness" or "not being on the team." This reaction solves nothing in terms of reducing resistance to change or gaining acceptance of it. Many managers do not accept that they are regarded as imposing "life-threatening" changes and establishing "no-win" adversarial relationships between management and those below in the organization.

Small-group theory is highly applicable in health informatics because of the way that medical environments are organized. The care of the patient or the education of students entails many small groups. These groups converse and share information and feelings, and strong opinion leaders can sway others to their way of thinking relatively easily.

Kurt Lewin's field theory allows a diagramming of the types of conflict situations commonly found in health care. In this way, the typical approach–

avoidance forces can be visualized (Lorenzi & Riley, 1994; Deutsch & Krauss, 1965). For example, if I accept this new system, what will it mean to me and my job? Will I have a job? How will it change my role? Will this new system lessen my role? These anxieties are very clear and very real to the people within the system. Remember: one person's microchanges are often another person's megachanges. So as the system designers think they are making a minor change to enhance the total system, an individual end user may see the change as a megachange and resist it vehemently. When designing the total "people" strategy for any system, it is important to involve the people from the very beginning and to clearly understand how groups function within the organization.

All of these social science theories assist the change management leader in understanding some of the underlying behavior issues as they bring health informatics technology into today's complex health systems.

Change Principles for Today's Organizations

Change may not be a strong enough word to fully express the challenge that organizations and the people in them face today. Writers such as Paul David (1989) and Nicholas Imparato and Oren Harari (1994) argue strongly that we are in the midst of a megachange from one social, economic, and cultural paradigm to another. Organizational strategies that worked under the old paradigm are no longer valid. Imparato and Harari describe this as "jumping the curve"—moving from an old growth curve to a new one rather than moving along the old curve as we have done for ages.

Imparato and Harari advocate four organizing principles for organizations wishing to jump the curve successfully (Imparato & Harari, 1994):

1. Look a customer ahead.
2. Build the organization around the software and build the software around the customer.
3. Ensure that those who live the values and ideals of the organization are the most rewarded and the most satisfied.
4. Make customers the final arbiters by offering an unconditional guarantee of complete satisfaction.

On the surface, the fourth principle may seem ridiculous for the area of clinical health care; however, given some thoughtful analysis and interpretation, it applies as much in health care as in any other organization. The crucial principle for health informatics professionals is the second one. New technologies must be organized around customer needs, not traditional bureaucratic boundaries. For progressive healthcare organizations, their largest assets will be the quality of their people, their software, and their databases, not their bricks and mortar or their equipment. Notice also a key implication of organizing around software; as the software continuously changes, so will the organization. This flexibility will be a characteristic of successful organizations in the new paradigm.

A Practical Change Management Strategy

Change management is the process of assisting individuals and organizations in passing from the old paradigm to new ways of doing things. Therefore, a change process should both begin and end with a visible acknowledgment or celebration of the impending or just completed change. According to James Belasco (1990),

Our culture is filled with empowering transitions. New Year's Eve parties symbolize the ending of one year and the hope to be found in the one just beginning. Funerals are times to remember the good points of the loved one and the hope for new beginnings elsewhere. Parties given to retiring or leaving employees are celebrations of the ending of the employee's past status and the hope for the new opportunities to be found in the new status.

Thach and Woodman (1994) define the three major informatics organizational change methods as follows:

- Technical installation model—this traditional model focuses on the technical challenges, largely ignoring organizational and human issues. This model has often been sarcastically referred to as the techies "drop shipping" the technology into the applications area. This model has often led to understandably high levels of organizational conflict.
- Systems approach—this more recent model is the balancing of the technical with the organizational considerations in achieving an implementation. In this model, user inputs are often solicited and integrated into the project plan. Issues such as training are not left as afterthoughts.
- Gap analysis—this model integrates informatics into the overall organization strategic planning process. This model, derived from Lewin's conceptual work, starts with an envisioning of the organizational future. Then, the steps necessary to reach that future are defined. The scope of the envisioning ensures that the informatics effort is well integrated into the necessary organizational changes.

Based on our research, there is no single change management strategy that is effective in every situation. It is essential for the change management leader to take the time to know the desired state (vision–goal) and the particular organization and then to develop the appropriate strategies and plans to help facilitate the desired state. Over the years we have evolved a core model that is a combination of the systems and gap approaches described above. There are many options within this model, but we believe that it is helpful for change leaders to have an overview map in mind as they begin to implement new information technology systems. The five-stage model has proven effective for reducing barriers to technology change (Lorenzi, Mantel, & Riley, 1990).

Assessment

The assessment phase of this model is the foundation for determining the organizational and user knowledge and ownership of the health informatics system that is under consideration. Ideally, this phase of the model begins even before the planning for the technological implementation of the new system. The longer the delay, the harder it will be to successfully manage the change and gain ultimate user ownership.

There are two parts to the assessment phase. The first is to *inform* all potentially affected people, in writing, of the impending change. This written information need not be lengthy or elaborate, but it will alert everyone to the changes in process.

The second part involves *collecting information* from those involved in the change by the use of both surveys and interviews. The survey instrument should be sent to randomly selected members of the affected group. One person in ten might be appropriate if the affected group is large. Five to ten open-ended questions should assess the individuals' current perceptions of the potential changes, their issues of greatest concern about these changes, and their suggestions to reduce those concerns. Recording and analyzing the responders' demographics will allow more in-depth analysis of the concerns raised by these potentially affected people.

In the personal face-to-face interviews with randomly selected people at all levels throughout the affected portions of the organization, it is important to listen to the stories the people are telling and to assess their positive and negative feelings about the proposed health informatics system. These interviews should help in ascertaining the current levels of positive and negative feelings; what each person envisions the future will be, both with and without the new system; what each interviewee could contribute to making that vision a reality; and how the interviewee could contribute to the future success of the new system. These interviews provide critical insights for the actual implementation plan. Often those people interviewed become advocates—and sometimes even champions—of the new system, thus easing the change process considerably.

An alternative or supplement to the one-on-one interviews is focus-group sessions. These allow anywhere from five to seven people from across the organization to share their feelings and ideas about the current system and new system.

Feedback and Options

The information obtained above must now be analyzed, integrated, and packaged for presentation to both top management and to those directly responsible for the technical implementation. This is a key stage for understanding the strengths and weaknesses of the current plans, identifying the major organizational areas of both excitement and resistance (positive and negative forces), identifying the potential stumbling blocks, understanding the vision the staff holds for the future, and reviewing the options suggested by the staff for making the vision come true. If this stage occurs early enough in the process, data from the assessment stage can be given to the new system developers for review.

When designing your model, this phase is important in order to establish that the organization *learns* from the inputs of its staff and begins to act strategically in the decision and implementation processes.

Strategy Development

This phase of the model allows those responsible for the change to use the information collected to develop *effective change strategies* from an organizational perspective. These strategies must focus on a visible, effective process to "bring on board" the affected people within the organization. This could include newsletters, focus groups, discussions, one-on-one training, and confidential "handholding." This latter can be especially important for professionals such as physicians, who may not wish to admit ignorance and/ or apprehension about the new system.

Implementation

This phase of our model refers to the implementation of the change management strategies determined to be needed for the organization, not to the implementation of the new system. The implementation of the change strategies developed above must begin before the actual implementation of the new system. These behaviorally focused efforts consist of a series of steps, including informing and working with the people involved in a systematic and timely manner. This step-by-step progression toward the behavioral change desired and the future goals is important to each individual's acceptance of the new system. This is an effective mechanism for tying together the new technology implementation action plan with the behavioral strategies.

Reassessment

Six months after the new system is installed, a behavioral effects data-gathering process should be conducted. This stage resembles the initial assessment stage—written surveys and one-on-one and/or focus-group interviews. Data gathered from this stage allow measurement of the acceptance of the new system, which provides the basis for fine tuning. This process also serves as input to the evaluation of the implementation process. It assures all the participants that their inputs and concerns are still valued and sought, even though the particular implementation has already occurred.

Conclusion

It is not always easy to know exactly why a particular person or group resists change. However, experience shows that an intelligent application of the basic five-step change model—coupled with a sound technological implementation plan—leads to more rapid and more productive introductions of technology into organizations. The process can be expensive in terms of time and energy but nowhere near the cost of an expensive technical system that never gains real user acceptance.

Perhaps most important, overall success requires an emotional commitment to success on the part of all involved. The people must believe the project is being done for the right reasons—namely, to further the delivery of higher quality, more cost-effective health care. If a project is generally perceived to be aimed at just "saving a quick buck" or boosting someone's ego or status, that project is doomed to fail.

An MCI television commercial depicts a book editor, faced with adapting to major informatics changes, commenting that "Art is constant; tools change." In the same vein, the ideals of all our professions are a constant; the tools change. The challenge facing health informatics is to successfully implement those new tools in organizations that often do not welcome them.

Questions

1. Using your own words, define change management.
2. What might be some ways to help people celebrate remembering the past and moving to the future?
3. In the "Cast of Characters," which roles might physicians at various levels in the organizational hierarchy be most likely to play? Why? Least likely to play? Why? Answer the same questions for nurses, administrators, and informatics professionals.
4. Why is the "feedback and options" phase so important in the change management model presented?
5. For the change scenario presented in this chapter, create a detailed change management plan that you think would lead to better results than those that were described in the scenario.

References

Bales, R.F. (1954). In conference. *Harvard Business Review, 32,* 44–50.

Belasco, J.A. (1990). *Teaching the elephant to dance: Empowering change in your organization.* New York: Crown Publishers.

Change for change's sake. (1994, September). *Management Review,* p. 9.

Conner, D.R. (1994, September). Bouncing back. *Sky,* pp. 30–34.

David, P.A. (1989). *Computer and dynamo: The modern productivity paradox in a not-too-distant mirror* (CEPR Pub. #172). Stanford, CA: Stanford Center for Economic Policy Research.

Deutsch, M., & Krauss, R.M. (1965). *Theories in social psychology.* New York: Basic Books.

Draft Proceedings of the International Medical Informatics Association Working Conference on the Organizational Impact of Informatics. (1993). Cincinnati, OH: Riley Associates.

Golembiewski, R.T., Billingsley, K., & Yeager, S. (1976). Measuring change and persistence in human affairs: Types of change generated by OD designs. *Journal of Applied Behavioral Science, 12,* 133–157.

Imparato, N., & Harari, O. (1994, October). When new worlds stir. *Management Review,* pp. 22–28.

Lorenzi, N.M., Mantel, M.I., & Riley, R.T. (1990, December). Preparing your organizations for technological change. *Healthcare Informatics,* pp. 33–34.

Lorenzi, N.M., & Riley, R.T. (1994). *Organizational aspects of health informatics: Managing technological change* (pp. 228–229). New York: Springer-Verlag.

Thach, L., & Woodman, R.W. (1994, Summer). Organizational change and information technology: Managing on the edge of cyberspace. *Organizational Dynamics,* pp. 31–33.

Watzlawick, P., Weakland, J.H., & Fisch, R. (1974). *Change: Principles of problem formulation and problem resolution.* New York: W.W. Norton.

16
The Legacy of Advancing Technology: Ethical Issues and Healthcare Information Management Systems

GAIL ANN DELUCA HAVENS

"Ethical issues are not founded on whether technology is acceptable to humankind, but rather on whether people have the humanity with which to make technology a true instrument of man's will." (Levine, 1980, p. 194)

The technical acumen and expertise that are a hallmark of our society have allowed us to make significant advances in the development of automated information systems. These advances have benefitted both institutions and individuals. Automated healthcare information systems have been characterized as the repository of the most sensitive, personal, and intimate information about an individual (Gostin et al., 1993). However, the processes of acquiring, handling, and retrieving healthcare information electronically raise multiple ethical issues. These issues must be addressed if such technology is to be a credible component in the delivery of health care that promotes consumer trust and confidence and that yields desirable outcomes cost effectively.

Traditionally, the examination of ethical issues related to healthcare information technology has focused on matters related to patient privacy (Bennett, 1991; Bruce, 1988; Chlapowski, 1991; Gostin et al., 1993; Hiller & Seidel, 1982; Maciorowski, 1991; Milholland, 1994; Romano, 1987; Westin, 1976), the confidentiality of information (Bialorucki & Blaine, 1992; Bruce, 1988; Fishman, 1994; Gostin et al., 1993; Hiller & Seidel, 1982; Milholland, 1994; Pheby, 1982; Romano, 1987; Westin, 1976), and data protection (Brooks, Semenuk, & Vaughan, 1988; Faaoso, 1992; Griesser, 1985, 1989; Hiller & Seidel, 1982; Mason, 1986; Milholland, 1994; Romano, 1987; Schmaus, 1991; Westin, 1976). Most of us would agree that maintaining individual privacy and the confidentiality of information and protecting personal data from misuse, destruction, or loss of use are desirable goals. Where we encounter problems in discussing such matters is in determining whether maintaining individual privacy and the confidentiality of information and protecting personal data always take precedence over competing claims that might be just as right and equally as good.

Are there situations where a competing claim might take precedence over an individual's privacy, the confidential nature of his/her personal information, or the protection of personal data? If so, what rationale grounds such decisions? Smith characterizes our society as having "lost its footing with respect to the specific boundaries surrounding the collection, use, and protection of personal information" (Smith, 1994, p. 209). Although an apt analogy, the message ought not to be construed as a negative one. Rather, we should regard it as a realistic assessment of societal attempts to address the legacy of ethical issues concerning healthcare information systems bequeathed to us by a rapidly advancing technology. The ensuing discussion is intended to provide information that will be helpful in identifying and examining several of these issues.

First, a framework for examining ethical issues is presented. This is followed by a discussion of several fundamental ethical principles, namely beneficence, nonmaleficence, and respect for autonomy, particularly relevant to the ethical concerns generated by healthcare information systems. Next, specific ethical issues related to confidentiality, privacy, information privacy, and data protection and healthcare information systems are examined. Observations about the ethical challenges presented by computerized knowledge systems follow. They are included for reflection and to remind us that ethical issues will be generated perpetually by healthcare information systems. Remarks related to moral obligations and healthcare information systems bring the discussion to a close.

A Framework for Examining Ethical Issues

Ethics and Values

Ethics is a form of thinking about morality, moral problems, and moral judgments (Frankena, 1973). The term *ethical* as it is being used in this discussion refers to pertaining to ethics. For instance, what ought to be a given institution's standard regarding the confidentiality of a patient's laboratory results? Without doubt, this is an important question when discussing ethical issues related to healthcare information systems. However, the overriding question is how to go about engaging in moral reasoning in attempting to define this standard? What are the goals, values, principles, and rules that ought to guide this process of moral judgment? A value has been characterized as a desirable or preferred way of acting or knowing something that, ultimately, governs one's actions or decisions (Giger & Davidhizar, 1991). Values are prescriptive or proscriptive beliefs upon which one acts by preference (Rokeach, 1973).

Moral and Nonmoral Values

It is important to recognize that values differ according to whether they are moral or nonmoral in nature. Moral values are things that may be morally good or morally bad. Similarly, nonmoral values are things that may be good or bad in a nonmoral sense. The subjects of moral values include persons, groups of persons, and character traits. Moral values also can be recognized by their grounds, including motives, intentions, or dispositions, that contribute to a judgment being formed about the moral goodness or badness of a particular person or action (Frankena, 1973). Nonmoral values usually are those that are associated with individual opinions and personal choices. Self-interest (Beauchamp & Childress, 1994) or personal preferences or aesthetics (Frankena, 1973) are among the reasons or grounds upon which nonmoral value judgments differentiate good nonmoral values from those that are not.

Ethical Principles and Rules

Principles are general action guides for judgment in specific cases. There are several principles that are regarded as basic guides in reasoning about ethical issues. These ethical principles include producing good or benefits and weighing these positive aspects against the risks and costs, also called beneficence; avoiding causing harm, referred to as nonmaleficence; and respect for the personal rule of self, that is, respect for autonomy (Beauchamp & Childress, 1989, 1994; Fry, 1994; Jameton, 1984; Veatch & Fry, 1987). A particular ethical principle ought to be followed unless overridden by another principle that might be weightier in a particular situation. For instance, returning to the example of the accessibility of a patient's laboratory results, should the principle of respect for autonomy dictate that all laboratory results are to be made available only on a need-to-know basis or might the principle of beneficence with its inherent balancing of benefits and risks provide guidance in the process of deciding to whom which laboratory results will be accessible? Principles provide essential guidance for the development of rules. Rules are more restricted in scope than principles. They imbue ethical principles with specificity and provide the foundation for the subsequent development of standards and organizational policies, for instance.

Morals and Morality

Jameton (1984) describes morals as values and principles to which individuals are committed personally (i.e., those that they follow and defend in daily life). Morals give substance to morality, which has been depicted as the moral institution of life (Frankena, 1973). It is helpful to think of morality as an amalgam, a combination of components, that includes

- Goals, values, rules, and principles,
- Points of view,
- Ways of feeling,
- Sources of motivation, including sanctions,

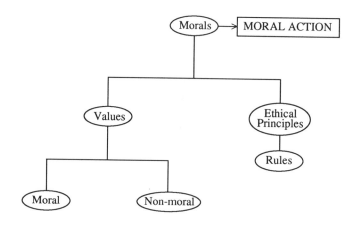

FIGURE 16-1. Components of moral action.

- Forms of judgment, and
- Reasons for these judgments.

How do ethics, values, ethical principles and rules, and morals relate to each other? One common characteristic of these concepts is their relationship to action, to behavior, to doing rather than to being. These relationships are illustrated in Figure 16-1. However, lest we think that acting in morally good ways is simply a matter of doing, it is important to understand that those performing the action also must be inclined to morally good acts by character traits or dispositions that are congruent with moral actions. These components of moral inclination are shown in Figure 16-2.

There is a danger, however, in this line of reasoning that principles and rules will be regarded as the ultimate determinants of good and bad moral actions with character traits and dispositions subjugated to them. Or, conversely, principles and rules could be considered extensions of character traits and dispositions and be defined by them. Frankena (1973), cautioning against this dichotomous approach, proposes that the morality of principles and the morality of traits are not different moralities; they should be re-

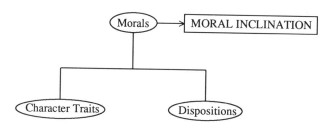

FIGURE 16-2. Components of moral inclination.

garded as complementary aspects of the same morality. This complementary morality is illustrated in Figure 16-3.

It is with this conception of morality as a conjoining of moral actions and inclinations that we continue our discussion of ethical issues and healthcare information systems.

Ethical Principles and Healthcare Information Systems

Beneficence

A useful way to think about beneficence is as a positive action. The ethical principle of beneficence refers to a moral obligation to act for the benefit of others, balancing the benefits and drawbacks of such action (Beauchamp & Childress, 1994). In addition to this conception of general beneficence is the obligation of specific beneficence attributable to particular societal roles. For instance, specific moral and contractual obligations of beneficence apply to the roles of healthcare professionals and of information system managers and technical experts, respectively. Each of these roles and the environments in which they operate stand in a special commitment, some in moral relationships by virtue of professional obligations, to patients. Indeed, the overriding moral obligation of healthcare professionals and institutions is the welfare of patients. These moral and contractual obligations, however, necessarily require balancing benefits, such as patient health, welfare, and safety, with risks and costs.

Nonmaleficence

The ethical principle of nonmaleficence provides the foundation for the moral obligation to avoid acting so as to inflict harm on another. We are

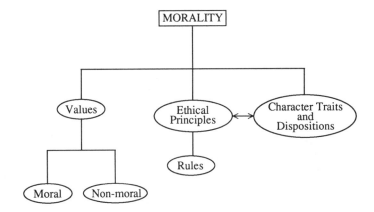

FIGURE 16-3. A morality of complementary actions and inclinations.

expected to intentionally refrain from actions that cause harm, including harm resulting from setbacks to multiple interests that might arise in acquiring, handling, and retrieving personal information in a healthcare information system. These would include setbacks to physical and psychological interests in addition to setbacks to privacy, property, or reputation resulting from the mishandling and/or unauthorized release of sensitive patient information (Milholland, 1994).

Bloustein characterizes the harm resulting from a setback to one's privacy by having private facts made public as "damage is to an individual's self-respect by being made a public spectacle" (Bloustein, 1964, p. 981). Healthcare information systems may inflict harm on individuals in two significant ways (Miller, 1971):

1. By disseminating information about the individual to a wider audience than the individual consented to or anticipated when he or she originally surrendered the information, and
2. By introducing factual or contextual inaccuracies in the data that create an erroneous impression of the individual's actual conduct or achievements in the minds of those to whom the information is exposed.

Respect for Autonomy

The ethical principle of respect for autonomy provides fundamental justification for the right of self-determination. Persons who are autonomous exhibit a personal rule of self that is free of the controlling interferences of others and of personal constraints, such as inadequate understanding, that prevent meaningful choice (Beauchamp & Childress, 1989, 1994). Confidentiality and privacy are associated autonomy rights. These particular rights generate significant concerns when examining ethical issues surrounding healthcare information systems.

Confidentiality

Discussions about confidentiality usually go hand-in-hand with understandings of obligations to keep secret information acquired in particular relationships. Healthcare professionals are morally obligated to maintain the confidential nature of the information shared with them by their patients (American Medical Association, 1981; American Nurses Association, 1985; Fry, 1994; Jameton, 1984; Veatch & Fry, 1987). For those individuals employed by healthcare organizations who are not obliged to confidentiality by professional codes or standards, a contractual duty to maintain the confidentiality of healthcare information must be created (Griesser, 1989). The following assumptions are reasonable premises of individuals seeking health care regarding their personal information:

1. Individuals reveal sensitive information about themselves to healthcare professionals because such information is necessary for the professional to intervene appropriately;
2. Individuals believe the healthcare professional will share the sensitive information with others only when needed to provide the required intervention;
3. Individuals trust that their personal information will be used only for the purpose intended, unless other uses are requested and consent is obtained; and
4. Individuals presume that no harm will follow from revealing the required personal information.

Indeed, a recent public opinion survey revealed that the vast majority of the public interviewed believe their healthcare providers maintain the confidentiality of their medical information (Harris and Associates & Westin, 1993).

The moral obligation to maintain confidentiality includes information that is acquired but not recorded, as well as recorded information, whether it be recorded manually or electronically. In a 1976 report on the investigation of the impact of computers on citizens' rights in healthcare record keeping, Dr. Willis Ware's definitions of confidentiality included (Westin, 1976, p. 348):

1. Status accorded to data or information indicating that it is sensitive for some reason, therefore needs to be protected against theft or improper use, and must be disseminated only to individuals or organizations authorized (or privileged) to have it;
2. By extension, status (sometimes assured by law) accorded to data or information that reflects an understood agreement between the person furnishing the data and the person or organization holding it that prescribes the protection to be provided and the dissemination and use to be permitted.

The concept of confidentiality is fundamentally different from that of privacy. Whereas privacy concerns relate to individuals, issues of confidentiality are pertinent to relationships between or among persons or institutions. Confidentiality relates only to the redisclosure of information previously disclosed. It is controlled by the person or institution to whom an individual's privacy is relinquished. In examining issues related to the rights of individuals and computerized healthcare information, Westin defined confidentiality as "the question of how personal data collected for approved social purposes shall be held and used by the organization that originally collected it, what other secondary or further uses may be made of it, and when consent by the individual will be required for such uses" (Westin, 1976, p. 6).

Winslade described confidentiality as "logically dependent upon loss of privacy" and stated that "it is important to recognize the priority of privacy and the derivative nature of confidentiality, especially in health care situations" (Winslade, 1982, p. 503). Information acquired in a special relationship (e.g., a patient/healthcare professional or a patient/healthcare institution relationship) obligates the recipient of the information not to disclose any information about the other party without that party's permission. In this way, while we grant others access to our personal information, we also retain, theoretically, some control over the information generated about us. Ideally, this ought to minimize the harm to us from information used for reasons others than those intended when it originally was revealed.

The challenges of maintaining the confidentiality of patient information in health care are compounded by electronic and telecommunications media and confounded by the number of people in a healthcare organization, as well as external to it, who have a legitimate interest in patient information in order to make their expected contribution to the continuum of patient care. Currently, the paper medical record is evolving into a computer-based patient record (CPR). The American Health Information Management Association (AHIMA) has stated that "The success of the CPR depends in part on patients' trust that their personal health information will be kept confidential" (AHIMA, 1992, p. 1). In a position statement on the confidentiality of the CPR, AHIMA recommends that "Safeguards concerning privacy and confidentiality address the healthcare providers duty to protect patients from unnecessary intrusion into their private life, and to safeguard the health information entrusted to them" (AHIMA, 1992, p. 2).

Unfortunately, the confidential nature of patient information continues to be compromised at times by behaviors of healthcare professionals that have little to do with the technological advances surrounding such information and cannot be rectified by technology. The most serious and common breaches of confidentiality are purported to occur during casual encounters in healthcare institutions (Bruce, 1988; Milholland, 1994). Activities such as discussions about patients among healthcare professionals in the public places of healthcare institutions (e.g., in elevators, hallways, and cafeteria lines) risk revealing information about patients to those who ought not to know it. This kind of conduct is a violation of the healthcare professional's moral obligation to keep such information in confidence.

Snooping in patients' records, particularly in the electronic version of patients' records, is a much more insidious practice than the breaches of confidentiality that occur in the context of casual encounters (Bialorucki & Blaine, 1992; Bruce, 1988; Curran & Curran, 1991; Fishman, 1994; Gostin et al., 1993; Maciorowski, 1991). Electronic snooping, that is, the practice of browsing through the patient's medical record, is a curious phenomenon. It appears that patient information that is stored electronically often is not treated with the same level of confidentiality as manually recorded patient information confined in a paper record. Perhaps this is a transitory phenomenon that will disappear when the basic education of healthcare professionals routinely addresses moral obligations related to the confidentiality of electronically stored patient information. The same degree of moral responsibility ought to be ascribed to the electronic medium as is now ascribed to patient information that is stored in the paper record. Although it is likely that breaches of electronic information systems often are not negatively motivated, it is naive to believe that these breaches can be thwarted effectively by security systems alone. Regardless of the medium used for storage, it is imperative that the education and training of all who work in health care conveys the moral accountability inherent in acquiring, handling, and retrieving patient care information.

Privacy

Privacy is a state or condition of physical or informational inaccessibility (Beauchamp & Childress, 1994). Interpreted as the exclusive access of a person to a realm of his own, privacy is depicted as an "extended part of the person" (Van Den Haag, 1971, p. 151). Simmel describes individuals as being in a "continual competition with society over the ownership of our selves" (Simmel, 1971, p. 72). During the process, each of us self-defines an area that is uniquely our own with others entering only by invitation. "This condition of insulation is what we call privacy" (Simmel, 1971, p. 72). Schoeman explains the notion of insulation more fully by noting that "the point of the restrictions on access is in large part not to isolate people but to enable them to relate intimately or in looser associations that serve personal and group goals" (Schoeman, 1992, p. 21).

Privacy also is depicted as a moral norm (Van Den Haag, 1971). Prosser conceives of privacy as "a composite of the value our society places on mental tranquillity, reputation, and intangible forms of property" (cited in Bloustein, 1964, p. 962). Hirshleifer describes privacy as "autonomy within society ... a particular kind of social structure together with its supporting social ethic ... a way of organizing society" (Hirshleifer, 1980, pp. 649–650). The notion of autonomy finds support in the principle of respect for autonomy that "includes the right to decide ... what will happen to one's person-to one's body, to information about one's life, to one's secrets ..." (Beauchamp & Childress, 1994, p. 410). To respect another's privacy is to respect that individual as a person, that is, to concede that one ought to take account of the way in which a particular individual's affairs might be affected by one's own decision (Benn, 1971).

Privacy is variously identified as personal, individual, informational, physical, or mental, all of which overlap by varying degrees. No definitive typology of privacy exists. However, Schoeman (1992) has ordered conceptions of privacy along a narrow to broad continuum, as illustrated in Figure 16-4, that serves to overcome some of the ambiguity in terminology that

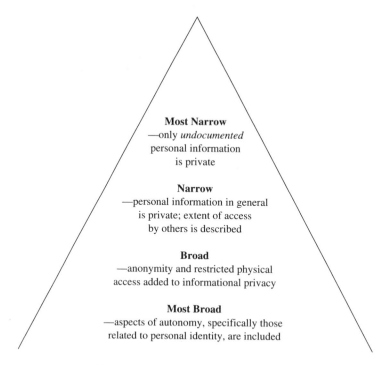

FIGURE 16-4. Conceptions of privacy.

currently exists. Because the ethical issues that arise related to privacy and healthcare information systems to a great extent are issues related to information privacy, the remainder of the discussion of privacy focuses on information privacy and on the concept of personal information as property.

Information Privacy

Information, especially that which has been interpreted in some way, is material in a form that is meaningful (Brown, 1990). Information is defined as the communication of knowledge (*American Heritage Dictionary*, 1985). Information privacy is described as "the ability of the individual to control the circulation of information relating to him or her" (Bennett, 1991, p. 67). In discussing information privacy, Gostin et al. (1993) portrayed information privacy as existing when information about an individual is beyond the range of others without specific authorization. A report of research on computerized medical records and citizens rights conducted in the mid-1970s included the following definitions of information privacy developed by Dr. Willis Ware (Westin, 1976):

1. The claim of individuals, groups, or institutions to determine for themselves when, how, and to what extent data about them is communicated to or used by others;

2. The protection of an individual against harm or damage as a result of the operation of a record system;
3. The protection of an individual (or class of individuals) against unwelcome, unfair, improper, or excessive collection or dissemination of information or data about himself.

As understood in the data protection field, privacy in the context of health care "is the patient's right of secrecy of his/her data and his/her protection against misuse or unjustified publication inside or outside the health care field and is the responsibility of the health care provider" (Griesser, 1989, p. 225).

A current definition of information privacy describes it as a condition of limited access to *identifiable* information about individuals (Smith, 1994). The significant term in this definition is identifiable, as it is the association of personal information with a particular individual that precipitates the ethical concerns. Simmel (1971), as discussed above, portrayed privacy as a condition of insulation that serves to protect our selves from being taken over by society. Bloustein, however, adopted a slightly different approach to examining the concept of privacy by discussing the principle of *inviolate personality* initially brought forth by Warren and Brandeis in the late 19th Century. "I take the principle of 'inviolate personality' to posit the individual's independence, dignity and integrity; it defines man's essence as a unique and self-determining being" (Bloustein, 1964, p. 971). This conceptual dyad of insulation-inviolability grounds the notion of personhood articulated by Chlapowski in his note about information privacy. "The sphere around each individual allows the individual to be a creature unto herself, a creature of her own *identity*, free from outside definition or other identity-altering influence" (Chlapowski, 1991, p. 151).

Personal information as property. To construe personal information as property seems a reasonable conception. Hirshleifer agues that it is our "internalized respect for property " that "permits autonomy to persist within society" (Hirshleifer, 1980, p. 657). Personal information has been characterized as "one of the products of an individual's person" (Chlapowski, 1991, p. 159). Although no explicit justification for this representation exists either in constitutional or case law, support for this conception continues to accumulate in the literature, especially since the term *zones of privacy* was introduced in the finding of Supreme Court Justice William O. Douglas in *Griswold v. Connecticut* (1965). The conception of personal information as property is much older, however, having been expressed in the seventeenth century by John Locke, a philosopher and a physician, "Though the earth, and all inferior creatures, be common to all men, yet every man has a property in his own person: this no body has any right to but himself" (Locke, 1689/1764, p. 216).

The conception of personal information as property that could not be taken or misused by government without due process of law is said to be an outcome of the legal and theoretical efforts to clarify the concept of privacy that occurred in the 1960s (Bennett, 1991). "Information privacy meant that personal data could only be provided to a public or private organization for the purpose of fulfilling a legitimate social task" (Bennett, 1991, p. 59). Shortly afterward, Miller argued that the market's treatment of personal information as a commodity supported the theory of privacy as property (Miller, 1971). A report on the study of computerized medical records and citizens' rights published in 1976, greatly expanded on the notion of personal information as property by examining the concept from the perspective of contract or exchange theory:

The concept here is that an individual, exercising his right to give or withhold personal information, releases valuable personal data either in order to obtain a specific benefit for himself (or his family or group, or to promote a social good he supports) or else to fulfill a legal duty (carrying the sanction of majority will under democratic theory). In return, the recipient (the data user) has two basic obligations: to use the personal information only for the purpose agreed upon (unless authorized by additional consent or by law), and not to treat the information so carelessly or maliciously that it harms the individual from whom it was obtained (Westin, 1976, p. 271).

The report continued:

Making informational privacy a property right as well as a human right does something useful in a capitalist society: it buttresses the individual's claim to assert (or at least to share) control over the uses made of his or her valuable property. It also explains why there should be a reciprocal duty on the part of the data user to live up to his side of the informational contract—not to be guilty of unjust enrichment at another's expense. Whether as a basis for legislation or judicial decision, or to explain to the public the implied-contract relationship that should be seen arising between data subject and data user, this concept has great merit for public policy (Westin, 1976, p. 271).

Although no particular item is intrinsically private, the value placed "on a condition of non-access determines how it comes to be categorized as private" (Beauchamp & Childress, 1994, p. 409). As with other property interests, however, although the property may belong to an individual, it holds a value independent of the individual. Miller warned that "as the importance of information increases, the central issue that emerges . . . is how to contain the excesses of this new form of power, while channeling its benefits to best serve the citizenry" (Miller, 1971, p. 259). Westin alerted us to the increasing value of personal information in the context of a society growing increasingly more dependent on data when he described our personal characteristics as "the vital raw material of business, governmental, and political decision-making. . . . Thus, whatever it may have been in earlier centuries, personal information has become, like clean air and water, a scarce commodity today, capable of being valued in an economic sense alongside its social worth in terms of protecting individual dignity and democratic values" (Westin, 1976, p. 271).

The characterization of personal information as a valuable commodity was echoed recently by Chlapowski (1991). Furthermore, an inexorable increase in the value of personal information currently is occurring (Gostin et al., 1993; Maciorowski, 1991; Mason, 1986; Milholland, 1994; Peck, 1984; Smith, 1994). "Community concern for the individual's dignity is at issue . . ." (Bloustein, 1964, p. 1006). "If we really believe that personal privacy is fundamental to our democratic tradition of individual autonomy, and that its preservation is thought desirable" (Miller, 1971, p. 259), the present rapidly escalating value of personal information requires increasing vigilance in order to protect individuals from society's claim of ownership of this property (Chlapowski, 1991; Westin, 1976).

Data Protection

Data protection is defined as an associated group of policies governing the protection of automatically recorded personal information (Bennett, 1991). More specifically, data protection is described as the sum of measures suitable to safeguard data and programs from undesired occurrences that, performed deliberately or unintentionally, lead to disclosure, modification, destruction, or loss of data (Griesser, 1985, 1989). A data protection system ought to exemplify a reasonable balance between honoring the moral obligations of healthcare professionals and organizations to patients and achieving the scientific, technical, and organizational advantages inherent in an automated healthcare information system. Ethical issues related to data protection most often coalesce around its components, namely program and data integrity, availability of data and resources, physical security measures, and usage integrity.

Data and Program Integrity

The integrity of data and programs depends on the accurate representation of source documents in automated form (Faaoso, 1992; Griesser, 1989; Mason, 1986; Romano, 1987) and on not being exposed to (1) accidental or malicious alteration, (2) unauthorized copying, (3) loss by theft, and/or (4) destruction by hardware failures, software deficiencies, operating mistakes, or physical damage by fire or water (Griesser, 1989; Romano, 1987; Schmaus, 1991). The accuracy, correctness, completeness, and validity of data are a matter of grave concern in healthcare information systems, as automated patient information is used with increasing frequency in clinical decision making. Information used in diagnosis and treatment that is not accurate, correct, complete, or valid could result in physical and/or psychological harm to patients. The training and education of users of healthcare information systems in the technology acknowledge the ethical obligation to avoid causing harm to patients by promoting greater accuracy of the information (Faaoso, 1992; Schmaus, 1991). Such training and education interventions also create opportunities to introduce users of healthcare information systems to their moral obligations pertaining to data and program integrity (Westin, 1976), as well as to reacquaint seasoned users with their moral obligations.

Availability of Data and Resources

The presumption in using a healthcare information system is that the data are available when and where needed and that the resources necessary to operate the system are available as well (Griesser, 1989). This requires a substantial commitment of the financial and human resources of a healthcare organization. Furthermore, it obligates the organization to a planning process for system design and data protection that involves all the principals, namely, nurses, physicians, administrators, and computer experts (Griesser, 1989), to ensure the health, safety, and welfare of the patients to be served by the system and to avoid squandering organizational resources.

Physical Security Measures

The potential for the loss of patient and organizational data, computer programs, and information system equipment obligates the healthcare organization to design physical security measures that will protect data, programs, and equipment from physical damage (e.g., by water or smoke, technical malfunctions, or sabotage) (Griesser, 1989). The patient, administrative, and financial information stored in the database of a healthcare information system is a significantly valuable organizational asset. Great harm could be inflicted on patients and on the healthcare organization by organizational neglect of the ethical obligation to protect data, software, and hardware from damage or destruction.

Usage Integrity

Usage integrity is a method of ensuring the privacy of patient information by implementing measures to protect against unauthorized access to programs and data and the unintentional or deliberate misuse of patient and healthcare organizational data (Griesser, 1985, 1989; Romano, 1987). A healthcare information system is used by many people for a variety of purposes from multiple locations. The introduction of microcomputers that are capable of enhancing patient care, research, and organizational operations into healthcare organizations has facilitated networks of patient information beyond the physical space of particular healthcare facilities. At the same time, however, as the number of system users increases (Brannigan, 1992), along with a commensurate increase in the potential for unauthorized access to personal information (Bennett, 1991; Fishman, 1994), the risk of harm to patients increases correspondingly. Usage integrity is promoted by categorizing data according to sensitivity (Griesser, 1989) and by applying a need-to-know standard when identifying classes of users (Brooks et al., 1988; Faaoso, 1992; Griesser, 1989; Hiller & Beyda, 1981; Hiller & Seidel, 1982; Milholland, 1994).

Categories of data sensitivity. Griesser (1989) offers the following typology for data sensitivity:

1. *Normal Sensitivity*—This level of information is available to all eligible individuals, subject to professional or contractual obligations of confidentiality, based on their need to know in order to perform their tasks. Personal, social, and statistical data usually would be categorized in this level. Exceptions would be made in the case of personal and/or social data that were linked to a diagnosis or admission to a particular inpatient unit that was socially stigmatizing, thereby necessitating special consideration of the data as sensitive in order to ensure usage integrity.
2. *Sensitive*—Information in this category is available only to defined groups of users. Included in this category would be health risks, rendered hospital services, financial data, and some activity data (i.e., ordered and carried out diagnostic, therapeutic, and nursing interventions).
3. *Very Sensitive*—This category contains information accessible only to selected and explicitly authorized groups who are in direct contact with the patient. Some diagnoses and activity data would be categorized at this level.
4. *Highly Sensitive*—Information in this category includes those patient care data that can endanger the patient's privacy and compromise his or her social life. These data are restricted solely to the use of the treating physician. Their retrieval and use by others may occur only with the patient's explicit consent. Some diagnoses and the clinical data associated with them are examples of the type of data that would be placed in this category.

Need-to-know standard. Satisfying the user's need to know and giving access to patient care information may be accomplished in a healthcare organization by initially identifying the users of the healthcare information system and, then, classifying the users into groups according to their organizational functions. Subsequently, access to particular patient care information is structured by user groups and determined by the (Griesser, 1989):

1. Workplace-related functions of users,
2. Inherent need-to-know of specific elements of patient care data,
3. Access rights of the various users to the different data categories with respect to their need to know for performing their professional activities, and
4. Competencies a user must have to receive the privileges that are required.

By employing this strategy in designing and implementing an information system, a healthcare organization facilitates the usage integrity of programs and data. In doing so, the organization also is making an effort to meet its ethical obligation to its patients to protect the data entrusted to it.

Knowledge Bases

The use of computerized knowledge bases in patient care decision making has the potential to raise a number of ethical issues related to the health, safety, and well-being of patients in the care of nurses and physicians. An approach to differentiating these ethical issues by the components that constitute knowledge bases, that is, by factual knowledge and by directives for action, has been suggested (Doroszewski, 1988).

Factual Knowledge

In considering the factual knowledge component, computerized expert consultation systems respond to the user's question with factual statements (i.e., laws) that describe relations between phenomena and processes taking place in the human organism, including results of therapeutic or other actions (Doroszewski, 1988). Ethical issues relate to the responsibility of the expert, a nurse or physician for instance, and the computer scientist for the truthfulness and adequacy of laws of a given fragment of knowledge represented by means of an artificial intelligence approach. This is an especially complex challenge, given the absolute requirement of the translation of patient care knowledge into a valid, correct, and accurate computer representation.

Directives for Action

The directives for action component of expert systems contains suggestions for the action to be performed in a given situation. The directives indicate how the patient care goal established by the knowledge system user may be achieved. The responsibility of the nurse or physician expert and the computer scientist pertaining to directives for action is similar to the responsibility related to factual statements, that is, for the truthfulness and adequacy of conclusions that incorporate large fields of patient care knowledge pertaining to the normal, as well as to the pathological, state of the organism and arrived at as a result of complex reasoning. It is important to note that the process of drawing conclusions necessarily includes an evaluative process. Therefore, the directives for action component of patient care expert systems contain a value element, as do most statements in natural patient care knowledge.

Natural Knowledge vs. Model Representations of Knowledge

The responsibility of a nurse or a physician in the role of a computer expert is the same as that of an author formulating opinions by means of natural language. One important difference exists, however, between computerized information and that contained in books. Written or spoken text embodies natural knowledge in the sense that it is customary, traditionally accepted, and easily intelligible knowledge, whereas computerized knowledge bases contain model representations of knowledge. The usefulness and limitations, as well as the possibilities and drawbacks, of such model representations are not yet fully estimated and understood. When coupled with the difficult nature of healthcare problems, knowledge, and reasoning encountered by specialists in artificial intelligence, it is evident that designing computerized patient care expert systems remains an experimental activity (Doroszewski, 1988). As such, it has the potential to raise ethical issues similar to those introduced by other scientific experiments and to generate corresponding ethical obligations for healthcare professionals, as well as for healthcare organizations.

Moral Obligations and Healthcare Information Systems

The overriding moral concern related to healthcare information systems is the health, safety, and well-being of patients. Meeting the moral obligation of protecting the information privacy of patients is respecting the patient as a person with a unique value system and identity. This individuality determines the degree of privacy ascribed to the patient's particular personal information by the patient. It is the moral obligation of healthcare providers and organizations to abide by the patient's self-determination of the privacy of his or her personal information in most cases. This obligation is inherent in the relationship between heathcare providers and organizations and patients. However, although it is a binding moral obligation, it is not an absolute obligation and, therefore, may be overridden by a competing moral claim. For instance, ensuring public health and safety requires the reporting of certain diseases to state and/or federal health agencies (Bruce, 1988).

Obligations in relationships are defined by the social roles and traditions that constitute particular relationships (Beauchamp & Childress, 1994; Brown, 1990). The social roles of healthcare providers (for instance, nurses and physicians) and healthcare organizations (hospitals as an example) stand in particular relationships with patients. These relationships morally obligate nurses, physicians, and hospitals to specific actions regarding the health, safety, and welfare of patients. Similar professional and/or contractual obligations hold for all individuals who provide direct or indirect patient care or who support the delivery of patient care.

The specific actions taken by nurses, physicians, and hospitals related to maintaining the inviolate nature of the personal information of patients are the results of weighing, of balancing, benefits, risks, and costs. Operating within the action–inclination framework of morality that was discussed earlier, the ethical principles of producing benefits over risks, avoiding causing harm, and respecting the personal rule of self guide a balancing of legitimate interests related to personal information. Included among these interests, in addition to the interests of the patient, are those of healthcare professionals, healthcare organizations, scientific communities, government, and healthcare payors, regulators, and planners. It is these competing interests that generate the ethical issues associated with healthcare information systems that challenge healthcare professionals and organizations alike.

Questions

1. How do the issues raised in this chapter affect you in your work? What can you gain from the study of ethics?
2. Dispute or defend the statement with which Havens begins her chapter: "Ethical issues are not founded on whether technology is acceptable to humankind, but rather on whether people have the humanity with which to make technology a true instrument of man's will" (Levine, 1980).
3. As we move towards a computer-based patient record, segments of the physician community continue to voice concern regarding privacy and confidentiality. How can these and related concerns be best addressed?
4. Consider the changing healthcare environment. Do health information networks intensify concerns regarding privacy and confidentiality?
5. Clinical decision support systems pose a special set of ethical questions. Can a practitioner choose not to use such systems? What does their use imply for individual professional judgment? If there is an error in a system, who is liable?
6. Assume that a decision support system used in intensive care sets forth a poor prognosis for a patient, supported by extensive data. Can a managed care organization deem continued interventions medically inappropriate?

References

American Health Information Management Association. (1992, July). *A position statement on the confidentiality of the computer-based patient record.* Chicago: Author.

American Heritage Dictionary (2nd ed.). (1985). Boston: Houghton Mifflin.

American Medical Association. (1984). *Current opinions of the Judicial Council of the American Medical Association.* Chicago: Author.

American Nurses' Association. (1985). *Code for nurses with interpretive statements.* Kansas City, MO: Author.

Beauchamp, T.L., & Childress, J.F. (1989). *Principles of biomedical ethics* (3rd ed.). New York: Oxford University Press.

Beauchamp, T.L., & Childress, J.F. (1994). *Principles of biomedical ethics* (4th ed.). New York: Oxford University Press.

Benn, S.I. (1971). Privacy, freedom, and respect for persons. In J.R. Pennock & J.W. Chapman (Eds.), *Privacy* (pp. 1–26). New York: Atherton Press.

Bennett, C.J. (1991). Computers, personal data, and theories of technology: Comparative approaches to privacy protection in the 1990s. *Science, Technology, & Human Values, 16*(1), 51–69.

Bialorucki, T., & Blaine, M.J. (1992). Protecting patient confidentiality in the pursuit of the ultimate computerized information system. *Journal of Nursing Care Quality, 7*(1), 53–56.

Bloustein, E.J. (1964). Privacy as an aspect of human dignity: An answer to Dean Prosser. *New York University Law Review, 39*, 962–1007.

Brannigan, V.M. (1992). Protecting the privacy of patient information in clinical networks: Regulatory effectiveness analysis. In D.F. Parsons, C.M. Fleischer, & R.A. Greenes (Vol. Eds.), *Annals of the New York Academy of Science: Vol. 670. Extended clinical consulting by hospital computer networks* (670th ed., pp. 191–201). New York: The New York Academy of Sciences.

Brooks, G.M., Semenuk, T., & Vaughan, V.S. (1988). Controlling information: Who, what, how? *Computers in Healthcare, 9*(1), 16–18.

Brown, G. (1990). *The information game: Ethical issues in a microchip world.* Atlantic Highlands, NJ: Humanities Press International.

Bruce, J.A.C. (1988). *Privacy and confidentiality of health care information* (2nd ed.). Chicago: American Hospital Publishing.

Chlapowski, F.S. (1991). The constitutional protection of informational privacy. *Boston University Law Review, 71*, 133–160.

Curran, M., & Curran, K. (1991). The ethics of information. *JONA, 21*(1), 47–49.

Doroszewski, J. (1988). Ethical and methodological aspects of medical computer data bases and knowledge bases. *Theoretical Medicine, 9*, 117–128.

Faaoso, N. (1992). Automated patient care systems: The ethical impact. *Nursing Management, 23*(7), 46–48.

Fishman, D. (1994). Confidentiality. *Computers in Nursing, 12*(2), 73–77.

Frankena, W.K. (1973). *Ethics* (2nd ed.). Englewood Cliffs, NJ: Prentice-Hall.

Fry, S.T. (1994). *Ethics in nursing practice: A guide to ethical decision making.* Geneva, Switzerland: International Council of Nurses.

Giger, J.N., & Davidhizar, R.E. (1991). *Transcultural nursing.* St. Louis, MO: Mosby Year Book.

Gostin, L.O., Turek-Brezina, J., Powers, M., Kozloff, R., Faden, R., & Steinauer, D.D. (1993). Privacy and security of personal information in a new health care system. *JAMA, 270*, 2487–2493.

Griesser, G. (1985). The issue of data protection in computer-aided health care information systems. In K.J. Hannah, E.J. Guillemin, & D.N. Conklin (Eds.), *Nursing uses of computer and information science* (pp. 113–117). North-Holland, Amsterdam: Elsevier Science.

Griesser, G. (1989). Data protection in hospital information systems: 1. Definition and overview. In H.F. Orthner & B.I. Blum (Eds.), *Implementing health care information systems* (pp. 222–253). New York: Springer-Verlag.

Griswold v. Connecticut, 381 U.S. 479 (1965).

Harris, L. and Associates, & Westin, A.F. (1993). *Health information privacy survey: 1993.* Atlanta, GA: Equifax.

Hiller, M.D., & Beyda, V. (1981). Computers, medical records, and the right to privacy. *Journal of Health, Politics, and Law, 6,* 463–487.

Hiller, M.D., & Seidel, L.F. (1982). Patient care management systems, medical records, and privacy: A balancing act. *Public Health Reports, 97,* 332–345.

Hirshleifer, J. (1980). Privacy: Its origin, function, and future. *The Journal of Legal Studies, 9,* 649–664.

Jameton, A. (1984). *Nursing practice: The ethical issues.* Englewood Cliffs, NJ: Prentice-Hall.

Levine, M.E. (1980). The ethics of computer technology in health care. *Nursing Forum, XIX*(2), 193–198.

Locke, J. (1764). *Two treatises of government* (6th printing). London, England: A. Millar, H. Woodfall, I. Whiston and B. White, I. Rivington, L. Davis and C. Reyners, R. Baldwin, H. Clarke and Collins; W. Johnston, W. Owen, I. Richardson, S. Crowder, T. Longman, B. Law, C. Rivington, E. Dilly, R. Withy, C. and R. Ware, S. Baker, T. Payne, A. Shuckburgh, and I. Hinxman. (Original work published 1689)

Maciorowski, L.F. (1991). The enduring concerns of privacy and confidentiality. *Holistic Nursing Practice, 5*(3), 51–56.

Mason, R.O. (1986). Four ethical issues of the information age. *MIS Quarterly, 10*(1), 5–12.

Milholland, D.K. (1994). Privacy and confidentiality of patient information: Challenges for nursing. *JONA, 24*(2), 19–24.

Miller, A.R. (1971). *The assault on privacy: Computers, data banks, and dossiers.* Ann Arbor, MI: The University of Michigan Press.

Peck, R.S. (1984). Extending the constitutional right to privacy in the new technological age. *Hofstra Law Review, 12,* 893–912.

Pheby, D.F.H. (1982). Changing practice on confidentiality: A cause for concern. *Journal of Medical Ethics, 8,* 12–24.

Rokeach, M. (1973). *The nature of human values.* New York: The Free Press.

Romano, C.A. (1987). Privacy, confidentiality, and security of computerized systems: The nursing responsibility. *Computers in Nursing, 5*(3), 99–104.

Schmaus, D. (1991). Computer security and data confidentiality. *AORN Journal, 54,* 885–890.

Schoeman, F.D. (1992). *Privacy and social freedom.* Cambridge, England: Cambridge University Press.

Simmel, A. (1971). Privacy is not an isolated freedom. In J.R. Pennock & J.W. Chapman (Eds.), *Privacy* (pp. 71–87). New York: Atherton Press.

Smith, H.J. (1994). *Managing privacy: Information technology and corporate America.* Chapel Hill, NC: The University of North Carolina Press.

Van Den Haag, E. (1971). On privacy. In J.R. Pennock & J.W. Chapman (Eds.), *Privacy* (pp. 149–168). New York: Atherton Press.

Veatch, R.M., & Fry, S.T. (1987). *Case studies in nursing ethics.* Philadelphia: J.B. Lippincott.

Westin, A.F. (1976). *Computers, health records and citizens rights* (NBS Monograph No. 157). Washington, DC: Government Printing Office.

Winslade, W.J. (1982). Confidentiality of medical records: An overview of concepts and legal policies. *The Journal of Legal Medicine, 3,* 497–533.

Unit 6
Choosing and Working with Systems

Unit Introduction

Unit Introduction

Within the networked environment, systems selection and installation remain critical processes. Despite the many changes in technology, the processes for choosing and implementing systems involve familiar activities, from needs assessment and planning, on through contract negotiation and education.

Sharrott outlines scenarios for distributed computing and characterizes them by degree of control. Selection involves both analysis and politics. In the distributed environment, integration and mainframe computing are still important; benefits accrue from improved departmental computing and functionality.

McAlindon outlines activities involved in choosing and installing an information system. After the vision is defined, other vital processes follow, including needs assessments, vendor system previews, education, testing, conversion, and evaluation.

Hammon urges healthcare organizations to work with information technology vendors. Plans for an integrated healthcare information environment should address technology-related decisions. Contracts should specify performance criteria and procedures for handling problems.

17
Centralized and Distributed Information Systems: Two Architecture Approaches for the 1990s

LAWRENCE H. SHARROTT

Centralized vs. Distributed Computing

Today there are two major ways of providing data processing services within most businesses, including hospitals. The first approach is centralized computing and involves the acquisition of a large computer typically known as a mainframe. To this computer are attached a number of dumb terminals that do not have any processing power of their own. All of the computing is done on the large machine. The results of the processing are presented either on the terminal or in reports. All of the data necessary for the work being performed are housed on one of the many disk drives that are attached to the mainframe.

The other approach is known as the distributed processing approach or client server approach. This technique uses a high-speed network to connect a number of computers, including machines usually referred to as personal computers or somewhat larger machines typically designated as minicomputers. Each of these machines is intelligent, that is, each has the ability to run programs and manipulate data.

The computers that a person will use to perform work are called workstations or clients. Data may be stored on the user's workstation or on a file server, that is, a computer with large amounts of disk storage that serves as a repository (or server) for significant amounts of data.

In centralized computing, all programs and all data are on one machine and all processing shares the same centralized resources. In the distributed approach, data and programs may be located on any of the machines that are connected to the network. In fact, the programs on one workstation may act upon data that are located on another workstation. Each of these approaches has its advantages and disadvantages. Each fills a need in the provision of data processing services.

Advantages of Distributed Computing

There are many reasons for selecting a distributed system to deliver data processing services. The two leading reasons are politics and cost. There are a number of other reasons that also enter into the decision-making process, including the best possible reason, functionality of the system.

In many medical centers, there are strong political entities that wield considerable influence and have significant needs for data processing resources. There are powerful reasons for acquiring and managing a data processing center within a department. Control of the budget dollars for data processing improves departmental stature. Departments may argue that locating data processing within their units will free floor space elsewhere in the institution. Most important, controlling the data processing function means controlling the information necessary for a strong negotiating position relative to the rest of the institution. Cost is also a strong motivator for acquiring departmental and distributed processing systems. Several scenarios are possible within a distributed environment, delivering different cost/benefit ratios to the institution.

Three Scenarios for Distributed Computing

Scenario 1: The Controlled Environment

In this scenario, which actually reduces costs, the processing environment is tightly managed and controlled. Departments may select the needed processing software and hardware that fit the functional needs of their departments, but the variety of vendors will probably be restricted.

The management information services (MIS) department may have established a standard hardware platform within which systems may be selected. Although interfacing technology has dramatically improved, it is still much easier and less costly to connect multiple machines from the same vendor than to connect a number of disparate machines. In this controlled environment, the networking probably comes from the same vendor as the computing hardware, and departmental processors tend to be on the small side.

This scenario yields most of the benefits of a fully distributed environment. Departmental users may select, within bounds, the computing system that they want for their department. They manage and control their own destiny and have the status, power, and control that they are seeking. In the near future, standards now evolving in the industry, such as HL/7, will facilitate interconnects that result in a truly seamless interconnect capability. This will permit any machine on the network to easily access data stored on another computer.

Scenario 2: The Uncontrolled Environment

The second scenario for distributed processing does not yield the same level of benefits and may incur a higher level of costs, though costs remain difficult to measure. In this scenario, there is basically no management of the selection and procurement process. No architecture, guidelines, or recommended approaches are outlined for system selection. Departments may choose whatever system they please without regard for factors other than their own requirements. The result can be a costly miasma of many types of computers from a wide variety of vendors.

Such an environment has a critical need for a widely available and standard networking scheme and a standard communication protocol for the interconnection of machines. However, the network hardware is likely to come from a third party and require the use of network software from an additional vendor. With computers from a wide variety of vendors, and hence few vendor discounts for multiple machines at one site, maintenance costs are high.

Support personnel becomes an issue, because a small staff cannot hope to be skilled on a large number of machines from varying vendors. Interfacing the machines and their applications can become more difficult, especially when the machines use different communications techniques. Moreover, if these machines are all located in their respective departments and in dedicated and environmentally controlled space, the institution incurs additional physical plant costs. Many of these costs are hidden and indirect, but they are real costs that drive to the bottom line of the health-care institution.

Scenario 3: The Partially Controlled Environment

The most realistic scenario is somewhere in between the two described above. Departments are permitted to select the systems they want, but have some constraints in the selection process. The number of vendors is restricted but not absolutely controlled. With equipment from no more than two to three vendors, support can be handled by a small staff.

Minicomputers typically do not require an extensive support staff, and many of the commercially available turnkey systems can be handled by a well-trained and interested end user. Operations may still require trained operators, but many of the system setup and technical operations are provided by the vendor under their maintenance contract. However, the issues of providing a proper environment, appropriate backup, maintenance, and service level all still exist in this environment.

As is true of the uncontrolled environment, costs may be hidden in the areas of staffing and of maintaining and operating the equipment. Because the costs of operations and systems administration are pushed into the user departments, the approach may be considered a form of financial accounting chargeback. It also causes departments to have some of their staff increase the breadth of their jobs, as they may be responsible for their normal tasks as well as the care and feeding of the computing system. This may be desirable and improve certain jobs within the institution. It potentially provides a new technically based career path for the department member who wishes to extend the practical use of computers within that particular department.

Selecting an Approach

Comparing the cost effectiveness of a distributed environment versus a centralized environment can be difficult. For an accurate comparison, all of the costs must be captured for both options. Costs will be highly dependent on the variety of computers, the number allowed, and the support requirements for each. The level of indirect costs will increase the difficulty of an accurate comparison between the two competing approaches.

In a distributed environment, costs are incurred across a number of departments and are associated with each computer. Large networks with multiple minicomputers and many workstations can be expensive. Although costs may approach those for a mainframe system, the distributed environment may allow for increased functionality. Costs for a centralized mainframe environment, with simple terminals connected to the mainframe, are easier to track or project. Once all of the costs are captured, the comparison is straightforward and proceeds strictly from a cost point of view.

Size is an important factor in selecting an approach. With increasing demands on computing resources, the requirements for processing power and storage are growing dramatically. It is becoming increasingly difficult for even large mainframe computers to handle all of the terminals and data storage required by an entire business enterprise. When this occurs, networks of mainframe computers may be called for. This is not a typical case in hospitals today, but it certainly could be so in the not too distant future. As reporting on the cost and care of patients increases and as the amount of data collected on each patient due to clinical systems increases, the computing resources required will demand increased numbers of mainframes or networked technology. Increasing need for power is also driven by the introduction of the windows graphical environment. This computing approach has improved both the processing and presentation of information.

The difficult issues to face are the perceptions of power, control, and seamless service. In large healthcare institutions, an individual ancillary department such as radiology or laboratory can be a very large operation. The heads of these departments generate significant revenues for the institution and will want to provide their services on a high-quality, low-cost basis. To satisfy these needs, these departments will demand that the computing solution for them fulfill their functional and business needs. Given the systems available, even the most centralized organization in a large institution will probably be faced with distributed processing in these two departments. The requirements in these areas are so unique and the interfaces so specific that the possibility of obtaining a high-quality solution from one vendor for the hospital as a whole, including these departments, is not very likely.

Thus, the location and control of the computing resource for these departments will become major issues, to be resolved mainly through the political process. The level of influence wielded by the head of the department will have as dramatic an impact on these issues as the leadership power and influence of the institution's highest management. Cost will be of some concern, but will not become the burning issue over which these questions will be resolved. The managerial and political culture of an institution will likely determine the approach to be taken.

Distributed Processing

Developments

Distributed processing has been a part of the data processing field for some time. The means for accomplishing it have changed during the past five years. Prior to the advent of the personal computer, most distributed computing environments consisted of several computers linked by wire or telephone lines. These connections were rather slow in speed. The logical connections were point to point, with one machine generally connected to only one other machine. Many of the configurations were in either a star topology, as shown in Figure 17-1 or a hierarchical topology as shown in Figure 17-2.

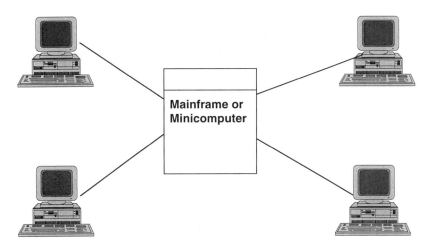

FIGURE 17-1. Star network.

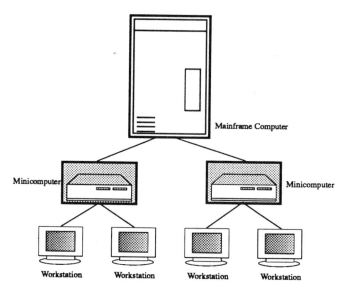

FIGURE 17-2. Hierarchical distributed system.

Personal computers have gradually rendered the traditional networks inadequate. At first, the users of personal computers were content to be isolated. They then demanded that they be connected to the corporate mainframe computers, so that they could obtain data without rekeying. This connection also allowed them to place data back on the mainframe after they manipulated those data with innovative tools on their personal computers. The next phase was to share data and high-quality printers or other resources with other personal computer users. Doing this through the mainframe was awkward and, depending on the type of connection, quite slow. When peer to peer communication and full data sharing became the next demand, the need for high-speed local area networks (LANs) became evident. The commonly installed LANs today are either ethernet or Token Ring types.

By providing high-speed communication over a limited distance, LANs extend new services and techniques. LANs make it possible for groups of personal computers to share data files or expensive components, such as laser printers. Software that is located on one computer can be retrieved and run on another machine located on the same network. When the LAN is connected to a minicomputer or a mainframe, the personal computer becomes a stand-alone processor, a terminal to the main machine, or a cooperative processor.

In the cooperative processor role, a program can be moved from the main computer and run on the personal computer. The data may still reside on the main machine but be brought to the desktop only as needed. The result is a very versatile environment that allows unique integration of data, processing power, high-quality display of information, and a graphical user interface. As the costs of personal computers and networking have dropped, the demand for Lotus-type spreadsheets and Macintosh style presentation graphics has increased dramatically.

The implementation of these new technologies will still be driven by corporate culture, leadership styles, and politics, but the direction based upon end user demand is clear. Distributed processing will continue to increase in all industries. In health care, as departmental needs become more complex and software solutions come closer to fulfilling those needs, the number of distributed systems is likely to grow. Continued pressure for more cost effective management and still greater computing power on the desktop will certainly feed the demand for distributed processing.

Issues

Distributed processing is not without its problems. Especially in large distributed environments, it is difficult to guarantee service levels, maintain common versions of programs, and resolve problems. Because LANs contain many active electronic components, a methodical approach to the isolation of the problem is required. In many instances, two technicians must work in concert to determine the source of the problem, which can range from a failing personal computer or network card to a segment of damaged cable.

In a centralized mainframe environment, processor failure is very clear. When the computer fails, everything is down. In the distributed environment, this is not the case. The failure of one CPU on the network may have very little to do with other processors on the network. This failure may be reported by end users in unclear and subtle ways. In all cases, however, end users will clearly state the one position that they understand: the network is down.

Integrated network management tools are sorely needed to manage heterogeneous networks that are developing in healthcare institutions. Many of the computer industry's leading firms now sell such tools. When widely supported by network and computer vendors, they will greatly enhance the ability to manage network, guarantee availability, and resolve problems.

One of the major advantages of a centralized system is the extent to which it makes possible the integration of information. When a system is designed, the analysts who are the architects of the system can define the data elements to be stored within the system. Through the use of advanced relational database techniques, these analysts can easily define relationships among data elements, such as length of stay and attending physician. These architects have many tools at their disposal, such as data modeling and prototyping, and can design the whole structure. As long as they design carefully, the ability to define relationships will not be narrowly restricted.

With a distributed system, developing and providing the ability to manipulate the data required for these relationships can be a difficult task. Distributed processing in healthcare institutions is in its infancy. Vendors are building the tools and techniques that allow for easy integration of data. Although integration will remain difficult to achieve until standards for data sharing are more firmly embedded in software applications, it is becoming easier with each new release of software products from vendors such as Microsoft. With careful analysis and an understanding of the available data, relational databases can be built on a distributed network system that allows the necessary manipulations. This approach is becoming more widely available daily. Some of the financial systems in use today can provide some of these capabilities in a networked environment. A good data storage and reporting facility can be built using windows tools and the historical databases fed by the patient accounting systems and used to provide length of stay and financial forecasting data.

Like any other complex business, healthcare institutions require the use of computing technologies to help manage their business. The general financial trends in health care call for the provision of services through fewer resources. If properly planned and implemented, computing can help to provide the services needed at lower cost. Whether the environment is centralized or distributed, the institution absolutely must prioritize its needs as part of its strategic and tactical plans.

Because of its large financial profile, mainframe computing typically has a higher visibility to the management of an institution. Replacing a mainframe may involve spending several million dollars. This level of expenditure will require the development of plans, much discussion, and approval from multiple levels of management, including the board of trustees.

In a distributed environment, the growth of the computing resource can take place with a much lower profile. The addition of a new system may involve adding a small number of personal computers or perhaps a small minicomputer. Because these expenditures may be made with the approval of only the department manager or the controller, there is greater danger of growing a system that does not meet the needs of the institution. A process must be created for developing, rank ordering, and managing to priorities. The temptation to placate a squeaky wheel department with a partial, low-cost solution is very real and can lead to chaos.

Mainframe Use

Distributed processing will not mean the death of large mainframe computers. Complex environments will continue to require large-scale, high-speed processing. High-volume billing is a problem for no less than a mainframe, and the same may hold true for the storage and manipulation of very large databases. If used to provide the administrative functions of admitting, discharge, and transfer, a mainframe can become a part of a distributed environment where the laboratory and radiology have their own machines. On such a network, the mainframe can broadcast the necessary patient demographic and location information to other machines, which in turn can transmit data back to the mainframe for the purpose of billing.

With the installation of a transaction-oriented database, the mainframe can also be used as a database management machine providing rapid access by graphical workstations to the data. As important patient-oriented events are captured, they can be transferred to the mainframe database for storage and later manipulation. This technique requires common definition and timely capture of the data elements, but potentially could become the foundation for automated clinical and financial patient records. If interactively available through a network, it could also be used in providing actual treatment to patients. (Despite its potential, such an approach will most like encounter resistance among traditional mainframe computing staff. Distributed databases, remote cooperative computers, and distributed control are not within their technological cultural background.)

In many cases, the model of choice will have the mainframe connected to departmental machines through a LAN, such as IBM's Token Ring. Departments that have traditionally used computers, such as billing, collections, and admitting, will be directly connected to the mainframe computer through ordinary terminals. Other departments such as nursing and clinical ancillary departments will connect their departmental computers to the mainframe through the LAN. Their own processing will be done on the departmental machine that provides the solutions to their particular needs. Data that must be used for institutional reporting will be housed on the mainframe, whereas data needed for the management of individual departments will be housed on departmental processors. Thus, the needs of the institution will be met by concentrating the appropriate data on the mainframe, and the needs of the individual department will be met through a dedicated departmental computing system.

Benefits

In a distributed environment, benefits will accrue from the improved computing available to departments throughout the healthcare institution. Specialized systems supported by niche vendors will offer individual departments higher functionality than systems provided by a large generic vendor attempting to meet heterogeneous needs. Although hardware acquisitions and software development remain expensive, buying or licensing systems may provide some cost relief from developing systems in-house. The only caveat is that purchased systems must in fact provide the services that are needed.

Computing will meet less resistance in the workplace as departments are included in the selection process and given a real choice in the system they are to use. As users participate in the installation process, they become invested in the success of the project. The probability of success will increase.

Increased functionality should have positive effects on the provision of treatment to patients. Using a single workstation in their office or at the point of care, clinicians will be able to retrieve all clinical data on their patients. With technological advances, it will soon be possible for clinicians to call the hospital on their car phones, and have a computer read to them the current lab results.

The Future

Distributed processing has come about for a number of reasons. Personal computers and the innovative software that runs on them have had a dramatic effect. The lowering of computing costs has made computing technologies more widely available. Computers are now so much a part of our society that we see them in many homes and think it unusual if businesses operate without them.

The result has been a reduced fear of computers and a more defined expectation of what computing should be like. It is not unusual for professionals to expect that their computing work have a video game look and feel to it. Ease of use and broad availability of information are the future of computing. The WIMPs (windows, icons, mouse, pointing) approach has already become common. This will continue the trend toward more intelligent and powerful workstations for people to use.

As image and voice technology improve, the need for higher-speed connections between the data (servers) and the users (workstations) will become more important. The implementation of standard protocols for communicating will increase. Transmission Control Protocol/Internetworking Protocol (TCP/IP), Open Systems Interconnection (OSI), Ethernet, Token Ring, Health Level 7 (HL/7), and American Standards for Testing Materials (ASTM) will all become common terms in the implementation of computing systems. Each of these will play an important part in allowing diverse computing systems to talk freely with each other.

Because a well-designed and implemented distributed system can make available to all users all of the data within the institution, control of the data and security become important issues. However, the factors that have the greatest effect on the implementation of these new technologies are now and will continue to be funding, change management, and institutional politics. Only if these issues and factors are addressed can health care realize in full the promise of the new technologies.

Questions

1. Can a network designed to support a distributed LAN architecture support the communications requirements of a mainframe environment?
2. What criteria should be applied to determine the cost effectiveness of a distributed LAN environment?
3. Currently the pharmacy is running on a mainframe-based application that has been in operation for some time. They are proposing to replace this application with one based on networked personal computers. What should your strategy be for implementing this new pharmacy system?

18
Choosing and Installing an Information System

Mary N. McAlindon

Choosing and installing an information system for patient care is an exciting and important process for healthcare agencies, especially when considering the two major changes affecting health care today: government regulation and industry-sponsored initiatives leading to managed care. In response to these changes, major system vendors are developing solutions to meet the needs of communities rather than single acute care hospitals by developing bargaining organizations designed to provide employers with the best healthcare coverage at the lowest cost. According to Johnson (1994), these organizations will force mergers to eliminate duplicated services, help providers become more efficient, and encourage hospital-owned clinics with physicians as employees. These "opportunities" have increased interest in the fully automated patient record, which in turn depends on an information system to gather the needed information at the point of care. The purpose of these information systems is to gather data and provide information for healthcare professionals in clinical practice, management, education, and research. They also provide information to satisfy reporting requirements of the government, health insurers, and the accrediting and licensing agencies.

There are three major phases to be completed in choosing and installing an information system: (a) defining the vision, (b) selecting the system, and (c) installing the system.

Defining the Vision

There are three major concepts to be considered in choosing an information system for the current and future needs of the institution: the aspects of information that form the basis for communication, networking, and a central data repository. These help to define the vision that guides the selection of a system that reflects the philosophy of the institution and its employees.

Aspects of Information

Information is a combination of three aspects of technology: data, information, and knowledge. Data are discrete entities that describe or measure something without interpreting it. Numbers are data, names are data; without further description or interpretation, they are meaningless. Information consists of interpreted, organized, or structured data, whereas knowledge refers to information that is combined or synthesized so that interrelationships are identified (Blum, 1986; Graves & Amos, 1990). For instance, we gather data when taking a blood pressure and we compare it to a previous blood pressure to provide additional information. We further combine the blood pressures of hypertensive patients taking medication to provide additional knowledge for the care of patients with this diagnosis. Data, information, and knowledge constitute the content of professional communication. Nurses deliver and manage patient care through continuous communication with families, other professionals, and staff. It is extremely important to challenge the types of data we gather, the way that we gather them, and the ways that we use them when selecting, installing, and using information systems, so that we can improve the way that we do things, and not replicate our inefficiencies.

Networking

The second important concept is that of networking. Networking is an information exchanging process between computers and individuals. Local area networks (LANs) tie users and computer systems together for sharing of information within an institution. Wide area networks (WANs) tie users outside the institution and their computer systems together, they go *beyond the walls*. Computers are networked to get information to the right person, in the right place, at the right time. In an age where communication has become almost instantaneous, computers have become an essential information tool because the ultimate vision is to tie communities into a national network of healthcare information.

People are networked for communication and the exchange of information. When choosing and installing information systems, networking must occur within and between departments, and often within and among institutions if they are part of a corporate enterprise. Networking also occurs vertically and horizontally, with those above and below on the organizational chart, and with peers across departments. A focus on patient or client care and not on departmental concerns can break down the walls between departments for true networking.

The Central Data Repository

Networking to provide information and knowledge is vital to the third concept, the central data repository (CDR). The centralized repository contains data from all client encounters gathered into one central location. This concept assures access to patient care information, and is necessary for the eventual success of a community health network.

The CDR must be integrated at five levels. The first level involves the user who needs a single interface to access the full range of available information. At this level, doctors, nurses, laboratory technicians, and therapists need to be able to enter and retrieve patient care information at workstations close to the source of the data to be entered. Demographic data, financial, and payor information, and results from tests and procedures should be available at these workstations.

The second level of integration occurs within the institution. This level requires a sharing of data between different applications. If software applications have been purchased from different vendors for laboratory, radiology, pharmacy, medical records, or nursing, it may be difficult for them to communicate with a central repository or database to be used *across the boundaries* of the different systems. This is a very important consideration when choosing an information system vendor.

The third level of integration for a clinical data repository is the corporate or enterprise level. At this level information communication occurs *outside the walls* and extends to all units of a multientity organization. The information from this level of integration provides productivity and cost analysis for all entities in the enterprise in addition to providing access to patient care information. For instance, a patient discharged from the hospital to an extended care facility for rehabilitation may then return home for care from a visiting nurse and then to outpatient physical therapy. All of this healthcare information would be recorded in the central data repository to provide access to the information for all healthcare providers. Seamless, convenient, and necessary for quality and continuity of care!

At the fourth level of integration, the communication of information occurs between payors, providers, and employers. Health information networks of the future will combine the information collected from regions and states and provide information for the fifth and final level of integration, the national level, where all healthcare information is shared across regions and states. In order to accomplish this integration the sources of patient care information must be automated, with all data gathered at the source and entered into the computer. Then, with integration of the sources of patient information into a seamless record, all information from all sources resides in a single repository. An understanding of these concepts is necessary for the definition of a vision that reflects the philosophy and strategic plan of the enterprise or institution, and this must occur before system selection can begin.

Selecting the System

In selecting an information system it is necessary to form a committee to (a) devise a strategic plan that reflects that of the institution, (b) conduct a preliminary survey, (c) preview vendor systems, and (d) develop a request for proposal for selecting a system. The process of selecting an information system begins with the formation of a multidisciplinary committee. Members should include representatives from the major patient care services such as nursing, laboratory, pharmacy, radiology, respiratory care, medical records, and physical therapy who know the inner workings of their departments. It is also important to have physician and financial representation on the committee. Committee chairpersons may be elected, or rotated among members of the group.

Devising a Strategic Plan

The first task in devising a strategic plan is to determine the committee members' knowledge and personal philosophy of information systems. Asking each member to write his or her definition of an information system is the first step in this process. A second step is the literature search and readings that help committee members become aware of different kinds of systems, their uses, and the terminology used in describing information systems. Discussion of the readings is a very good tool for consensus building in a disparate group thinking only of their own departments. Completion of this step is the beginning of the visualization of an information system that correlates with the institution philosophy and strategic plan.

Conducting the Preliminary Survey

The second step in the process is the preliminary survey or needs assessment. This is done to determine the existing paper flow and communication patterns. Where does the information come from? Where does it go? How is it handled within the department? Communication patterns include voice mail, faxes, and pneumatic tube systems. The purpose of the needs assessment is to determine what processes should be redesigned; information systems present an opportunity for improving the process of providing health care; to replicate a costly, time-consuming paper system would be counterproductive.

Previewing Vendor Systems

The third step in the information system selection process consists of vendor presentations and site visits. Vendor products are chosen for presentation by reading "top-vendor" lists in the journals, attending the trade shows and

TABLE 18-1. Questions Asked During Vendor Presentations

- Name and location of the parent company
- Number and location of completed installations
- Modules available (laboratory, pharmacy, radiology etc.)
- Type of hardware
- Software language underlying the system
- Approximate cost for an institution our size
- Availability of communications networks
- Levels of security
- Numbers of personnel and resources needed for maintenance
- Stability and reputation of the parent company
- Resources committed to research and development

Source: Adapted from McAlindon, M., Danz, S., & Theodoroff, R. (1987).

TABLE 18-2. Criteria for Ranking Presentations

- Philosophy compatible with that of the institution
- Good reputation
- Financial stability
- Commitment to the healthcare industry
- Ability to develop missing modules or to interface to those that would have to be purchased separately

professional meetings where vendors exhibit, and calling peers in other hospitals in the area. Vendors chosen in this manner are asked to make presentations to the committee. Each vendor representative is asked a series of questions (Table 18-1) that the committee has devised so that there is consistency in rating the presentations.

Additional questions might be asked about the capability for making changes in the database, whether new data fields can be added to the system, and whether the system is easy to use. Ask about the types of hardware used and other special equipment that might be needed; some proprietary terminals are expensive to buy and maintain.

Following the vendor presentations, the committee ranks the vendor presentations by comparing what they had seen to the selection criteria illustrated in Table 18-2. The vendors closest to matching the selection criteria are asked to identify installed systems for site visits. Following the site visits, the information systems are again ranked according to the selection criteria, and the top four or five are chosen to receive requests for proposal.

Developing a Request for Proposal

The request for proposal (RFP) is often written with the help of a consultant. This document is developed by the purchaser to define the information system service and products desired. The vendor then provides a written response describing how the request will be met. Table 18-3 lists the broad

TABLE 18-3. Items to Be Defined in the Request for Proposal

- Need for a clinical data repository
- Capture of data at the source
- Interinstitutional focus
- Intrainstitutional focus
- Ability to be interactive

---

aspects of the system to be defined in the RFP. The RFPs are sent to four or five vendors so that there are several systems from which to choose. An RFP evaluation plan is necessary in order to make comparisons for final system recommendation The two or three top choices are invited to contract discussions. It is important to have more than one choice to leverage the discussion and encourage competition so that costs of the system can be negotiated. Having a second choice also provides a backup in case the first choice fails to sign a contract. Cost of the systems is not usually brought into the decision-making process until the contract phase.

Installing the System

System installation begins with a change in committee membership, and includes (a) development of an installation plan, (b) committee education, (c) database framework completion, (d) the system testing process, (e) staff education, (f) conversion, and (g) evaluation. The installation committee is formed of personnel from the various clinical departments. It is important to retain a few members of the selection committee because they have the *vision* with which the system was chosen and this needs to be carried forward. The members of this committee are often the project managers for their departmental systems.

Development of the Installation Plan

In developing the installation plan, the first decision to be made is the order in which the various components of the system will be installed. Depending on the modules purchased, a schedule for installation must be determined. For instance, if an order management system is part of the package, it makes sense to install the departments that receive orders before installing the departments that send orders. In this instance, the laboratory, pharmacy, radiology, and other areas that have information systems internal to these departments would probably be installed early in the process. The departments that send orders (nursing and others) are then installed so that orders can be sent and results returned by computer. Departments that do not have internal computer systems usually receive requests for service on printers in the department, and manually enter their results in the computer.

The plan is the same for all modules and departments: determine the process, prepare a timeline of tasks to be completed, and determine the order of task completion. This timeline is updated periodically, with an overdue task list published with names of the person responsible for completing the task. This imparts accountability, and allows for early recognition of miscalculated timetables or difficulties with the completion of tasks.

Committee Education

Education of the development team is very important and occurs early in the process. The vendor usually provides the education necessary for understanding the database components and the framework used in the development of the database. Departmental directors and staff are interviewed to determine the process of information flow in their departments. How information enters the department, how it is processed, resulted, completed, or charged, and where it finally resides are questions that must be answered. With this process mapped for each department, the installation team can begin to build the framework for placing and resulting each procedure that will be entered in the system, as well as any associated security, charging, and routing.

Database Framework Development

As soon as the departmental interviews have been completed, the installation team begins to build the database. Internal departmental system databases are built by individual installation teams headed by the departmental project managers. The order management module is usually built by the nursing installation team.

Each procedure or test that can be ordered from any department must be built in the system. The vendor provides a framework for entering synonyms, security codes, charge codes, and routing codes. These are necessary for the proper functioning of the system and are transparent to the user who does not realize that these exist. If procedures have been built in other modules such as laboratory or radiology, they must be imported to the order management system and adapted for use by nursing and other departments through the addition of synonyms and routings. There are thousands of procedures and tests ordered in healthcare institutions every day; each of these must be built in the system so that they can be ordered, resulted, routed, and charged.

Testing to ensure accuracy takes place at certain stages in the process beginning shortly after the database building is begun. As illustrated in Table 18-4, there are six types of testing that take place during the installation process.

TABLE 18-4. Six Types of Testing That Occur During Installation

- Database
- System
- Integration
- Parallel
- Charge
- Pilot

The System Testing Process

The database is tested when it is partially complete to be sure that the development work is being done correctly. During the database test, the procedures that have been built are tested to ensure that the synonyms, charge codes, routing, and security are correct. If this test is successful, the database is completed. Department directors are asked to verify the completeness of their portion of the database, signifying that all of the tests and procedures associated with the department are correct.

The second testing period is concerned with system functionality and occurs during database completion. It determines whether the information is sent correctly, in the proper form, to the correct printers, in the designated format. This test allows for correction of any issues found in the system software.

Integration testing occurs after the database framework is completed. This test assures that the database, system, hardware, and software are working together properly. Orders entered from every terminal to every printer in each department assure that security and routing are correct, and the hardware and system software seem to be operating correctly. Security can be set at several levels. This is verified during testing to assure that authorized users can perform certain functions and others cannot. Routing is also an important determination that must be tested to assure that information gets to the right person, in the right place, at the right time. The testing of every device and every procedure in the system is extremely important for eventual success of the project.

Tests are also done to determine whether or not the charging process for each procedure is correct. The parallel test uses actual patient names and care orders so that the computer system is tested in a live environment with the paper system being used as a backup for patient care. A pilot test occurs just before conversion. In this instance, one or two patient care areas begin entering orders without a manual backup as a final test of the system. Each of the testing periods is followed by correction of the problems found during the test.

Staff Education

As the testing cycle nears completion, staff education begins. Education involves the development of teaching manuals and scripts for instructors, and user manuals and help sheets for system users. Manuals that provide a learn-it-yourself format contain screen prints of information that reinforce the learning process. These provide support for the staff in conjunction with the help sheets that are abbreviated versions of the manual.

Support of the staff is essential for a successful conversion. There should be expert users available in each department and patient care area during the times that the department is open. Staff should take their questions to the shift support person, who then refers them if necessary. Information systems and vendor support are usually the highest levels of user support. For several weeks after conversion to new systems, 24-hour support is often necessary.

Development of Policies and Procedures

Many processes will change with automation of the communication and information flow and users must know what is expected of them before they are asked to use the system. Policies and procedures must be developed to describe the changes in processes occurring with the new system. These occur within and among departments and institutions depending on the scope of the system. Meetings over a period of several months are needed as various departments determine how they will enter procedures and tests, and result and charge them. Policy and procedure manuals are maintained in a central location and are distributed to all areas using the system.

Conversion

When the testing is successfully completed, education finished, and the policy and procedure manuals distributed, it is time to *convert* the system. There are two schools of thought about conversion. Many vendors advocate the simultaneous or *big-bang* theory of conversion in which all areas are converted at once. This has the advantages of concentrated support from the vendor for a shorter period of time with the disruption and change affecting everyone at once.

The phased theory of conversion advocates the conversion of a few patient care areas at once. This is less traumatic for the institution, and allows for concentrated support of the areas converting to the new system. Vendor support is lessened after the first phase, the institution support staff is more likely to become tired of the process, and new findings must be taught to those who are already converted, but there is less disruption to patient care.

System Evaluation

Evaluation of the system, the users, and the education process is important for cost–benefits analysis. There must be documented advantages to support the expenditure of monies for information systems. Time and motion and paper-flow studies done before system installation and repeated 6 to 12 months after conversion are excellent ways to determine the effectiveness of the system. Customer and staff satisfaction may also be useful evaluation measures.

Conclusion

Choosing and installing an information system is an interesting and frustrating process that will inevitably be a source of satisfaction for all involved in the project. It is important to remember to

- Define the vision,
- Choose wisely,
- Build carefully,
- Test thoroughly,
- Educate fully,
- Support kindly,
- Evaluate continuously,

and you will be successful!

References

Blum, B. (1986). *Clinical information systems.* New York: Springer-Verlag.

Graves, J., & Amos, L. (1990) Knowledge technology: Costs, benefits, ethical considerations. In: J. McCloskey & H. Grace (Eds.), *Current issues in nursing* (pp. 592–600). Baltimore: Mosby.

McAlindon, M., Danz, S., & Theodoroff, R. (1987). Choosing the hospital information system: A nursing perspective. *Journal of Nursing Administration, 7*(10), 11–15.

Johnson, R. (1994). Forces shaping the HIS industry. *Healthcare Informatics, 2,* 15.

19
Understanding the Purchasing and Installation Process

GARY L. HAMMON

In the current technological environment, a healthcare organization can and should work with vendors of information technology. Planning is key to producing a climate conducive to the successful integration of products. The management of the information resources department must be aware of the pitfalls to be avoided or overcome. Also, the steps involving the review of product offerings, the selection process, procurement procedures, site visits, demonstrations, contract negotiations, and final award must be handled in a professional manner. Faced with a plethora of vendors and products, the information systems manager has to choose wisely in order to meet the needs of the organization and to achieve the integrated information solution at the least cost and with the greatest benefit.

The selection, acquisition, and purchase of the product or products may be the easiest part of the task. Contract negotiations can be difficult, but the healthcare organization must be firm and reasonable. Once the hardware and/or software is delivered, the real challenge begins. Will the new technology work in a stand-alone mode? Will the new technology work with existing technology (hardware/software integration)? Will the new technology, in conjunction with the existing technology, meet the needs as expected (data and information integration)? Will the vendor perform (both delivery and installation) as specified in the purchasing documents? There are no ironclad guarantees.

The integration of new software with existing mainframe software poses fewer hardware issues than the installation of a complete stand-alone hardware/software system utilizing a network for communications with existing system(s). However, the same concerns over in-house personnel capabilities, vendor personnel, contractual terms, and relationship with the vendor(s) apply and need to be addressed.

The information resources department must work with the vendors, both current and new, to ensure success. They must forge a partnership arrangement with the vendors for the good of the healthcare institution.

Preliminary Considerations

In a few cases, a healthcare organization has a staff that is large enough and possesses the requisite training and experience to meet the management and technical requirements for a successful (on time and within budget) selection and integration of technologies. Some information resources managers underestimate the size and complexity of the task. An institution is ill advised to rely on a vendor to safeguard the institution's interest, and unrealistic to have this expectation.

Most healthcare organizations do not have staff with the requisite training and experience for a successful selection, management of the process, and integration of technologies. What do they do to protect the organization's investment and deliver the service to the end user?

The preliminary work sets the stage for a successful or unsuccessful installation. If the details of the various activities are not monitored and verified, the probability of difficulties in the future increases.

Planning Considerations

Once the healthcare organization makes the decision and commitment to move toward an integrated healthcare information system environment, a plan must be developed to chart the necessary steps and budget implications of each step to meet the goal. Evaluation points should be identified within the plan to ensure a timely and on budget completion of the project. The healthcare institution should share this information with potential vendors so they understand the organization's expectations. This step will not remove all the substandard vendors, but can be used in the event of nonperformance or other difficulties.

As part of the planning process, the senior management of the healthcare organization must determine whether the existing data processing (information resources) department has the quantity and quality of staff to meet the technological and managerial requirements of the undertaking. This is an important step, and an unduly optimistic or unwarranted positive evaluation can be harmful to the success of the project and the bottom line of the institution.

For the implementation of an integrated system to succeed, important technical decisions must be made prior to selection and acquisition of hardware and software. If the expertise is not available in-house, the institution should employ an experienced integration consultant to assist with this phase of the effort. This will save time and money for the institution.

Some of the technology-related data gathering and performance decisions to be made early in the process are the following:

- What are the requirements of the currently installed systems regarding an interface (one way and two way) to another system?
  Electrical signal?
  Bit stream?
  Use of start and stop bits?
  Packet switching available?
  Handling of and requirements for received information?
  Procedure(s) and requirements for transmitting information?
- How should the existing and planned systems be physically connected?
  Direct connect?
  Protocol converters?
  Peer to peer?
  Local area network?
  Telephone switch?
  A combination of the above?
- What is the targeted response time for attached terminals or PCs?
- What is considered a reasonable amount of overhead per interface within the network? How much overhead can the network and the user tolerate?
- What is the desirable approach or methodology to balancing throughput within the network without unfairly loading one or more of the component machines?

There are other considerations, but the detail in these areas alone documents the need to have or engage personnel with the expertise to address technology choices and to protect purchasing organizations and their users. Responses to technical questions are invaluable, assisting in the evaluation of vendor offerings during the purchasing process and later in the assessment of vendor performance.

If the in-house staff does not have the expertise to install the new system and make it operational, a budget should be allocated to employ a third party to handle this responsibility. In the long run, this will be considered an investment and not an expense. Both the timely installation of the new system and the integration of existing systems will benefit the institution and the end users.

Contractual Considerations

It has been said that a contract is like a good fence—it makes better neighbors. A contract cannot guarantee that the vendor will perform as expected, but it can define the institution's expectations, requirements, time schedules, and monetary considerations. A responsible vendor will want a contract that spells out this information in order to prevent misunderstandings. A lawsuit will not ensure the system will be installed on schedule and within budget and should be the last resort, after all other efforts have failed. Delay dollar penalties, on the other hand, can offset some of the monetary losses of the organization and place pressure on the vendor to perform.

Purchase documents should be explicitly cited in the contract and should contain the specifications and performance data used in the selection process. The institution should state

- Expected date of delivery and installation,
- Expected date of system turnover to the information resources department for acceptance testing, and
- Expected system operational (go live) date, following acceptance testing and correction of errors and bugs.

For each of these three items, the healthcare institution should require the assessment of dollar penalties in the event the vendor cannot meet or exceed these requirements. Because the vendor will probably require the institution to accept the same penalty in the event the delay is the fault of the purchaser, the institution should carefully evaluate possible exposure. Other contract sections should stipulate

- Performance criteria as outlined in the purchasing documents attached to and cited in the contract.
- Procedures for the vendor to clear up performance discrepancies, correct malfunctions, and address other shortcomings, including an escalation procedure (names and telephone numbers for several levels of management above the local office) in the event local staff is not responsive.
- Procedures to handle fingerpointing when problems arise, assigning responsibility to the major contractor or vendor for conflict resolution and involving the institution as an interested party, but not in the middle of the problem.
- A provision to ensure that the integration scheme follows a current standard and not a one-of-a-kind vendor-oriented standard, protecting future upgrades.

A checklist for contract negotiations is reproduced in Table 19-1.

Another Consideration

The local representative and the immediate manager of the vendor with the preferred system should have made a favorable impression prior to the start of the final selection process. In the event that the vendor personnel are not professional, responsive, and likeable, the institution should reconsider the vendor's product. As far as the institution is concerned, the local personnel are the vendor. If the information resources manager and/or the departmental personnel do not respect and/or like the vendor's personnel, the chances of success are diminished. When misunderstandings and difficulties occur, as they will, relationships will not have the foundation of trust

TABLE 19-1. A Checklist for Users

According to Touche Ross & Co. analyst Lee Gruenfeld, once you've done a comprehensive requirements analysis for a systems integration project, and you're ready to sign an agreement that parcels out the responsibilities, liabilities and risks, make sure you:

- Include as many important system performance specifications as possible in the contract. The integrator may not like it, but usually he'll agree to it.
- Insist on seeing the contracts between the primary integrator and any secondary equipment suppliers he may be using. Prices should be specified. And make sure the primary integrator has access to source code and a license that allows him to modify and upgrade software as required. Consider signing a separate agreement with each vendor on the job.
- Review the contract's liability limitations. Who's going to pay if something goes wrong or if the project turns out to require more, or more expensive, hardware?
- Consider ways to expedite dispute resolution. Approaches such as out-of-court arbitration can reduce legal expenses and allow work to continue while disputes are settled.
- Plan for what will happen if your integrator is gobbled up in a merger or acquisition or if he goes out of business. Who becomes responsible for finishing the job? Can you get the source code?
- Make sure the integrator and his employees are specifically prohibited from disclosing any confidential, competitive information they may pick up on the job.
- Prohibit the integrator from raiding your shop for IS talent. Experienced analysts are the lifeblood of consultants and integrators. And they usually get them from you-know-who.

Source: Excerpted with permission from *DATAMATION,* May 15, 1989, Cahners Publishing Company.

to allow a reasonable, timely solution. The healthcare organization cannot and will not benefit from an adversary relationship. A carefully drawn purchasing document and contract are important, but the gray areas and misunderstandings can be handled in a professional manner for rapid closure. People and not companies make things happen!

If the desired system is the only system that meets the expressed needs of the institution, there is an alternative. Depending upon vendor organization and the level of personnel who are cause for concern, the healthcare institution can empower an executive level officer and the information resources manager to meet with the vendor's local or regional manager. The next step depends upon the results of the meeting. If the vendor agrees to replace the personnel in question, the institution should take some time to become acquainted with the replacement. Only then should the institution decide on the selection issue. However, if the vendor will not make a replacement, the institution should reconsider the vendor's system and look at other alternatives.

After the above process, if the institution decides to acquire the vendor's system in spite of the personnel assigned to the account, then the purchasing document and contract become even more important. The institution must meticulously delineate each and every specification, because the working relationship with the vendor personnel will most likely not be of a nature that allows the institution to recover from items omitted in error.

Ongoing Considerations

During installation, acceptance testing, error correction, and time periods for going live, the manager of information resources should meet with the senior on-site vendor representative at least daily. This should be a formal session, formally recorded by a designated notetaker. Proceedings should be published for all participants and used to check the status of project activities to review open items from previous meetings, and to discuss new items and other project-related questions or concerns. Two-way communication is vital; effectively handled, it can establish rapport and prevent misunderstandings or the build up of hostile feelings. The daily sessions should focus on both information exchange and problem solving.

After the operational system has been accepted, the manager of information resources should meet with the vendor's local manager and/or senior maintenance technician and software specialist on a monthly basis. It might be useful to invite the sales representative also. Again, this should be a formal session, formally recorded. The published record should be used in reviewing maintenance history for hardware and software over the previous 30 days and open item maintenance lists from previous meetings. The record should also assist in the discussion of new hardware and software upgrades and of any questions or concerns. Again, effective two-way communication with vendor personnel is vital for the healthcare organization.

If the open item list continues to grow without apparent resolution, the institution should contact the manager of the person with whom the ongoing meetings have been held and request a meeting to review the situation and resolve it. If resolution is not forthcoming in a reasonable time, the next step is to escalate the problems to the next level of management, and all the way to the president of the company if necessary. Such escalation is unfortunate, but probably will not have to occur a second time with the same local management staff. A word of caution, however: to preserve a working relationship with local vendor staff, the institution should not call the president until all the other levels of management have had a chance to act, or unless the situation is so desperate that immediate resolution is needed.

By building rapport with the assigned vendor personnel, the information resources manager can benefit from shared brainstorming and planning sessions. Of course, these sessions will reflect the vendor's bias, but can provide useful information for comparing products and developing alternative strategies. This is one more resource for the manager to use in meeting continuing planning responsibilities.

Conclusion

The manager of the information resources department begins to set the stage for dealing with vendor personnel at the initial contact with a sales representative. Then the review of products activity, selection process, contract negotiations, installation, and acceptance testing build upon this base. Good vendor relationships are not accidental. They are carefully constructed and are vital to a successful project and to ongoing installation.

Questions

1. If an institution can find the right system, the vendor will be happy to take responsibility for the successful installation. [ ] Yes [ ] No
2. The institution will not have to be involved with the implementation process once the contract is signed. [ ] Yes [ ] No
3. The information resources department will not have to be concerned with the preparation of a contract because the vendor usually has a standard contract. [ ] Yes [ ] No
4. If the information resources department does not like the vendor's contract, then the healthcare organization's legal staff or firm can handle the development of a suitable contract without assistance from Information Resources. [ ] Yes [ ] No
5. If the assigned vendor personnel are not cooperative and supportive, then just run them off and do all the work in-house. [ ] Yes [ ] No
6. In the event the in-house staff is not experienced with the proposed technology, it is better to make some mistakes while learning and save money by not hiring a consultant. [ ] Yes [ ] No
7. The selection and installation of a network is a good time to train the staff in the new technology. [ ] Yes [ ] No
8. The institution can turn over all the planning, selection, acquisition, and installation of a new system to the consultant and forget the problems. [ ] Yes [ ] No
9. The vendor of the selected new system will be concerned over the possible impact of interface overhead on the existing systems. [ ] Yes [ ] No

Suggested Periodicals for Further Reading

Serial publications are the best source today for continuing to learn more about the area of integration. There may be textbooks published in the future, as the methodology for integration is undergoing definition. Some current serials to read are:

Monthly Journals
Datamation
PC Resources
PC Computing

Weekly News Publications
Computerworld
InfoWorld
Network World

Unit 7
Changing the Professions

Unit Introduction

Unit Introduction

As information technology transforms health care delivery, it also changes the various healthcare professions. Nursing has fostered the discipline known as nursing informatics. Clinical pathology is increasingly dependent upon laboratory information systems, and diagnostic radiology has changed dramatically with imaging and radiology information systems, among others.

Mills describes computer applications that support operations and information flow in nursing and looks to future developments. Nursing information specialists will set priorities and develop standards for systems integration and networking, the patient record, quality management, managed care, and resource utilization.

Newbold provides an overview of research in nursing informatics. Over 40 studies have examined nursing attitudes towards computers; studies in other areas have been limited. The National Institute for Nursing Research has identified six major goals. Opportunities abound.

Genre discusses laboratory information systems (LIS) in the clinical pathology lab. Benefits of a new LIS include improved reporting and delivery, test result archive, and audit trail data. LIS can support change in such areas as utilization management/patient care, order entry, and outreach/affiliation/merger efforts.

For Shannon, radiology is an "information business" and the major function of diagnostic radiology is quality consultation. With developments like computed radiography (CR), systems are needed to handle the volume of images, including radiology information systems (RIS) and picture archiving and communications systems (PACS). Technology assessment and functional enhancements will offer more.

20
Computerization: Priorities for Nursing Administration

Mary Etta Mills

For nurse administrators, the availability, management, and representation of data for decision making are critical. As healthcare organizations invest major financial and human resources in computer support systems, the challenge for the nurse administrator is how best to

- Identify organization-wide and nursing-specific information and technology needs, and
- Organize, coordinate, and develop information system management.

Initiatives for cost reduction, service diversification, and managed competition create new demands for decision support. In the changing world of health care, information is driven by many sources of data. Healthcare organizations must comply with information standards used for accreditation, and healthcare legislation will inevitably establish information requirements which are dependent on computerization.

Information Requirements

Accreditation

The Joint Commission for Accreditation of Healthcare Organizations (1994) has implemented information standards directed at the coordination and integration of information. Broadly, the required ten information standards fall into five categories: planning, patient data, aggregate data, knowledge-based information, and comparative data.

Planning entails that the processes of information management meet the organization's needs, provide for data security, use uniform data definitions (such as minimum data sets), be managed by appropriately prepared individuals, provide efficient and effective data transmission, and enable broad data linkage across the organization. The expectation is that the information system will enable the collection, transformation, and communication of data addressing individual *patient data* specific to processes and outcomes of care. Furthermore, the information system must provide *aggregate data* to support managerial decision making and operations. In support of patient care and organizational processes, there must be availability of *knowledge-based information* such as reference information. Finally, *comparative data* on which to evaluate performance must be provided.

Information standards under development by the Joint Commission (Corum, 1994) will address healthcare networks, focusing on systems integration, continuity of care, and coordination of services. A "network" in this regard is considered to be composed of multiple healthcare delivery organizations. The direction is toward one-time data entry and immediate accessibility of data to all users. This approach is consistent with that of the Computer Based Patient Record Institute, which seeks a uniform single patient record.

Legislation

Draft legislation of the American Health Security Act (1993) provided a framework for health information. This framework included national standards for forms, health data sets, electronic networks, and data transmission. Integral to the system were expectations for consumer information, measurement of health status, health security cards, links among healthcare records, analysis of patterns of health care, health system evaluation, and data confidentiality and security. Regardless of the fate of this legislation, integrated information systems supportive of interactive decision making will be developed.

Applications for Key Management Functions

Organizational Structuring

Integrated databases and analytic models can open up new options for structuring and operating nursing departments. Nurse executives will be less insulated from operations because executive information systems will assist in acquiring information needed to monitor, coordinate, and control the activities of the nursing department. The result will be flattened organizations, with fewer middle managers to analyze and relay information.

Standard reports and functional reporting systems will be replaced by streamlined qualitative reports on key performance indicators. Available in real time, not solely at the end of standard reporting periods, these reports will allow for timely feedback to firstline supervisors, supporting decentralized decision making and encouraging the practicing nurse to invest in the goals of the organization.

R858.S773
2005

Strategic mans.

r today. Use this

O UTSA Professional Staff
O High School Student
O Other

any reasons for your level of
r Dissatisfaction
k of this form

ents?
YES
NO

For Library Use Only

BLNK	FND	INI	ACQ	CAT	CIRC	LIB	USER	SHLF	MISS

Operating the Organization

The primary responsibility of administrators is to ensure that the organization and its resources are managed with efficiency and effectiveness. Three fundamental systems support nursing department operations: workload management systems, workforce management systems, and financial management systems.

Workload Management Systems

Today, nursing administrators are compelled to determine the level of care needed in a given area at a given time by analyzing patient acuity levels and applying patient classification systems. The delivery of quality nursing care and the justification of costs incurred in providing it require the accurate quantification of workload.

Automated patient classification methodologies facilitate the collection, storage, manipulation, and retrieval of large volumes of workload data. Used in planning for the allocation of human resources, these patient specific data can also be used to

* Identify workload by diagnostic category or product line,
* Facilitate analysis of workload trends per hospital stay, and
* Support costing of nursing services per patient.

The information generated by automated patient classification systems can assist managers in the allocation of resources, both daily and long term, and in the preparation of budgetary requests.

Workforce Management Systems

Used in matching personnel to workload in the most cost-efficient manner, workforce management systems generally include components for nursing personnel management and staff scheduling.

Nursing personnel systems track all human resource planning information necessary to manage the nursing workforce, with a database architecture created specifically for that purpose. Personnel databases can include information regarding every position (availability, specifications) and each individual (employment history, performance tracking, wage and salary history, professional registration, credentialing, educational history). Comprehensive, up-to-date information facilitates effective management of nursing personnel, assists in their recruitment and retention of nurses, and documents their career paths. Nursing personnel systems can also assist in providing career counseling, monitoring licensure and continuing education attendance, meeting hospital accreditation requirements, and developing manpower contingency plans in the event of disaster.

The staff scheduling system uses the database provided by the personnel management system and functions in conjunction with the patient classification system to generate staff schedules based on specific patient care requirements. Because they are driven by the personnel management and patient classification systems, staffing systems can take into account patient need, staff expertise, staff scheduling preferences, and personnel policies. However, the complexity of such systems varies widely, with intelligent systems capable of adjusting staff schedules in an interactive manner on a shift-by-shift basis.

Scheduling systems assist the nurse manager in maintaining records, monitoring attendance, ensuring compliance with personnel policies, and scheduling time off for personnel. Information is readily available to document work patterns of all nursing personnel.

Financial Management Systems

Operating budgets for nursing departments account for approximately 40 percent of the typical hospital's operating budget. Computers are essential if managers are to effectively control the nursing department budget and accurately plan for new programs. The primary advantage provided by financial management systems lies in their ability to organize, manipulate, store, and retrieve data in preparing departmental budgets and analyzing budgetary variances.

Budget preparation for nursing departments is often a tedious, time-consuming, number-intensive process. By linking patient classification data and staffing requirements to a budget methodology, the preparation of an annual operating budget can be expedited. Necessary reallocations and adjustments for new programs are facilitated by the use of spreadsheets. "What if" scenarios can be tested to ensure that the budget provides a realistic plan for managers.

Financial management systems provide managers with up-to-date reports that focus their attention on major variances and potential problems. Nursing financial management systems allow a great deal of flexibility while linking reports to responsibility centers. Reporting can be tailored to organizational level and individual nursing units. These capabilities are critical in today's competitive environment; they make it possible for nursing to respond effectively to the demands for cost control.

By integrating patient classification data, personnel management data, and budgetary data, managers are able to analyze variances and explain budgetary deviations due to price, volume, or acuity variances. Nurse managers are able to target management interventions, designed to produce the desired performance results and to achieve organizational goals.

Information Access and Dissemination

Electronic bulletin boards, calendaring, filing, and mail provide a means by which nursing administration can communicate basic announcements, notices, and sets of information to a broad array of nursing managers and staff as well as to support departments. This means of rapid information transfer has provided an ability to manage basic systems communication rapidly, in the short term, and without expensive and lengthy paper generation and distribution.

Administrative computing further encompasses word processing, graphics, and database management. At this time, most businesses consider word processing basic to their office routine as a means to rapidly produce documents that can be modified without redundant work effort. Graphics capabilities allow the administrator to manipulate and display data. They are especially useful in determining and depicting trends relative to budget management, productivity, and resource flow. For example, critical data elements such as key expenditures, productivity figures from automated management systems, and personnel recruitment and turnover can be routinely input. Using this base, the administrator can visually depict both experiential and predictive trends for use in planning and management.

Local area network technology that links micro/mini/mainframe computers can further enhance both computing and communication technologies by integrating departmental healthcare computing systems to allow use of distributed data management techniques. This system can help meet informational needs by providing access to clinical research databases, patient management systems, and patient charges.

Telecommunications such as voice messaging services, interactive video conferencing, and external linkages to the health science library further expedite administrative functions. Time available to plan and creatively conceptualize is often a luxury making the availability of these types of technology an asset.

Integrated Systems

The collection, coordination, and communication of information to support complex patient care, organizational, and regulatory requirements are of growing importance. Integration provides a cost-effective approach to systemwide coverage and an effective way to access and manage information that supports complex decision making.

In an era of resource limitations, including both financial constriction and personnel shortages, efficiency and effectiveness have become increasingly important. Having data automatically distributed into multiple programs for analysis specific to given output generation and perhaps redistribution into still other programs becomes an essential conservator of valuable staff time. Elimination of duplicative information recording, collection, and analysis by nursing staff can reduce the almost 40 percent of nursing time currently spent on paperwork. This in itself will facilitate the use of professional staff in directly delivering or supervising patient care.

In a truly integrated system, all of the functions are designed from the outset to work together. Whether or not this is technically feasible is still a subject of debate by vendors. Although development continues in this area, interfacing that connects unrelated automated systems has had more success. As a result, some nursing management systems such as patient classification, staffing requirements, scheduling systems, and productivity analysis have been interfaced for automated sequential analysis. The interrelatedness of these programs provides the nurse administrator with information specific to correlated administrative issues. In addition to providing an immediate image of key operational issues, this type of program networking allows planning and forecasting with the use of data based simulations.

System Design Goals

Eight system design goals are important to the development or selection of computer systems that support integrated data management.

A Single Patient Database. First, there should be a single patient database. This single database should be exclusive of the geographic location in which the patient is seen clinically. With data in a single central repository, redundancy of documentation will be reduced; care and treatment plans will be cohesive across episodes of health care.

Integration of Clinical and Financial Data. Second, integration of clinical and financial data should be accomplished so episodes of care can be reflected in a single, integrated picture.

One-Time Entry of Information. Third, there should be one-time entry of information. For example, a patient's demographic data should be entered into the admitting/registration system.

Easy Retrieval of Data from the Database in a Form Defined by the User. Fourth, easy retrieval of data from the database in a form defined by the user should be possible.

Flexibility. Fifth, the system should be flexible. It should be easily modified to meet changing user needs and regulatory requirements and should allow users to easily tailor the input and output components of the system.

Easy Expansion. Sixth, the system should be easily and cost effectively expandable to accommodate increasing terminals, users, applications, and data, including those in diverse geographic locations.

Reliability. Seventh, the system should be reliable and operational 24 hours per day, seven days a week. Contingency backup should be available for all online patient care applications.

Security. Eighth, the system should provide for extremely tight data, program, and terminal security and should be able to restrict access on multiple levels.

Data Needs

Data must be provided that are required to plan, analyze, monitor, and control individual departments, divisions, and the organization as a whole. Computer systems should support and reflect integrated and related functions in the following broad administrative and financial areas:

Patient billing, review reports, volume statistics;
Budget, purchasing, general ledger;
Personnel, payroll, fulltime equivalents, cost center reports;
Capital planning, expenditure;
Quality improvement, utilization review, case mix, severity, acuity;
New systems to support data analysis as a routine effort;
Budgeting process (planning, development, control);
Financial statements and all related reports;
Cash report, inventory reports, investment report;
Census/patient volume report;
Project management reports;
Productivity.

Clinical data not addressed here also need to be integrated with financial and administrative data to provide a complete system information base.

Full information access for the nurse administrator enhances systemwide planning. The administrator generates decision support questions for data retrieval and display by information managers or personally accesses the database to obtain information. Given the paucity of planning time available in most daily administrative schedules, it is unrealistic to expect the nurse administrator to directly generate analytic reports. Information systems coordinators are especially useful in this role in addition to systems design, implementation, and operation toward optimally supporting nursing.

Future Directions

Leadership Influence on Information Systems

In recognition of the importance of nursing's influence on healthcare information systems development and implementation, associations such as the American Organization of Nurse Executives (AONE, 1994) have articulated priorities for nursing leaders in the evolution of information systems. The emphasis is on nursing leaders being knowledgeable about nursing informatics and responsible for ensuring that information systems support administrative and clinical decision-making processes that are truly patient centered.

Health information systems will be influenced by nurse leaders as they:

"1. Identify institutional, patient, and caregiver elements that, if collected, would provide the necessary data for comparisons within one institution and across healthcare settings.
2. Evaluate administrative and clinical decision-making processes that would benefit from technology and the ability of healthcare information systems to support these processes.
3. Collaborate with key departmental executives and constituencies throughout the phases of development, implementation, and evaluation.
4. Identify appropriate personnel who will act as resources to nursing clinicians and administrators as the information system is operationalized.
5. Collaborate with senior executives as contracts for information system vendor and consultant services are negotiated.
6. Influence the development of guidelines to ensure privacy and confidentiality for both patient and staff information.
7. Utilize collected data for decision-making and strategic planning purposes." (AONE, 1994, p. 5)

These roles will be critical to the establishment of information systems supportive to future healthcare delivery systems.

Organizational Priorities for the Nursing Information Specialist

The challenge for the nurse administrator is how to best organize, coordinate, and develop information system management. A national study (Mills, 1994) surveyed chief nurse administrators and nursing information specialists (NIS) in the same tertiary care hospitals, all over 500 beds in size. Over 100 of the specialists indicated that they were most heavily engaged in the areas of project management, staff training, implementation of clinical systems, and advisory and coordinating capacities. Chief nurse administrators identified their priorities for the next five years as focused on the following areas:

- Systems implementation,
- Strategic planning,
- Systems development, and
- Coordination of information systems.

Results suggested that communication between the chief nurse administrator and NIS was least well developed surrounding the areas of systems planning, implementation of clinical nursing systems, and strategic planning. For the nurse administrator, this implies a need for clear articulation of priorities, resource support, and involvement of the NIS in meetings that establish information expectations.

Systems Development

Systems Integration and Networking

The future standard against which administrators judge computer systems will be the ability to acquire information that optimally represents the status of each of a large number of interacting variables, the outcomes of these interactions, and the probability of future outcomes based on changes in the variables. Ultimately, system integration must go beyond systems internal to the organization to include network capability linking those internal systems to external environments (i.e., care providers, social and support services, and regulatory bodies). These expanded systems will serve to increase resources available for healthcare service and administration.

Data compilation and integration are critical to the rapidly growing managed competition concept. Community health management information systems (CHMIS) have been discussed as a vehicle to gather and communicate data necessary to setting medical practice standards for both quality and reimbursement (Scott, 1993). CHMIS is expected to link healthcare providers, purchasers, payers, and patients, using a system built around integrated hardware and software.

Other opportunities exist to link networks to external information bases, including statistics on staffing levels, mix, and cost analysis; compensation for distinct local and regional areas; and turnover and employment. The comparison of such data will be critical to the formulation of program plans and strategic directions.

Patient Record

Input to the patient record will combine automated patient physiologic monitoring and manual or voice data entry of clinical information. Key physiologic indicators will be monitored against preestablished standards and analyzed for trends and interactions predictive of health status intervention needs. This information will become part of the integrated patient record.

Information specific to patient care orders and process and outcome of care documentation will be entered into the record. This primary database will automatically service programs designed to generate required corollary information. This includes patient classification and acuity analysis, staffing requirements, personnel scheduling, productivity, payroll data, specific patient service charges, practice patterns, quality of management, and risk management monitoring.

Quality Management

As a key program component for clinicians, administrators, and regulators, quality management will focus increasingly on automated monitoring of predetermined variations (thresholds) indicative of trends in patient care.

These trends may be positive or negative and may be specific to individual patients or reflective of patient group experience (e.g., diagnostic categories).

Providing a qualitative base (quality) against which quantitative experience (resource use and expenditure) can be assessed is important. Even more valuable is the early identification of problems, creating the opportunity to intervene to achieve optimal patient care.

Eventually much qualitative data will be formatted to be compatible with regulatory reporting requirements such as those of the Joint Commission for Accreditation of Healthcare Organizations and federal legislation. This will include programming software to systematically collect, track, analyze, and report clinical and organizational data.

An increasing emphasis on organizational and management effectiveness will expand the current concept of quality to include organizational variables as impacting patient care. The development of integrated systems will facilitate automated collection and reporting of these variables for internal and external use.

Managed Care

Major restructuring of the healthcare system will continue to create expanded options for patient care delivery. This has already led to the development of managed care as a means of coordinating services and controlling cost for individuals and groups of patients. Networks that allow systems to interface will be developed to ease patient movement through various types and levels of care providers. This includes such features as appointment systems, progress tracking, clinical paths, outcome measurement, and cost reporting and analysis.

Decision makers will need data-based guidance in evaluating and reconciling cost and quality considerations. Current new decision support products suggest that developers are addressing the issue of managed care contracts relative to financial analysis. This development effort will need to be more definitively expanded to encompass direct patient service planning and delivery.

Resource Utilization

Every system entails costs and benefits. Many hospital administrators assume automated systems will pay for themselves by reducing costs, mostly from changes in workforce requirements (either in numbers or in function). Many of these same administrators further assume enhanced patient care and increased provider effectiveness.

Future development of computer systems, however, will need careful study of the impact of automated systems on workers. The results may provide guidance for job restructuring before the system is implemented. This approach would enable the manager to effectively reduce costs while improving productivity and patient care.

Summary

Information management, as a field, is growing increasingly sophisticated and complex as applied to health care and healthcare organizations. Nurse administrators are responsible for meeting increasingly stringent accreditation standards and legislative requirements in the area of systems integration.

Integrated system elements are critical to optimal administrative functioning. Single entry data sets that directly support multiple reporting requirements (some analytically based) will conserve valuable staff time. Programs supported by integrated systems include, for example, patient classification, acuity, productivity, quality of care, and financial analyses.

In the future, computer systems will support both intraorganizational systems integration and interorganizational networking. Computerized patient records will serve as a primary generation point for data required by administrative systems. Quality management at the patient and organizational level will be an area of increased emphasis. Computer systems will be developed to coordinate services offered in the diversified care settings created by healthcare restructuring. Systemwide analyses will extend to include the cost/benefit of computer implementation and the effectiveness of job restructuring in reducing costs while improving patient care.

Questions

1. What are the primary information management concepts embodied within accreditation standards and legislative initiatives?
2. What are the three fundamental systems that support nursing department operations?
3. What system design goals are important to the development or selection of computer systems that provide information specific to correlated administrative issues?
4. How can nurse administrators ensure that organizational priorities will be addressed?
5. What expectations should nurse administrators have for future information system design?

References

American Health Security Act of 1993. Washington, DC, 110–120.
American Organization of Nurse Executives (1994). AONE Board of Directors adopts white paper on nursing leadership influence on information systems. *AONE News, 6,* 5.

Corum, W. (1994). JCAHO standards and systems integration. *Healthcare Informatics, 1,* 22–28.

Joint Commission for Accreditation of Healthcare Organizations. (1994). Management of information. In: *Accreditation manual for hospitals, 1994* (pp. 35–44). Chicago: JCAHO.

Mills, M.E. (1994). Organizational priorities for the Nursing informatics Specialist. In: S.J. Grobe & E. Pluyter-Wenting (Eds.), *Nursing Informatics: An international overview for nursing in a technological era* (pp. 12–16). New York: Elsevier.

Scott, J.S. (1993). Community health MIS. *Computers in Healthcare, 7,* 22–28.

Bibliography

Simpson, R.L. (1993). *The nurse executive's guide to directing and managing nursing information systems.* Ann Arbor, MI: The Center of Healthcare Information Management.

Zielstorff, R., Hudgings, C, & Grobe, S. (1993). *Next generation nursing information systems.* Washington, DC: American Nurses Publishing.

21
Nursing Informatics Research: The National Agenda

Susan K. Newbold

Nursing research is a method by which nursing knowledge is generated, tested, and validated. Nursing research helps to answer nursing questions ultimately related to improved patient care. This chapter describes what research is being conducted in nursing informatics to answer nursing questions. Recommendations for a national research agenda are derived from several sources.

What Is Nursing Informatics?

Nursing informatics is a specialty area of practice that integrates computer science, information science, and nursing science and is designed to assist in the management and processing of nursing data, information, and knowledge to support the practice of nursing and the delivery of nursing care (Graves & Corcoran, 1989). Nursing informatics is an emerging field, only having been recognized by the American Nurses Association (ANA) as a discipline in 1992.

Preparation for Conducting Nursing Informatics Research

Conducting nursing research requires professionals who are educated to perform research. Doctoral and some master's level educational programs prepare nurses to carry out research. There are a few programs emerging with a special emphasis on informatics.

At the University of Maryland at Baltimore, the doctoral level curriculum is unique in that nurses are prepared as scholars and researchers with an emphasis in informatics. In addition to theory and dissertation credits, students take 17 semester credits of research and statistics. The research study is both quantitative and qualitative in nature. Students also complete 21 specialty focus credits in information science and nursing informatics.

The University of Maryland and the University of Utah are the only two programs in the United States offering a master's degree specifically in nursing informatics. These programs are discussed in more detail in *Nursing Informatics: Where Caring and Technology Meet* (Gassert, 1995). The U.S. Department of Health and Human Services National Library of Medicine (NLM) offers predoctoral and postdoctoral training in the broader field of medical informatics. This training, which encompasses nursing informatics, is offered at 10 universities in the United States. At this writing three nurses have completed postdoctoral education in medical informatics through the NLM programs. The Massachusetts General Hospital offers a post-master's degree fellowship in nursing informatics.

Nurse researchers who focus on nursing informatics can be employed in academic settings and in joint positions between medical centers and universities. Nurses can also conduct research in a consultant role either employed by a consulting firm or in independent practice.

Current Areas of Interest for Nursing Informatics Research

Waltz, Strickland, and Lenz (1991) comment that early in the development of a discipline is when research is conducted on affective measures. This may help to explain why the largest body of nursing informatics research conducted by the greatest number of people in nursing is in the domain of attitudes of nurses toward computers. Literature on nursing attitudes towards computers was first published in the late 1970s and early 1980s and is still being conducted today. The research is primarily quantitative in nature, although there has been at least one qualitative attitude study conducted (Abbott, 1993).

The fact that there are over 40 published studies of nurses' attitudes toward computer use, however, does not preclude further research. Of the 40 studies located, not one takes place in the long-term care facility setting where the use of automation is emerging. Few studies specifically examine clinical nursing systems, but rather focus on order entry or computer-assisted instruction. No studies investigate the attitudes of nurses toward a particular brand of computer software. Of even more concern is the fact that reporting of measurement concerns is spotty or absent. Few studies reveal the theoretical underpinnings, the theoretical and operational definitions of the variables, and/or the approaches to establishing reliability, validity, and item analysis.

Today there are a number of nurses conducting research in informatics. Recent publications contain research studies on the following topics:

- Cognitive learning, learning styles, knowledge acquisition, clinical reasoning, clinical decision making,
- Machine learning, expert systems,
- Nursing intervention lexicon and taxonomy,
- User interface for novice and expert nurses,
- Attitudes of nurses toward computerization,
- Impact of computerization on nursing,
- Benefits assessment,
- Meta-analysis of published research on computer-based instruction,
- Qualitative study of interactive video from the perspective of the nursing student,
- Secondary analysis of data for nursing diagnoses,
- Comparison of computerized and manually generated nursing care plan,
- Computer-based diagnostics systems,
- Unified medical language systems,
- Integrated advanced information management systems (IAIMS),
- Design and construction of health professional workstations,
- Health outcomes,
- Multimedia systems for education and clinical applications, and
- Impact of technology on patient care.

Although this appears to be a lengthy list, the total number of nursing projects is actually small. This could be due, in part, to a lack of programs that prepare nurse researchers in informatics and/or a funding problem.

Dissemination of Nursing Informatics Research

Nursing informatics research conducted to enhance clinical practice and to understand the practice of the informatics nurse is reported primarily in the proceedings of nursing informatics conferences, the *Computers in Nursing* journal published by J.B. Lippincott, and nursing research journals.

In order to obtain information on research studies, the reader is advised to seek out proceedings such as those of the Symposium on Computer Applications in Medical Care (SCAMC, 1992–1994, 1995). Proceedings have been published yearly since 1976, although nurses as a group were not involved until about 1981.

Every three years, an international nursing informatics conference is held and proceedings are published. Previous conferences have been held in England (1982), Canada (1985), Ireland (1988), Australia (1991), and the United States (1994). The Sixth International Conference on Nursing Use of Computers and Information Science will be held in September 1997 in Stockholm, Sweden. Information about the conference can be obtained from the country representative to the International Medical Informatics Association (IMIA). In the United States the contact is the American Medical Informatics Association (AMIA), 4915 St. Elmo Avenue, Suite 402, Bethesda, MD., 20814. This address can also be used for information on the aforementioned SCAMC.

Until recently, the most up-to-date information on the activities of informatics nurses has been via the SCAMC proceedings. Now there is the potential for even more current information to be at the fingertips of nurse researchers. The Sigma Theta Tau International (STTI) Electronic Library is designed to be a comprehensive collection of databases of nursing knowledge resources. The Virginia Henderson International Nursing Library of the Sigma Theta Tau International Honor Society of Nursing currently has five databases:

- Registry of Nursing Knowledge
  This listing includes information from the Directory of Nurse Researchers that has been previously available only in printed form. Here a nurse may find other researchers who are interested in a specific topic.
- Research Conference Abstracts Database
  Surveys and abstracts of papers and posters presented at nursing meetings and conferences are included. This author submitted a paper to the Sigma Theta Tau International Conference held July 1994 in Sydney, Australia. If a nurse was not able to attend the conference, the abstract is available to access electronically.
- Sigma Theta Tau Grant Recipients and Projects Database
  This database includes demographic, research information, and abstracts about projects funded by Sigma Theta Tau International.
- Information Resources Database
- Table of Contents Database
  The tables of contents from *IMAGE: Journal of Nursing Scholarship* and Sigma Theta Tau monographs comprise this database.

An individual or library can purchase a subscription, which allows for access from home or the subscriber library.

Another STTI initiative is the Sigma Theta Tau *International Online Journal of Knowledge Synthesis for Nursing.* This is the second online journal in existence. The editor is Jane H. Barnsteiner, RN, Ph.D., FAAN. One purpose of the journal is to disseminate nursing research.

There are limited funding sources available to assist the nurse researcher. The National Institutes of Health (NIH) disperses documents regarding federal grants and contracts through the Internet. Other nursing and health-related organizations may offer funding. Avenues to check for funding include the Sigma Theta Tau International Honor Society of Nursing, the Health Care Financing Administration (HCFA), the Agency for Health Care Policy and Research (AHCPR), the National Institute for Nursing Research (NINR), and the American Nurses Association American Nurses Foundation (ANA ANF). Partnerships with vendors of computer systems should be explored as another potential source of funding.

On an informal basis, information about dissemination of research related to nursing informatics can be found in the informal conversations that take place on the Internet (Holtzclaw, 1994). This is an electronic communication highway that can be accessed either by way of a university connection or by a commercial online service. Special-interest groups can develop forums called listservers. There are several listservers related to topics of interest for informatics nurse specialists including one specifically on nursing informatics. Other topics include quantitative research, qualitative research, the computer-based patient record, healthcare informatics, and global nursing issues. Currently the nursing informatics listserver has over 600 subscribers from many countries around the world.

The National Agenda for Nursing Informatics Research

The National Institute for Nursing Research (formerly known as the National Center for Nursing Research) has identified six major research program goals (1993). The goals can be thought of as a national agenda for nursing informatics research. The goals are to:

- Establish nursing language, including lexicons, classification systems and taxonomies, as well as standards of nursing data.
- Develop methods to build databases of clinical information (including data, diagnoses, objectives, interventions, and outcomes) and management information (including staffing, charge capture, turnover, and vacancy rates) and analyze relationships among them. It is proposed to exploit the databases to discover new clinical knowledge, including descriptions of diagnoses relevant to nursing practice and to test relationships among diagnoses, objectives, interventions, and outcomes; also to discover relationships between management variables and patient care, for example, to determine how nursing care is affected by staffing; and to develop methods of assessing cost effectiveness, cost benefit, and productivity that take into account the quality of care, including structure, process, and outcomes; and institutional outcomes, including nurse turnover and vacancy rates.
- Determine how nurses use data, information, and knowledge to give patient care, and how care is affected by differing levels of expertise and by organizational factors and working conditions, and to design information systems accordingly.
- Develop and test patient care decision support systems and knowledge delivery systems that are appropriate for nurses' needs, with consideration for expertise, organizational factors, and working conditions.
- Develop prototypes and eventually working models of nurse workstations equipped with tools to provide for nurses all the information needed

for patient care, research, and education, at the point of use, and linked to an integrated information system.

- Develop and implement appropriate methods to evaluate nursing information systems and applications, particularly as to their effects on patient care.

These goals for health informaticians were developed by a cadre of nurses and others including Marion J. Ball and Kathryn J. Hannah. There are many opportunities for nurse researchers who wish to pursue work in this arena.

Using the Computer to Assist Nursing Research

Along with research *about* automation and nursing, nurse researchers are using computers to help with the increased complexity of design and analytical strategies inherent in any nursing research. Nurse researchers can use computers to assist with the following:

- Data collection, tracking and transmission,
- Identification of potential problems (as in quality improvement),
- Statistics,
- Presentation mechanisms and reports,
- Case identification,
- Random selection of criteria for evaluation, and
- Transferring of files between software packages.

Nurse researchers have a basic requirement to learn and use software packages for:

- Statistical analysis,
- Spreadsheet calculation,
- Database management, and
- Word processing.

Using computers for literature searches is an application familiar to many nurses. Computerized databases allow the researcher to rapidly search and retrieve abstracts of pertinent literature. The Cumulative Index of Nursing and Allied Health Literature (CINAHL) is available online through universities and college libraries. Many large teaching hospitals provide searching service to their staff, faculty, and students. A detailed list of the many other databases that may be of interest to nurse researchers is beyond the scope of this chapter. A more detailed list is available in *Introduction to Nursing Informatics* (Hannah, Ball, & Edwards, 1994).

The American Nurses Association *Scope of Practice for Nursing Informatics* (1994, p. 11) speaks to the role of the informatics nurse as it relates to research. The document reveals that informatics nurses are needed to "conduct the research that underlies the design and development of information systems" and "conduct research using data aggregated and made available by nursing and other information systems."

Another role is to "develop theory and methods of inquiry into nursing informatics." Studies have been done using the theoretical base of self-efficacy, systems theory, diffusion theory, adult learning theories, and the theory of planned behavior, among others. Nurse researchers are encouraged to look outside of nursing to disciplines such as psychology, data processing, and education to find other theories to guide research endeavors. In addition to the ANA, other national and international groups with nursing informatics special interest groups should be encouraged to have a research agenda as part of their goals.

Conclusion

Some research is being conducted in the arena of nursing informatics. There are still many avenues unexplored for the emerging profession of informatics nurse specialist. Nursing informatics research should be done in collaboration with other healthcare and information systems disciplines to contribute to the growing body of knowledge of healthcare informatics.

Questions

1. What other theoretical bases, besides the ones listed, would be appropriate for nursing informatics research?
2. Name at least four areas where research has been conducted in nursing informatics.
3. List at least four target areas where more nursing research is indicated.
4. What agencies are potential sources of funding for nursing informatics research?
5. Some believe that in order to exploit computer technology for improved patient care, nursing informatics specialists must achieve a greater level of technical knowledge in information science. Do you agree or disagree? Discuss your viewpoint on this issue.

References

Abbott, K. (1993). Student nurses' conceptions of computer use in hospitals. *Computers in Nursing, 11*(2), 78–89.

American Nurses Association. (1992). *Computers in nursing research: A theoretical perspective*. Washington, DC: Author.

American Nurses Association. (1994). *The scope of practice for nursing informatics.* Washington, DC: Author.

Gassert, C.A. (1995). Academic preparation in nursing informatics. In M.J. Ball, K.J. Hannah, S.K. Newbold, & J.V. Douglas (Eds.), *Nursing informatics: Where caring and technology meet* (2nd ed.). New York: Springer-Verlag.

Graves, J.R., & Corcoran, S. (1989). The study of nursing informatics. *Image: Journal of Nursing Scholarship, 21*(4), 227–231.

Hannah, K.J., Ball, M.J., & Edwards, M.J.A. (1994). *Introduction to nursing informatics.* New York: Springer-Verlag.

Holtzclaw, B.J. (1994). Communication networks: A tool for nurse researchers. In S.J. Grobe & E.S.P. Pluyter-Wenting (Eds.), *Nursing informatics: An international overview for nursing in a technological era* (p. 763). Amsterdam: Elsevier.

National Center for Nursing Research. (1993). *Nursing informatics: Enhancing patient care.* Bethesda, MD: U.S. Department of Health and Human Services.

Symposium on Computer Applications in Medical Care. *Proceedings.* New York: McGraw Hill (1992–1994) and Philadelphia: Hanley & Belfus (1995).

Waltz, C.F., Strickland, O.L., & Lenz, E.R. (1991). *Measurement in nursing research* (2nd ed.). Philadelphia: F.A. Davis.

22
Using the Computer to Manage Change in the Clinical Pathology Lab

Charles F. Genre

The current medical economic scene has changed and has in many cases expanded the traditional role of the laboratory information system (LIS). To realize the medical and administrative benefits that an LIS offers, health-care institutions need to evaluate the strategic role of an LIS and then enter carefully into the selection and implementation process. Functional advances that laboratories can realistically expect to see in the near future should influence their choice of systems today.

Selection

The selection of a LIS raises questions that have no absolute answers, but, rather, vary according to institution. The first question is simply, "Does the laboratory need a computer at all?" It may be counterproductive to impose a computer system upon laboratories in small- to medium-sized hospitals that are able to process orders, analyze specimens, and issue and store reports required for patient care without an LIS. Given that labor savings often prove illusory, the expense may not be warranted. No mathematical formula identifies the point at which size and complexity mandate an LIS, but the time comes when every institution should investigate the need for such a system. When the hospital laboratory needs to process specimens faster and to provide its departments with cumulative and specialized reports, whether by paper, peripheral printer, or computer screen in real time, an LIS may be warranted.

As laboratories grow, the billing process grows more cumbersome, charges get posted later, and some charges are lost through human error or even human intent. Despite prepaid health care, many hospitals continue to do significant fee for service work, especially in the outpatient area. Larger laboratories may acquire a computer to process billing rapidly, completely, and accurately.

Today many hospitals are launching laboratory outreach programs to generate additional revenue and to strengthen the bonds with their medical staff. These outreach programs must provide the same amenities as large commercial laboratories, including in-office result printing, clean and legible computer printouts of results, and, most importantly, correct and timely billing. Because this type of outreach program demands computer capability of some complexity, an institution's business plan may mandate acquisition of an LIS.

The plan to acquire an LIS should be approved by the hospital's administrative and financial officers. Always important, cooperation between the laboratory and hospital administration is critical when a major system is selected and implemented, especially if progress does not meet expectations, as often happens.

System Components

Using a consultant if resources allow, the laboratory staff should define the type of system needed, including the number of laboratory sections in the system. Basic systems generally include general chemistry, special chemistry in all its permutations, hematology, urinalysis, parasitology, and immunology.

Blood bank and anatomic pathology were not included in many vendors' initial offerings. These laboratories processed comparatively small volumes and physically and/or administratively were often separate from the main lab. Moreover, they had a level of complexity that the early systems could not handle easily. As a result, some vendors offered large computer software packages that were less sophisticated in these areas or subcontracted with specialized vendors to provide these products in some form of integrated or interfaced package.

Most vendors addressed microbiology in their initial offerings, but were not generally successful. Newer large system products have much more acceptable microbiology packages. Also, some microbiology instrumentation vendors offer freestanding systems with strong instrumentation, data handling, and reporting capabilities. To avoid duplication of effort, these must in some fashion be integrated into the mainframe system, according to each laboratory's needs.

Scope should be defined early in the selection process. Scope of an LIS influences work flow, billing, result reporting, and the completeness of computerized patient data retrieval and analysis. A decision to support outreach programs now or in the future calls for greater computer power as well as more sophisticated billing functions and specimen routing routines.

System Alternatives

Although large hospital chains sometimes select and implement an LIS for all the facilities they control, most hospitals must choose where their LIS should reside. Four alternatives usually exist; the system can be

- Freestanding,
- Linked to the main admission/discharge/transfer (ADT) and billing systems but issuing its own reports,
- Linked to the main hospital system by ADT, billing, order entry, and reporting, but still doing all its own processing internally, or
- Resident on and a function of the main hospital computer, even as part of a multifacility system.

The first three choices are not mutually exclusive and, in fact, may be stages of a single implementation line as the interaction between the laboratory and the main computer function matures. All three give the advantage of the rapid response times provided by stand-alone systems and the possibility of using the vendor's "bells and whistles" to enhance production. Adopting the third alternative, the linked system that does all its own processing, allows the laboratory to have the best of both worlds.

Placing the laboratory system on the mainframe offers few of the advantages provided by the most integrated stand-alone options. Mainframe systems are not generally designed to provide the rapid response times that high-volume laboratory sections need and expect, and are often run by personnel unfamiliar with the operational needs of a laboratory, such as scheduling, maintenance, and backup to provide uninterrupted service. However, the mainframe (HIS) system should, at least, be able to provide disseminated order entry, result reporting, and billing.

Evaluation

Selection of an LIS should be assigned to a small committee, including the medical director or director's designate, the laboratory administrator, and several other key individuals. The director should head the group and be committed to being involved throughout the selection and implementation phases. Throughout the process, open and honest communication is essential. The hospital's main information systems department must have input to ensure that the LIS can be integrated with the main institutional systems. If central billing is to be done, the finance department must be involved.

Though sometimes controversial, a consultant may be added to the team, for the selection process only or for the implementation and special projects phases as well. The consultant's role is to bring divergent ideas into a coherent whole, know available and suitable vendors, add technical knowledge, and interact with the hospital's information systems division (ISD).

In this role, the consultant can help avoid considering a system or configuration with power insufficient to support the current laboratory and its projected expansion. To add credibility to a diffuse and complicated process, the consultant must know laboratories intimately and work closely with the laboratory director and the selection committee.

A member of the committee or the consultant should draft a request for proposal (RFP) describing the laboratory and its present and future needs. Attention should be paid to special projects or needs and unusual circumstances. If the laboratory is attached to a hospital that has or expects a very large outpatient test volume or a special care unit that would skew a vendor's calculations, these should be explained clearly.

The RFP should be sent to all reasonable vendors. A single day should be designated to review the laboratory and its needs with all interested vendors. This review should occur on site, ideally with the vendors as a group. After the predetermined date for return of the responses to the RFP, the committee should identify candidate vendors for site visits.

Site Visits

Visits to all sites should be scheduled to include all members of the selection committee. Critical questions should not be left unanswered because a key visitor is absent. The laboratory should demand that the sites visited equal or exceed its own in size and complexity. More than one site per vendor should be visited, as should all the vendors who appear to meet the laboratory's needs. Given the length of the selection process, the site visit team should record all observations immediately on return from each visit. The site visit team should also involve the hospital's information systems department so that technical questions concerning the LIS and mainframe may be identified and addressed on an ongoing basis. The consultant is also a valuable resource on site visits.

After visits to all sites, the team should identify the finalists. The primary criteria used should center around the way in which the candidate systems satisfy the needs of the laboratory. If the scope and need were adequately identified at the outset, the choice of finalists should be easy. The finalists should be brought in separately to answer questions and to make detailed presentations of their systems to all laboratory sections, including the support areas of venipuncture and specimen receiving. This may take up to three days per vendor and should be performed on site.

A technical investigation of the hardware vendor should be undertaken separately. The hospital's information systems department should be of significant aid in this regard. Meetings with the hardware vendor and its local representatives should be held to discuss the hospital's unique needs for uninterrupted 24-hour service. Of course, the hospital should conduct financial reviews of both the software and the hardware vendors.

A meeting directed by the laboratory and including the information systems department along with administrative and financial officers should be held to jointly review all the finalists. The meeting should be as broad based as possible because broad-based support will be necessary for implementation and for future support. Although a winner is usually relatively evident, the laboratory should have the final decision if the finances and system interactions with the hospital's other systems are approximately equal.

The LIS selection committee must understand that vendors are salespersons. The committee should run financial checks on the vendors and investigate all their claims. If the vendor claims the system can be interfaced, the committee should ask to see the interface on a site visit. Under no circumstances should the committee accept the vendor's claims without investigation. The selection committee must use lawyers and hospital administrators to write a contract explicitly stating the terms and expectations. A clear, precise contract benefits both parties. The lab will know when it will receive its product and the vendor will know in no uncertain terms what it will be paid. At that time, the installation will be complete and maintenance can begin.

Implementation

Implementing an LIS for the first time is an almost once in a lifetime chance to make long desired systems changes. The challenge is not to computerize an existing manual laboratory, but to use the computer as a new and powerful tool. Throughout the process, one person should clearly be in charge; timetables should be reasonable and definite.

The laboratory needs to analyze everything it does, understand its component steps, and systematically map out its specimen ordering, processing, and reporting flow and billing functions. The laboratory must determine what it wants done. Ordering must be analyzed and tests grouped in a logical sequence. Laboratory tests may be grouped by performing sections, such as hematology or chemistry; request numbers may be given in blocks large enough to accommodate future expansion. Specimen draw requirements must be carefully quantitated so that venipuncture will not be requested to exsanguinate patients for whom numerous tests are ordered.

A computer should not recreate a poorly designed manual system, especially one based on a high exception rate. Sample dispersement throughout the laboratory must be analyzed and appropriate aliquot systems and labels designed. To assist in this process, those laboratory members who will be intimately involved with the decisions should visit several up and functioning laboratories. Only after the choice of an LIS do section supervisors really appreciate the problems associated with conversion.

Sample processing predominantly involves internal laboratory functions, but reporting involves several of the laboratory's prime customers, especially the requesting physicians and floor nurses. It is essential to pick a representative cross section of them to help design the timing and format of the reports and the needs for result reporting by printer or computer screen, especially in high-intensity areas. All reasonable requests should be met. Physicians and nurses who have had their input honored will be more tolerant of the inevitable disruptions caused by implementing a new system.

The decision to hire a computer supervisor often revolves around whether to get a "laboratory person" or a "computer person." If one candidate has credentials in both areas, is energetic, likes to spend nights at the hospital, and will be there at least two years, the choice is easy. Otherwise, trade-offs are necessary. If both the hardware and the software vendors can provide good support and training, most directors tend to prefer a laboratory person. They feel it is easier to teach adequate computer skills in the context of good support than to try to teach a computer person about the requirements for cultures, coagulation, ionized calciums, and so forth. This is particularly true for laboratories installing their first LIS, because for them production and specimen flow are critically important.

For any LIS, a backup system is an absolute necessity. It will be needed, most likely, early in the computerized era. The system should include order back up, accessioning and production, specimen identification numbers, and manual report forms. Most results can be stored automatically on interface buffers with the patient identification assigned. When the system goes live, the results can be automatically uploaded to the accessioned samples. In any case, a protocol must be written and practiced before going live, including requirements for entering results manually if the automatic upload fails.

Replacement Systems

Laboratories implementing replacement systems need to guard against duplicating the old with the new. They should see the process as a golden opportunity to correct past inadequacies. By now, systems have been set and laboratory personnel are familiar with computers. This is the time to reconsider the skills required of the laboratory's computer supervisor. Perhaps computer skills should be considered over laboratory knowledge.

Once all systems have been designed, both the original and the replacement LIS should run in parallel with their existing systems. In this era of cost control, hospital administrators must understand that additional person hours will be needed. The parallel run must include all laboratory personnel on all shifts, including weekend part-timers, and all nonlaboratory personnel who will interact with the system, including the physicians, nurses, and clerks. The parallel run should be intense and should last only long enough to get all personnel trained. Prolonged parallel runs simply bore people and use up work hours. These runs should not overlook result inquiry on the screen or printer. Not knowing how to work the printer properly will cause havoc, especially at peripheral locations.

The date to go live should be chosen so that the software vendor can provide support and ensure that last minute changes are made quickly. The hardware manufacturer should have on hand a good crew who understand the 24-hour needs of a hospital laboratory. The laboratory director must be present to coordinate the scenario and to make those decisions that inevitably need to be made and made quickly. One person should be present on site for as long as it takes and should have the authority to make decisions when necessary. Few real-time projects succeed if no one or if a committee is in charge.

For both first time and replacement systems, scheduling going live mid-week when volume is lower allows corrections to be performed on the weekend and fine tuning to be done before the high-volume time of the early week. For replacement systems, all samples entering the laboratory are accessioned into the new system at midnight. The two run parallel for several days, allowing the old system to complete all data through a particular date and the new to start on that date. Within the first two days, the majority of results from the old system have been reported. Each laboratory must decide when to cancel the unprepared tests in the old system and reenter them into the new. After one week's duration, these tests are usually in microbiology or have been sent out to a reference laboratory; reentering them is a relatively small task. Letting the old system complete its tests simplifies seeking results weeks later; tests up to a certain date are known to be in the old system and can be found with minimal confusion.

Benefits

For laboratories of sufficient size and complexity, an LIS is essential if they are to survive and prosper. The system affects literally every subsystem of the laboratory as well as numerous other patient care areas of the hospital. Care must be taken to ensure that these areas are positively affected; a review process should confirm desired outcomes and warn of possible negative effects.

The LIS should organize the inpatient specimen collection process and print patient collection labels in order of rooms to be collected. By specifying the type and number of tubes and the amount of blood to be obtained, the labels assist personnel and speed up collection. Most laboratories find it advantageous to set up a central specimen processing area to receive, verify, and/or accession samples into the laboratory system. Well-trained personnel in this area can prevent bottlenecks and detect specimens that are incorrectly labeled or requested. Although they tend to be blamed for misaccessioning specimens, they are often the unsung heroes who guard the system from mistakes generated elsewhere in the hospital system.

Larger laboratories may need more than a single processing area. Because of the diversity and complexity of specimen type and the need to generate numerous plate labels, microbiology often accessions its own samples. Critical care areas such as surgery, intensive care units, and the emergency room may benefit from special accessioning areas and/or dedicated specimen delivery systems, such as a tube system. These are generally less expensive than satellite labs spread throughout a facility.

The computer's impact on specimen analysis will vary by area. Sections that predominantly analyze in a batch mode will benefit from automatically assembled batches and printed worklists for specimen arrangement and result entry. The analyzer may be interfaced, but probably should not be unless definite economic gain is realized. In most hospitals, the batches are small enough to be entered manually almost as easily.

In the areas of high-volume analysis like automated chemistry and hematology, the impact of the computer can be revolutionary. When interfaced with the LIS, instruments can upload results as soon as they are verified. The traditional worklist simply delays the process of analysis; no longer should technologists be required to wait and load specimens in a particular order.

Bidirectional interfaces especially linked to the current high-capability, random-access chemistry and hematology analyzers should eliminate repeat accessioning of the test requests at the laboratory instrument. They should also significantly decrease reporting errors if positive specimen identification, such as bar codes, has been affixed to the specimen tube. Also, the design and number of aliquot labels can save considerable time in a busy laboratory. Automatically generated, different colored labels can signify specimen priority ("stat").

At some point during the analytical process, depending upon the analyzer and the number of times it needs to run controls, the result is checked for quality control referable to the specimen. Some of the newer random access analyzers retain calibration for extended periods of time, and results can be verified by a technologist as they are produced after consulting appropriate controls. Though laboratories may accomplish this in different ways, the rule should be to set up a system that will

- Avoid duplicate accessioning of tests as much as possible,
- Release properly controlled and verified results to the floors as rapidly as possible, and
- Implement automated quality control and result review whenever possible.

Reporting and Delivery

Report formats and optimal times of delivery should be determined in conjunction with the physicians and the nursing staff. At a minimum, an LIS should provide a cumulative report for all inpatients, updated daily and color coded to eliminate charting difficulties. The need for interim reports varies; high-intensity units should have printers and computer screens to provide access to results as soon as they are verified in the laboratory. In most hospitals, the laboratory can generate reports for early morning rounds if compilation time is short. If the LIS is interfaced to the HIS, reports can be generated at the nursing station on demand.

Teaching hospitals offer unique problems. Many physicians are involved and physician ordering patterns are not matured. The first morning paper reports are often pocketed by the earliest house officer to arrive on the scene. Tests are requested throughout the day rather than at normal intervals, effectively nullifying the usefulness of standard paper reports. Acutely ill patients must be moved frequently, making it difficult to route the paper reports to the appropriate location. In such hospitals, paper should not be the sole means of reporting.

An alternate way to transmit the information in its most updated form is electronic reporting on the computer screen. If there is a simple program for patient data inquiry, physicians, nurses, and medical students will all view the computer screen. The ability to print the screen is most helpful. Physicians and house staff often become very proficient at this and can easily and quickly determine what tests have been ordered and their production status.

Test Result Archive

If a consistent medical record number is used for both inpatient and outpatient visits, the LIS can easily retain all laboratory data for a patient for up to a year, as determined for each facility. Data retention benefits patients, such as the one who appears in the emergency room at 2 a.m. and whose chart cannot be located for any of a legion of reasons. With access to the LIS, the ER physician instantly retrieves the patient's laboratory results for the last year and puts together a pretty good picture from the results and the original laboratory requests. When paper reports are lost from the chart, real-time archive inquiry is often the most rapid way for a clinician to solve a problem. The ideal solution would be an electronic chart or patient database where all results (lab, x-ray, pharmacy) would be stored. In the interim, the test result archive is an excellent use of an LIS.

The benefit to laboratory physicians exclusive of production benefits resides in increased access to information. Anatomic pathologists should have at their fingertips all the previous results from cytology and biopsy for every case on their microscope. Similarly, they should have all the clinical laboratory results for the difficult case that requires anatomic and clinical data correlation for the best diagnosis. Clinical pathologists will constantly make use of past patient data in evaluating current results or in signing out interpretative tests. All laboratory physicians should be able to get result statistics (antibiograms, results of Pap smears, normal values) from the LIS or from data downloaded from the LIS to a microcomputer. A well-functioning LIS is an incredibly powerful tool for improving the quality of laboratory physicians' daily work and research and, as will be discussed later, is essential in utilization management.

Laboratory administrative performance is immeasurably aided by an LIS. For example, billing can be tailored to the institution and run either as a stand-alone function or, more commonly, interfaced to the main hospital billing department. Bills can be generated at the time of request or result, leaving only the question of what to do about tests for which results take a long time to become available.

Audit Trail Data

With an LIS, laboratory administration has an audit trail on each test through the entire process. This provides turnaround time data from request (if interfaced), collection, and verification to result reporting. These data are extremely important in quality assurance and in running the department. If a physician questions the time to acquire a test, the department can investigate the specific incident, including the personnel involved and the actual times involved. In more advanced forms, audit trail data can be used for workload recording and productivity, down to an individual level. The LIS can provide ordering patterns by physician and by medical section; these data can be useful in identifying and changing patterns for purposes of quality assurance or cost containment. Both quality control routines and maintenance schedules can be automated.

Risks

All the benefits of an LIS come with some risk. Hospitals often computerize in fits and starts. LISs have been available for a reasonably long time, and many hospitals have computerized their laboratories early in the process of automating hospitalwide. Other areas of the hospital may have little or no knowledge of computers and may not really understand the global consequences of an incorrectly written patient medical record number. They may not understand that the result may go to the wrong chart and the bill will go to someone else who may not be in the hospital at all. Computerized billing is a great advance, but constant review of the billing process is necessary because small changes by someone who does not understand the whole process may have amazing ramifications. In production, particularly when using manually entered batch methods, worklists may be moved over by one name in a particular direction and the potential for dissemination of many incorrect reports will exist. The laboratory must constantly monitor its processing and reporting and immediately and vigorously investigate all potential misadventures.

The Future

What do the next few years hold? System reliability will continue to improve and storage capacity will increase. Laboratory systems will probably use more and more local networks, increasing reliability and versatility. Many of the stand-alone systems such as those in anatomic pathology and blood banking will be effectively networked into the main LIS. Local area networks on PCs will operate individual production areas. Laboratory systems will concentrate on the laboratory and will make more extensive use of the hospital information system to report and store data, often in conjunction with the other support services.

Reporting will improve significantly. The standard cumulative report will continue because it serves most of the cases. New report formats will be used with increasing frequency. Graphs and trend reports and formats personalized for individual physicians or services will be used. Physician offices and homes will be linked to the computer, either the LIS or the HIS, and data will be more accessible. Meaningful duplicate order checking systems will be set up to curb unnecessary test requests. Cost data on test requests and on therapeutic choices could be given in real time with potentially significant cost savings for the hospital.

In the near future, test processing will be immeasurably aided by real specimen positive identification, the Achilles' heel of all clinical laboratories. This, coupled with the next generation of bidirectional interfaces for the highly automated instrumentation, should vastly decrease test turnaround time and help reduce personnel requirements or allow better use of different personnel skill mixes. The use of computer-generated, machine-readable labels will allow the laboratory to automate its specimen saving and retrieval functions. As a result, the test add on function will be more feasible, allowing the original hematology and chemistry screening and admission testing to be reduced in size, another area for possible reagent and personnel savings.

In the near future, the laboratory will automatically accept an order generated by the physician at the patient's bedside and receive a positively identified specimen to put in random fashion on an analyzer that has received the individual test requests downloaded from the LIS. The specimen tube stopper will not have to be popped, eliminating aerosols. After analysis, the tube will be placed in a robot to read the label and construct a save rack. Clerical staff will be able to retrieve the specimen if additional tests are requested.

Expanded Role

Within the clinical laboratory itself, the traditional chief concern is the production of data as individual units, the compilation of that data in a patient file, and then its presentation to our long-time chief client, the requesting physician. The result format may vary but it is usually destined for a chart in an office or at the bedside. The laboratory now has, in this new world of medical economics, many clients and all are interested in some data but much more information, not all of it of the traditional type or in the traditional format. This concept must be understood by those who are contemplating a first LIS purchase as well as by those who are current proud owners.

The LIS has matured and now has entered a new phase of life. No longer is the laboratory computer group spending the majority of its time in the maintenance of the system hardware and software. Most systems are so reliable that unscheduled downtime is not a problem and, ironically, most have really forgotten how to effectively use the backup plan.

In most large medical institutions with computer experience the majority of the LIS support effort should now be focused on outside expansion, utilization management, and interactions with new customers such as hospital management and outside affiliates. The laboratory and its parent institution should see the laboratory in an ever-expanding role as they both face new economics and ever-changing alliances.

Utilization Management/Patient Care

Payment for medical services of all types has radically changed. Although there remains significant regional difference in payment type, the emphasis in most areas is shifting toward increasing awareness of utilization management. This has had an obvious effect on the laboratory, most notably in the numbers and types of tests ordered.

It is the increasing responsibility of the medical staff to address the appropriateness of number and type of tests ordered. The LIS is a critical force in this effort. Resident in the system should be all the information necessary, such as test type and ordering physician, for real-time or cumulative monitoring of test utilization. The data can be used separately or merged with additional data such as diagnosis, acuity, or length of stay for better interpretation. This monitoring is essential to any program of cost containment and the LIS is vitally important.

The LIS can help test utilization by presenting patient results as true information, formatted in the most user-friendly way possible and inclusive of as much information as possible. The report should include all the production centers of the laboratory and even those remote centers perhaps not administratively within "Laboratory" (such as a blood gas laboratory run by Anesthesia or Pulmonary medicine) in the same report and on the same inquiry menu at the computer terminals. Administrative borders and departmental lines may have to be breached; but, to survive in today's economics, that is a small price. Every effort should be made to keep as much information about each patient in a single viewable screen or readable report for the physician regardless of the site of origin of the report. This is the laboratory's version of a unified medical report. Whether the report resides on the LIS or the institution's main computer system is irrelevant for the physician and should be functionally transparent. If the process is successful, patient care should markedly benefit and the process of utilization management can be pursued with a more positive image.

Order Entry

Integral to the concept of efficiency and utilization management is the process of automated order entry. It has many intellectually appreciated and obvious values but so many practical pitfalls that it warrants some individual attention. The primary pitfall is that which affects so many conversion processes; namely, the urge to quickly "convert" and thereby mimic an existing manual system. In many institutions manual systems selectively alter or skirt written procedures to make the final combined process a workable one. Examples of this folly are attempts to routinely duplicate manual order sheets on computer terminals screens without analysis of real needs and the failure to understand duplicate order placements, test cancellation, and standing orders. The lesson to be stressed is that computerized order entry is a wonderful tool for efficiency and utilization management if designed intelligently before enactment. It is a potentially frustrating example of inefficiency and name calling if done quickly and without prior needs analysis.

The second question concerning order entry is the opportunity it offers for test ordering management. The correct way in which to initiate this is to involve the medical staff and to concentrate initially on a few high-volume and high-visibility tests. Computerized order entry blocks can be placed to limit the number of these tests that can be ordered per day or per admission and not jeopardize patient care. The real question is where to put the computerized block. The ideal situation would be to have the block available in real time at the computer terminal or peripheral device at which the ordering and responsible physician is placing the request. Thereby he would get immediate feedback and could even override the block if he felt it to be medically necessary (a process itself that could be audited). Anything less than this is less effective. If a physician writes orders on a chart to be manually entered at a later date by a ward clerk or nurse, an order that is contrary to the policy may be blocked but the ordering physician is "long gone." This places the ward clerk in an untenable position.

There is another question involving the location of the block. If a HIS is used for order entry and it then passes the order to an LIS, the block should reside on the HIS, not on the LIS. Many laboratory systems have sophisticated ability to block or alter orders, but the block is most effective at the site of order entry.

These problems are not stated to defeat a process. The concept of test order management is excellent, but it must be carefully planned and tailored for the physician staff practicing in that location, and it should only be done after consultation and communication with that staff.

Outreach/Affiliation/Merger Efforts

In current medical economics virtually all hospital laboratories are involved in or planning some form of outreach efforts to offset decreased test volume from changed inpatient management and reimbursement. Affiliations and mergers are bringing together more and more institutions, many of which were previous competitors. Computerization is key to this effort.

Numerous community hospital laboratories are now pursuing the market of the surrounding physician offices traditionally courted by the commercial laboratories. The strategy involves closely matching a commercial laboratory in pricing, specimen pickup, billing, and reporting, and surpassing them in continuity of patient data (both in- and outpatient), professional consultation, and even in turnaround time. Pricing policy and specimen pickup are not topics for discussion here. For success in this venture physician office result reporting by remote printer is essential and can be done easily by an LIS, and this ability should be a requirement of any new system RFP. Billing should also be available through the system, although this is not always easy considering the bewildering numbering of payment schemes currently present. In certain accounts, depending upon size and local competition, in-office online order entry and result inquiry must be furnished for competitive reasons. In this case the LIS or HIS becomes involved intimately and easily in outreach and marketing, both for the laboratory and the parent institution. The important point is that hospitals are seeking affiliations with physicians, and laboratory services can be easily visible and quickly installed and serve not only as revenue sources but also as marketing vehicles. An LIS is essential for the process.

In certain locations several to many hospital laboratories are currently affiliating to more economically utilize excess laboratory production capacity. This strategy has certain merits, but a practical problem encountered is that of different and "incompatible" laboratory computer systems. Although these systems can be linked, the important concept is to try to make the linkage as transparent as possible to the users. Several large commercial laboratories that have realized this are currently considering linkage products to accomplish the transparency, but that solution requires commitment for reference work and rarely is a project like this really "free."

An alternate and more radical solution might be to determine which LIS of the affiliated hospitals offers the best match of capacity and utility, "turn off" the other systems and use the best one to run all the hospital laboratories of the group. If the chosen LIS is used primarily for test production and the management functions of test requesting and result reporting are uploaded to the affiliates' hospital computer systems, significant maintenance cost could be eliminated. This does, however, presuppose that the marriage of the affiliated hospitals will remain a good one.

In summary, the "outreach and affiliation" business in all its iterations has come of age. The LIS, either alone or in partnership with the HIS, has become an indispensable part of the equation not only from the perspective of test production but now, most interestingly, as a quickly reacting, far-reaching and versatile marketing tool for its owner. How the LIS is used, how it is interfaced with physician office PCs or network, and how it interacts with the large commercial laboratories vary by location and need, but the opportunities are immense.

Questions

1. What factors favor a laboratory's decision to acquire a laboratory computer system?
2. Who are the key players in the decision-making process for a laboratory computer system? Discuss their responsibilities.
3. What are the major benefits of a laboratory computer system for:
   a. the laboratory?
   b. the physicians?
   c. the parent hospital and its network?

Bibliography

Aller, R.D. (1994). Software links labs to physician office clients. *CAP Today, 8*(5), 21–25.

Aller, R.D. (1994). The future is now for electronic medical databases. *CAP Today, 8*(9), 48–52.

Ball, M.J. (1971). *Selecting a computer system for the clinical laboratory.* Springfield, IL: Charles C Thomas.

Braley, G.F. (1994). Laboratorians climb aboard the online bandwagon. *Health Management Technology, 8,* 30–36.

Chow, D. (1993). Down and out: Understanding and addressing laboratory network and computer failures. *CAP Today, 7*(11), 63–65.

Korpman, R.A. (1994). The role of suppliers and laboratories in the new information environment. *Clinica Chimica Acta, 224*(2), S23–37.

McDiwakk, R.D. (1993). An update on laboratory information management systems Guildford, UK. *Journal of Pharmaceutical & Biomedical Analysis, 11*(11–12), 1327–1330.

O'Desky, R.I. (1985). Is there a pathology department computer system apropos to your organization? *Healthcare Computing and Communications, 2,* 4.

O'Desky, R.I., & Ball, M.J. (1988). Clinical laboratory computerization: A glimpse at the system vendor community and some thoughts on the impact of technology in the next ten years. *Clinical Laboratory Management Review, 2*(2), 68–76.

Shires, D.B. (1974). *Computer technology in the health sciences.* Springfield, IL: Charles C Thomas.

Siemaszko, F. (1978). *Computing in clinical laboratories.* Kent, England: Pitman Medical Publishing.

Skjei, E. (1993). New look at how systems are linked. *CAP Today, 7*(11), 36–62.

Thompkins, W.J., & Webster, J.G., Eds. (1981). *Design of microcomputer-based medical instrumentation.* Englewood Cliffs, NJ: Prentice Hall.

23
Computer-Enhanced Radiology: A Transformation to Imaging

ROGER H. SHANNON

Introduction

Radiology is an information business. It is one of the core specialties of scientific medicine. In a sense, it is also a part of every direct care specialty, but it has differentiated into a separate field because of the special skills and knowledge that are required to correctly create and interpret images. Many other physicians have also become skilled in aspects of radiology, but few have the fundamental training to appreciate the context in which radiology is practiced or have a command of the subject sufficient to enable them to choose the most efficacious, cost-beneficial course of study from a full set of alternatives. Even skilled clinical subspecialists rarely see the number and variety of cases that a radiologist encounters in serving many such referring physicians.

Diagnostic radiology, therefore, is best practiced in an environment of good communication between radiologists and referring physicians, however skilled at image interpretation the latter may be. Good communication in this technical world consists of intercomputer exchange in addition to the many forms of interpersonal exchange to which one has become accustomed. These two aspects of communication will receive further attention in this chapter.

Computers are used in two distinctly different ways by diagnostic radiologists. First, computers are central components of imaging devices such as computed tomographic units (CT), ultrasound (U/S), gamma cameras, computed radiography (CR), and others. Second, computers are increasingly important in managing a wide variety of information germane to radiological practice. They are the hub of radiology information systems (RIS) which enhance management of administrative and medical information, and they make possible the management, storage, and communication of electronic images (IMAC or PACS).

This chapter focuses on the second use of computers as support systems, commenting on computers integral to acquisition devices only in order to clarify the important and expanding application of computers for radiology support.

The Major Function of Diagnostic Radiology

The core function of diagnostic radiology is quality consultation. Service is thereby rendered to both referring physicians and patients.

The ideal consultation incorporates several processes. First, one must choose what study or studies to do. Commonly the choice is straightforward, but often it is not. Choosing may require evaluation of complicated clinical information with preliminary consultation between referring physician and radiologist. Weighing of benefits, risks, and costs is frequently difficult. The sequencing of tests and determining when they should be done may be issues. Second, the selected examination(s) must be excellently performed. Good equipment, competent personnel, and individually validated procedures are each critical factors. Third, images resulting from a study should be assembled with all relevant supporting material. Clinical information, previous similar examinations or other concurrent studies, and reference materials are frequently important. These comprise what may be called the Selective Clinical Radiology Information Package (SCRIP).

Finally, a timely report should be produced and communicated to the physician(s) who will incorporate the radiological results into the clinical decision stream. The report has traditionally been rendered in hardcopy text, but it is becoming more common to make it available in electronic form with the possibility of including annotatable graphic material and voice notes just around the corner. Regardless of final report form, communication of results, opinions, correlations, and suggestions for resolving conflicting conclusions may require immediate personal communication on the part of the radiologist. Phone and e-mail are commonly used. Formal daily conferences between radiologists and clinicians have also become a highly successful way to achieve rapid, quality communication.

Consulting in its various forms is the professional heart of diagnostic radiology. It is a complex process that occurs in a complex setting. There are two parts of that setting that must be appreciated by the manager, or administrator, of radiology. The radiology department itself—an involved, extremely technical, capital intensive portion of the hospital—is the core system that constitutes the first part of the setting. Included in the conception of the radiology department are the main department and satellite operations in locations such as the emergency room, outpatient clinic, and surgery.

However, radiologic practice is not confined to the department, but permeates the entire hospital and the clinics of associated practitioners. This classic configuration is being extended further by electronic imaging that allows consultation and coverage of remote affiliates and enables radiologists on call to view images at home. Viewing stations, either light box or cathode ray tube (CRT), are scattered throughout wards, conference rooms, surgery, and other service areas. These are all elements of the second part of the setting—the "environment," or context, in which radiology is practiced. Procedures and discussions involving radiologic images and reports are legion. Clinical decisions and procedures are continually influenced by radiology. New information leads to new radiologic studies. It is largely outside of the formal radiology areas that consultations are assimilated by the clinical process and acquire meaning for the patient. The better the communication, the more powerful a tool radiology becomes.

In review, the formal radiology system is embedded in the medical environment. The radiology manager must be fully sensitive to the implications of the general systems principle that it is only in the environment that any system acquires its meaning. The clinical process belongs to the essential environment that gives birth to and makes use of radiologic consultation (Grobstein, 1973).

Trends and Transition

Rapid Growth

The proliferation of computer support for radiology has been stimulated by two trends. First, radiology has been one of the fastest growing medical specialties for many years. Mushrooming medical knowledge and new, often time-consuming, procedures have added volume and complexity to radiology's armamentarium. With growth have come subspecialties and larger, more complicated groups of professionals. Most medium size and larger hospitals have spread radiology to several satellites, and the supporting staff has become numerous and varied. Coordination of radiology has become immensely difficult. Manual procedures are no longer sufficient to deal with the volume of detail. Consequently, computer operations have been developed to supplement or replace older methods. The resulting systems are referred to as RIS.

Changing Technology

The second trend bringing computers into radiology began with the introduction of CT in 1972 (Hounsfield, 1972). CT relies on a computer to capture and analyze thousands of measurements that are arrayed in planes, or slices, that portray cross sections of the body parts examined. These pictures are electronic and are first displayed on CRTs, devices like television screens. It is still conventional, however, to transfer these images to film for final interpretation and storage. The methods and technology of CT have been applied to a host of other modalities so that even before the current incursion of CR on portable filming, between one-quarter and one-half of the number of actual images obtained in current practice originated in electronic form (Lodwick, 1986).

Computed radiography, the recent arrival, is a technology that holds the promise of converting all general film radiography to electronic form. It uses a light-stimulable phosphor that can be read by laser, erased, and re-used many times. The electronic image so obtained can be presented on a CRT or printed on film. It is CR that makes it possible to eliminate film altogether (Saarinen et al., 1989).

Support Systems

To handle electronic images in volume, additional computers appear to be a necessary adjunct to the classic radiological equipment inventory. Several synonyms designate the resulting systems. Four in popular use are PACS (picture archiving and communications systems), DIN (digital imaging networks), IMACS (image management and communication systems), and MDIS (Medical Diagnostic Imaging System).

RISs were developed earlier than PACS. The former are fairly mature and are in wide use. The latter are becoming more common for specialized applications such as Intensive Care Unit (ICU) support, remote over-reading, consulting, and home call. Since the previous edition of this book, there has been a major breakthrough in PACS installation to cover full departments. The military, the Baltimore Veterans Affairs Medical Center (VAMC), and Hammersmith in London all have established contracts with an American firm for full PACS systems. The Baltimore VAMC has achieved the goal of providing full electronic operation, including routine interpretation from CRTs. The Army is substantially on its way toward that goal at Madigan Army Medical Center with other installations following. During this same period, the Viennese have been mounting a full PACS system in conjunction with a European firm, and others are moving to follow these early examples. Current efforts are directed at further development of PACS and at interfacing a variety of existing RISs with the emerging PACS technology. Baltimore has been largely successful in interfacing its PACS, RIS, and hospital information system.

In the early 1980s, the American College of Radiology and the National Electrical Manufacturers Association formed a joint committee (ACR-NEMA) to develop standards for interfacing digital acquisition devices to PACS networks. These standards are now being incorporated in industrial design, and contracts frequently specify the standard interface as a requirement. [The new version 3.0 is to be known as "DICOM 3" (Best et al., 1992).] Numerous other groups are dealing with the problems of data definition and compatibility (Megargle, 1989). New findings and controversies frequently appear in the literature. And the state of the art moves forward. Radiology computer support systems have felled several barriers in the past two or three years, but much remains to be done before the new accomplishments can be considered standard fare. Radiology is in a state of dramatic transition that can make choices difficult and the lives of both practitioners and administrators frustrating. However, some difficulty now is justified by the promise of simplified, computer-supported management in the future.

RIS and PACS Functions

Radiology Information Systems (RIS)

The typical RIS offers several sets of functions. These include (1) registration of patients, (2) scheduling, (3) patient tracking, (4) film library management, (5) reporting of results, and (6) department management. Electronic mail, teaching applications, and research functions may be added. Various forms of decision support are also beginning to appear. Although the basic RIS is fairly mature, these systems continue to expand and evolve.

Registration

Registration is the process of initiating the patient RIS record. This is the demographic module. If the RIS is interfaced to the hospital information system (HIS), demographic information is passed to radiology from the hospital master record. If not otherwise available, patient information is entered directly.

Scheduling

Scheduling examinations may vary from a simple computer version of standard paper forms requiring a maximum of clerical effort to sophisticated systems with numerous automated functions that, after checking for conflicts and hazards, automatically schedule at appropriate times. They record examination-specific material, notify relevant action centers in the department, produce forms, allocate resources, and create pull notices to retrieve previous studies from film libraries, or implement archive retrieval procedures for PACS storage systems.

Patient Tracking

The patient tracking module follows each patient from arrival to departmental discharge, showing at any moment where the patient is and how close the examination is to being completed. Often technical factors, number and type of views acquired, and other operational and resource use data are coincidentally collected.

Film Libraries

Film libraries are notoriously complicated and difficult to control. These are the centers of coordination for all medically important patient information. Not only are all images, past and present, retrieved, matched, sometimes duplicated, distributed, loaned and recovered, stored, and perhaps displayed; but also associated information that may include demographics, clinical findings, work up consultations, formal interpretations, codes, and follow up with quality assurance (Q/A) information must be assembled together with the images. Film libraries collect and link the record elements that fully informed radiologists should have at their fingertips in order to perform the highest quality professional work. It is convenient to think of these image and information items as the selective clinical radiology information package (SCRIP) (Shannon, 1989). As each item is created, it ideally should be integrated into the SCRIP. Because material is acquired during the sequence of work up, examination, interpretation, decision, and follow-up, the professional user would never receive less than the current SCRIP with which to work.

Reporting

The notion of clinical information packages naturally leads to consideration of the classic end point of diagnostic radiology—the written report of the radiologist's findings and interpretation. In traditional manual operations, the report is typed on the requisition form, thereby retaining whatever demographic and clinical information has been entered by the requester. With the advent of electronic systems, many combinations of automated and manual functions were implemented. Independent word processors gained popularity early. Some of these used the submitted paper requisitions, just as did typewriter operations. Others used continuous forms requiring that information on the requisition be reentered. As medical information networks have proliferated, it has become clear that work volume and error rates rise if identical information must be entered more than once.

To take advantage of source entry and to ensure continuity of patient data, it has been advantageous to interface various information systems throughout the hospital or medical complex. Possible sources of demographic and clinical information for a radiology reporting terminal include the HIS and the RIS into which patient information has already been deposited.

Early RISs lacked the power to support word processing without unacceptable slowing of the entire RIS response time. However, modern systems include good word processing modules and often provide electronic means of distributing reports to wards or other remote request sites. Through a variety of means, progressively more complex and satisfactory integration of functional modules, like word processing, with departmental and hospital-wide systems is becoming commonplace. More sophisticated reporting has been followed by such ancillary functions as communication with billing systems, case coding, interesting case cataloguing, and capture of departmental management data.

One solid entry into the clinical arena during the past several years is speech recognition for reporting. Systems of the late 1980s (Robbins et. al., 1988) have been considerably improved and are in regular clinical use. These are interfaced in some cases with the hospital information systems.

Management

The final basic RIS module deals with management information. These modules vary widely in their sophistication, but usually provide examination volume and distribution, resource utilization, statistics on timeliness of important functions, and financial information to including revenues. Sorting of reports by source, referring physician, or interpreter can be used in support of quality improvement and privileging requirements.

These six functions—registration of patients, scheduling, patient tracking, film library management, reporting of results, and department management—together with electronic mail, constitute the basic RIS.

Picture Archiving and Communications Systems (PACS)

As RISs have matured in response to the growing need to keep track of materials and events and to manage written records, PACS have been evolving from somewhat different roots. However, both types of system appear to be converging on membership in an integrated multimedia information complex that will be a seamless combination of specialized medical devices and computer-based utilities.

One origin of image management systems can be found in the increasing use of digital acquisition devices, which have demanded that systems be developed to store, manipulate, and communicate electronic images throughout the radiology department and a growing variety of other sections of the medical community. A second origin of image management is found in the development of multimedia HIS (Dayhoff et al., 1992). These have been important for distribution of images and for integration of the medical record. PACS, however, are highly specific to and the major interest of radiology. PACS and electronic imaging devices are an inseparable combination that has become recognized as an integral and essential component of the coming computer-based communications environment on which health care of the future will rely. PACS will do a number of interesting things that derive from antecedent image acquisition systems.

Image Manipulation

In a sense, individual digital imaging devices like CT have always embraced the rudimentary functions of PACS. Computer-generated images are displayed on television-like CRTs where they can be manipulated and altered in a variety of ways. For instance, one can adjust exposures or choose only a portion of the full range of exposure and expand it to examine the segment in detail. Edges can be sharpened, or black and white can be reversed to produce a negative image. Future possibilities seem endless. Some will be important new diagnostic tools, others will prove merely curiosities. Display stations foreshadowed the full blown PACS workstations entering the workplace today.

Communication

Frequently, a second display station that communicates with the main viewing device can be found in a nearby room, allowing monitored image acquisition to continue while previous examinations are reviewed simultaneously at the second site. These multiple viewer configurations constitute rudimentary communication systems, a second element of PACS.

Archiving

Image storage, or archiving (a third element of PACS), has been achieved with magnetic discs in display stations in order to provide rapid retrieval of a limited number of active cases or with magnetic tape for longer-term retention of images that did not need to be so accessible. Although these images are fully manageable electronically, convention, an initial need for portability, diminishing but real technological limitations, and a cautious approach to new methods have resulted in recording these same images, for interpretation and storage, on film. The practice is redundant and expensive, and is becoming ever less justifiable in the face of competitive cost for quality electronic images. As the number and types of individual digital acquisition devices have increased, and as more complex and expensive storage technology, such as optical discs, has become available, sharing of support devices and expectation of easier access to images at distributed sites have been natural consequences. PACS consolidate these functions for entire departments.

Computed Radiography

With the recent development of reusable, electronically scanned media to replace conventional film radiography, transfer from an environment of physical records to one of total electronic management has much appeal. With this filmless process, images need never be inaccessible or lost. Records can be organized and combined in the best manner to suit a clinical need, and they can be used simultaneously at different sites served by institution-wide networks. Retrieval time is minimized, and one can perform a wide variety of image adjustments and manipulations not possible with film. Furthermore, a redundant system duplicating electronic and film images is expensive, making the transfer to a filmless system economically as well as functionally attractive to many PACS proponents.

Transition

In spite of pressures to transfer from film to digital electronics, PACS have encountered some resistance from the workplace for several reasons. First, properly exposed and developed films are very good (Vizy, 1989). Second, the ever active tendency for people to avoid change generates resistance that is in part justified by the knowledge that to learn even the best of new ways requires a period of degraded performance until the old skills are sufficiently supplanted by the new. Third, until recently there was not a fully developed filmless medical practice environment, but PACS have advanced to a point where the quality of patient care can be protected, and several filmless hospitals or departments exist or are in the process of implementation. In the meantime, sections of PACS—certain storage devices, simple work stations, image transmission networks, etc.—are also entering the market and seeing clinical use.

Finally, the economics and best strategy of transition is still not clear, but much is being learned from the pioneer installations. Although costs will likely be greater than hindsight will indicate they might have been, evidence suggests that once the transition to filmless departments has been accomplished, costs of the new image support systems will be competitive with the old (Seshadri et al., 1988). The transition will require the addition of a well-developed program for technology assessment (T/A) and a strategy for dealing with human factors, operations, and economics. The fairly recently recognized need for "technology management" will become of major importance (see Management Issues later in this chapter).

Technology Assessment

The problem of assessing whether or not a technology accomplishes what it is purported to do is relatively simple. To detect its unforeseen effects, particularly those that are indirect, is more difficult. Replacement economics also can be microcosted and adequately compared. Here, too, the indirect economic effects are more elusive. Perhaps the most difficult, but in the last analysis most important, is the assessment of a technology in terms of its impact on outcome of care to the patient (Lohr, 1988). This concept of technology validation in terms of the quality of results has achieved general recognition only recently. Support technology is particularly difficult to assess in this manner because, unlike the direction connection between the patient and individual tests and treatments, the effects of support technology are mediated through many channels, and, therefore, are more general and stochastically more subtle (Shannon & Allman, 1988).

PACS in diagnostic radiology, as currently conceived and segmentally implemented, consist of shared digital storage devices, communications networks ranging from local connections to wide area use of satellites, workstations for image manipulation and display, and well-managed databases for facile handling of images and associated information. The conception is intriguing, but the future holds more.

The Future

Even as PACS mature, a vision is developing that will serve as the organizing principle for information systems. PACS will become integrated with the other forms of information systems in the healthcare setting. There will be qualitative enhancements of their functionality. And management concepts regarding information systems will become better understood and implemented in sophisticated ways.

Integration

Many current systems are converging toward a synthesis through which they will become powerfully synergistic in an integrated, computer-supported information environment that recognizes the whole patient.

Technical Integration

Systems are coming together in three ways. First, now separate systems with similar functional characteristics will be intricately interfaced. Personal computers and their workstation cousins will interact with departmental systems. These in turn will communicate with HIS and the last will participate in still wider area networks that reach out to other offices and institutions with much the same ease as telephone and telefax systems. Particularly influential in development of wide area support are the progressing activities generated by the High Performance Computing Act of 1991 written by the then Senator Gore (Lindberg, 1994). Ten federal agencies participate in the High Performance Computing and Communication Program (HPCC). In 1993, legislation called for a National Information Infrastructure (NII) that would influence not only networks but the enhancement of functionality to be discussed below in the section on Functional Enhancements. Second, standards developments of the last several years have been encouraging in providing a basis for *open systems.* By opening systems, integrators are supported in combining diverse technologies and multiple vendors in seamless harmony. A third trend that is well established in the PC market is multimodality computing. We can expect to see a growing application of these techniques of bringing together symbols, images, and voice in professional settings (Schramm & Goldberg, 1989).

Domain Integration

The second type of system convergence involves systems that are functionally separated because they address different application domains rather than having similar domains but different developmental origins. Ordinarily the domains, or applications, alluded to must be accessed independently, often on dedicated terminals at a limited number of sites. Literature and other reference services, decision support systems, statistics packages, and programs to do specialized analysis and graphics are examples of important functions currently inaccessible through most RIS or HIS systems.

Integration of systems in each of the described ways is beginning, but no well-developed model is yet available in a clinical setting. Integrating these systems requires research and development in cognition, linguistics, logic, and both software and hardware technology. Some of the work can be accomplished by planning and analysis, but other portions of the necessary knowledge can be gained only from experience. The path to integrated systems is neither short nor easy to travel, but it is destined to be traversed.

Clinical Integration

For diagnostic radiology, assuming that its niche in clinical practice remains substantially intact, integrated systems will provide the opportunity to enter the mainstream of practice in a way that has never been possible. The SCRIP, or information package, can be a practical reality. Participation in workup strategies, performance of examinations and interpretations with full access to relevant information, and the ability to be part of the clinical decision team will bring the full talents of the radiologist to bear on patient problems. The developed potential of radiologic diagnosis and management will contribute to maximizing the clinical efficacy of the medical team.

Functional Enhancements

Beyond the promise of integrating existing systems, there lie some promising, new functional developments.

Image Guided Surgery

Much work has been done in developing the technology necessary to fuse and reconstruct images from a wide variety of sources. Work continues and is being further encouraged by the NII program. Research has reached a point where it is feasible to impose the virtual reality of images on the reality of the human body. Fusion of different presentations of reality enable physical procedures for diagnosis and therapy that were not imaginable just a few years ago. *Image-guided surgery* describes one of the most dramatic applications of these new developments, carrying with it a promise of new levels of collaboration among now disparate specialties (Jolesz & Shtern, 1992).

Imaging Databases

A long-standing interest of many in being able to develop a database of visual information has been rather well examined and set forth by an National Institutes of Health group (Zink & Jaffe, 1993). The extension of databases beyond alphanumerics promises great enrichment of the integrated environment described in the previous section. Service, research, and education should all benefit.

Intelligent Systems

PACS have crossed the watershed to prove the feasibility of the "filmless" hospital. The contribution to image and information management is immense, but success in implementation immediately shifts the focus to improving operations. The application of techniques of "computer intelligence" to operations and image presentation is underway (Stewart, 1994).

Management Issues

The notion that information systems are incidental to the real business of healthcare delivery must be replaced by full understanding that an integrated information system is a pervasive system, but also that it seamlessly insinuates most of the operations in the healthcare environment. On one hand, a managerial understanding of the full system will be necessary. On the other hand, because of its complex relationship to operations, different portions of the information system necessarily have different significance and different roles in relation to human affairs and responsibilities. These differences have implications for "ownership," management, funding, development and maintenance priority, and legal and regulatory status. For example, PACS in radiology are an essential element of the functions through which the radiologist fulfills his or her primary responsibility. The PACS role in this sense is qualitatively different from its utility function of remote image distribution. The latter function is more nearly like that of the telephone. If these differences are trivialized or ignored, managerial headaches will be legion (Shannon & Allman, 1992).

Conclusion

Diagnostic radiology is currently so specialized and complex that it has become significantly differentiated from the mainstream of medical practice. Both the practice and the management of diagnostic radiology are too complicated to function properly with manual methods. RIS have provided excellent assistance with organization, monitoring, and communication. PACS are emerging as a byproduct of digital imaging modalities and are becoming support systems of importance in their own right. The "filmless hospital" has been demonstrated as a model for the future. Integration of computer-driven information systems is now recognized as a general need of medical practice. Integration of RIS with PACS is receiving much attention. More recently, general recognition that the RIS/PACS combination must be folded into hospital information systems with access to other information domains has become established (Shannon, 1989; Stewart, 1994). This technology, of proven value to patient outcome, can restore and enhance the patient's confidence in medical organizations. This will be an accomplishment of great importance as this nation embraces the notion of managed care. At the center of the medical complex, however, imaging will remain a critical contributor to patient welfare.

Questions

1. What are the major components of computer support systems in diagnostic radiology? Include major system interfaces.
2. What are the components of the clinical radiology information package (SCRIP), and what is the source of each? How can we expect it to be enhanced in the future?
3. How would the SCRIP be assembled and maintained in a film-based system? In a filmless, digital electronic department?
4. As a radiology manager, what would be your prioritized list and the rationale for choosing which information system segments and interfaces to install? As a medical center manager, how would your list and rationale change? Do the lists conflict significantly?

References

Best, D.E., Horii, S.C., Bennett, W., & Parisot, C. (1992). Update of the ACR-NEMA digital imating and communications in medicine standard. *SPIE Medical Imaging VI: PACS Design and Evaluation, 1654,* 356–360.

Dayhoff, R.E., Maloney D.L., Kenney J.T., & Fletcher, R.D. (1992). Providing an integrated clinical data view in a hospital information system that manages multimedia data. In: P.D. Clayton (Ed.), *Fifteenth annual symposium on computer applications in medical care* (pp. 501–505). New York: McGraw-Hill.

Grobstein, C. (1973). Hierarchical order and neogenesis. In *Hierarchy theory: The challenge of complex systems* H.H. Pattee (Ed.), New York: George Braziller.

Hounsfield, G.N. (1972). A method of and apparatus for examination of a body by radiation such as x or gamma radiation. Patent specification 1283915. London.

Jolesz, F.J., & Shtern, F. (1992). The operating room of the future. Report of the National Cancer Institute Workshop, "Imaging-guided stereotactic tumor diagnosis and treatment." *Investigative Radiology, 27,* 326–328.

Lindberg, D.A.B. (1994). Global information infrastructure. *International Journal of Bio-Medical Computing, 34*(1–4), 13–19.

Lodwick, G.S. (1986). Radiology systems of the 1990s—meeting the challenge of change. *The Western Journal of Medicine, 145,* 848–852.

Lohr, K.N. (1988). Quality of care and technology assessment, R.A. Rettig (Ed.). Washington, DC: Institute of Medicine, National Academy Press.

Megargle, R. (1989). The healthcare information standards coordinating committee. In W.E. Hammond (Ed.), *Proceedings of the AAMSI Congress 7* (pp. 400–402). Washington, DC: AAMSI.

Robbins, A.H., Vincent, M.E., Shaffer, K., Maietta, R., & Srinivasan, M.K. (1988). Radiology reports: Assessment of a 5,000 word speech recognizer. *Radiology, 167,* 853–855.

Saarinen, A.O., Haynor, D.R., Loop, J.W., Johnson, L., Russell, J., Mitchell, K., & Nemerever, M. (1989). Modeling the economics of PACS: What is important? In R.H. Schneider, S.J. Dwyer, & G. Jost (Eds.), *Medical imaging III—PACS system design and evaluation 1093* (pp. 62–73). Bellingham, WA: SPIE, International Society for Optical Engineering.

Schramm, C., & Goldberg, M. (1989). Multimedia radiological reports: Creation and playback. *Journal of Digital Imaging, 2,* 106–113.

Seshadri, S.B., Arenson, R.L., DeSimone, D., & Hiss, S. (1988). Cost-savings associated with a digital radiology department: a preliminary study. In R.L. Arenson (Ed.), *Proceedings of the Ninth Conference on Computer Applications in Radiology.* Philadelphia: RISC.

Shannon, R.H. (1989). IMACS and radiology: Defining the problems. In S.K. Mun, M. Greberman, W.R. Hendee, & R.H. Shannon (Eds.), *Proceedings of the First International Conference on Image Management and Communication.* New York: IEEE.

Shannon, R.H. (1991). Computer enhanced radiology: A transformation to imaging. In: M.J. Ball, J.V. Douglas, R.I. O'Desky, & J.W. Albright (Eds.), *Healthcare Information Management Systems* (p. 85). New York: Springer-Verlag.

Shannon, R.H., & Allman, R.A. (1988). Technology assessment using an informatics framework for medical imaging. In R.L. Arenson (Ed.), *Proceedings of the Ninth Conference on Computer Applications in Radiology.* Philadelphia: RISC.

Shannon, R.H., & Allman, R.A. (1992). Picture archiving and communication systems (PACS): A medical device. In W.R. Brody & G.S. Johnston (Eds.), *Computer applications to assist radiology. Proceedings of the Society for Computer Applications in Radiology (SCAR).* Symposia Foundation, pp. 48–54.

Stewart, B.K. (1994, June). Next-generation PACS focus on intelligence. *Diagnostic Imaging,* pp. 81–84.

Vizy, K.N. (1989). The roles of film in an increasingly computerized world. *Investigative Radiology, 24,* 503–506.

Zink, S., & Jaffe, C.C. (1993). Medical imaging databases. A National Institutes of Health Workshop. *Investigative Radiology, 28,* 366–372.

Unit 8
Developing and Purchasing Expertise

Unit Introduction

A changing environment demands new expertise, and new tools require new skills. One way of addressing such needs is through training; such training can be on personal productivity tools or on systems. Yet another way is through retaining consultants. Administrators, including chief information officers, understanding how consultants work, bring their efforts in line with information systems plans, and manage them once on board.

For Hales, the computer is a personal productivity tool for healthcare executives. Literacy begins with self-assessment. After describing different types of training and offering rules of thumb, Hales reviews applications of interest to executives, from windows and spreadsheets to networks and decision support software.

According to Marr, the training of users should be as advanced as the systems themselves. Based on adult learning theory, training is offered via computer-based interactive learning modules; quality control targets accuracy, timeliness, and completeness. Seasoned users have special needs and can serve as change agents.

Childs offers insights into the healthcare consulting marketplace, projected to reach $600 million by the year 2000. Firms occupy distinct niches and cultures. A minisurvey shows that hospital administrators have an improved perception of consultants since 1991. Still, organizations must buy into using consultants and work at educating them.

Concordia reviews how consulting firms work, what services they provide, and what functions they are often retained to perform. To derive the most value from consultants, organizations must manage the process; definition of tasks, dates, and cost is critical.

One of the roles of the chief information officer (CIO), according to Marley, is to be a prudent buyer of consulting services. The CIO must align need and resources, identify risks, and identify future needs. Selection and management are critical.

24
Computer Skills Needed by Healthcare Executives

JOSEPH W. HALES

In anticipation of health reform in the 1990s, the business of health care is rapidly changing. These changes are pushing hospitals toward even smaller operating margins than resulted from the introduction of prospective payment in the 1980s. In order to remain viable, hospitals and other healthcare organizations must focus on the business of business. The collection and manipulation of the data required for sound decision making are growing increasingly complex. Even though the number of hospital beds is shrinking, many healthcare organizations are expanding as they attempt to increase their referral base and their market share. This expansion is leading to a greater need for data and the ability to process those data. For example, the information that forms the basis for a managed care contract or the purchase of an office practice cannot reasonably be derived in a competitive market from estimates or insufficient data.

Historically the business side of a hospital, or any healthcare enterprise, has relied on information systems for much of the input to the decision process. However, financial systems today often lack key information required for business decisions. Clinical and departmental information systems now provide vital information regarding case mix, staffing and workload, and efficiency. Even as the demand for information is increasing, the growing use of increasingly sophisticated clinical systems means the amount of information available is nearly overwhelming. Without adequate experience or training, it is easy to be inundated by, and unable to process, data that are now available. Further, poor planning can leave an institution without easy access to information it is already collecting or without access to information altogether.

Personal Computing Literacy

In the midst of a need for still more data, healthcare executives are left to find a path through the morass created by too much data. This path requires a rudimentary understanding of what computers can do for an institution (i.e., what is possible), in what time frame it can be done, and at what expense.

Not entirely independent from the literacy required to make decisions relative to institutional computing is the need to understand what the computer can do for an individual executive as a personal productivity tool (Harlan & Magraw, 1991). The latter category may build upon detailed technical expertise that is part of the former: networking, operating systems, databases. At the least, today it must include an operational understanding of personal computers. This chapter addresses the issue of skills required to make the computer *a tool to improve personal productivity.*

Specifically, this chapter focuses on desktop personal computing (e.g., IBM PC compatible and Apple Macintosh computers), identifying what skills are important, and what steps are required to obtain these skills. Additionally, the chapter considers the value of obtaining these skills. It is important to note that the skills and techniques discussed here are not limited to desktop microcomputers. Some tasks may require more powerful computers or databases that reside on a mini- or mainframe computer. The key to personal computing literacy is to develop a strategy to

- Identify the need to turn to the computer, and
- Assemble the necessary resources in terms of data and programs to manipulate the data.

Self-Assessment

An important first step in developing personal computing literacy is for the executive to assess his or her knowledge of the computer. Unfortunately, there is no simple test to assess personal computing literacy. Even if such a test existed, the healthcare executive is further challenged by the number of things that can be learned about personal computing. Therefore, a second step in self-assessment is to determine what of all that can be known needs to be known about personal computing. Unfortunately, there is no simple test for this either. It is essentially impossible to predict what a given healthcare executive does not now know, or what that executive will need to know soon. However, it may well be possible to establish a framework that will form the basis for what can (and perhaps must) be learned about personal computing.

One possible approach to assessing where to begin is to look at other executives and ask, "What are they able to do with the computer that I should be able to do?" It may be helpful to identify small clerical tasks that are repeated frequently or are tedious. These tasks are ideal candidates for automation through computerization. Further, by answering this question, the executive specifically identifies a manageable step, a goal, that can become the focus of reducing personal computing illiteracy.

The example stated is only one way for the executive to start assessing her personal computing literacy. In the end, the executive needs to be able to determine

- What the computer can do for her, and
- What must be learned to make the computer do it.

Knowing what can be done, what is possible, may be as important as knowing how. The remainder of this chapter provides an overview of the ways the computer can make the executive more productive. The level of skill or understanding the executive desires may not require learning all that is suggested in this chapter. However, he should be able to make that decision deliberately and with a knowledge of what is possible.

A final thought: once an initial self-assessment is done, it is important to conduct periodic reassessments. Dramatic changes have occurred since the personal computer was introduced by IBM in 1982 or the first Macintosh was introduced by Apple in 1984. In 1982, an IBM PC with one 360-kilobyte floppy disk drive, 256 kilobytes of memory, and a monochrome monitor cost nearly $5,000 (Williams, 1982). Today, an 11-ounce handheld computer of similar capacity (Andrews & Reinhardt, 1991) can be purchased for less than $700. Similar but more accelerated changes are anticipated in the next decade. Frequent reassessment and redefinition of computing literacy will be required in order to keep pace with the changing environment.

Areas of Knowledge

Computer literacy can be divided into three specific areas: hardware, operating system, and application programs. The first two areas can be problematic. For many users, literacy extends only so far as to answering the question, "What kind do I have?" Still others may use computers daily without knowing what type of "Intel inside" they have. This lack of understanding can lead to frustrating hours lost trying to make a computer work. Unfortunately, however, many problems with hardware and software require a level of experience or training that the average computer user would seldom use and quickly forget.

Hardware

Computer hardware typically refers to the chassis, the monitor or display, and the keyboard. The chassis contains the central processing unit (CPU), the brain of the computer. The chassis also contains memory: both high-speed, volatile (requires electricity in order to retain its contents) random access memory (RAM) and nonvolatile, magnetic disk memory. The chassis typically contains expansion slots that provide electrical circuit connections from generic connectors to the CPU. The most common hardware expansions include modems (for communication with other computers over phone lines) and network interfaces (for communication with other computers over dedicated wiring). Hardware may also include a pointing device, such as a mouse, and one or more removable disk devices, such as a floppy disk drive or CD-ROM (compact disk-read only memory) drive.

Operating System

The operating system is a program that controls the way application programs (like a word processing program) interact with the hardware. When a computer is turned on, the operating system is copied into RAM memory from the more permanent disk memory. The operating system worries about differences in types and sizes of RAM, disk memory, while displaying and providing a uniform interface to which application programs can refer. (Otherwise, application programs would have to be much more complex in order to accommodate the variety.)

Having established the basis of the hardware and operating system, the remainder of the chapter will consider only the variety of application programs that make the computer useful.

Training and Education

A variety of methods is available to the executive for learning about the computer itself. Today computer training is a burgeoning field. There has been rapid growth in professional courses and seminars, video and computer-based instruction, as well as books and audio tapes. These methods cater to the needs across the spectrum from novice to advanced user and cover the gamut of topics including introduction to the computer, computer hardware, operating system basics, and training in specific application programs.

Professional Training

One of the quicker ways to learn about the computer is through professionally prepared and administered computer training courses. These courses are offered at many community colleges, universities, public libraries, or computer stores. In fact, many institutions may have a computer training program. Training courses typically include hands-on instruction at the computer and assignments that are relevant to the executive's work. Professional instruction has the added advantage of providing interaction with a knowledgeable instructor.

Despite their advantages, structured courses may not move at the right pace or may cover material that is too elementary or too advanced—and may be the most expensive method. It may be difficult for the executive to assess in advance how well a course meets his needs. Additionally, the busy executive may not have enough time to commit to structured courses. However, in such cases, it may be possible to arrange for personal instruction. Finally, professional training may not be available in smaller communities.

Television and Video

Similar to professional training courses are video and television instruction. One public television offering covers specific application programs with step-by-step examples. A wide variety of video instruction programs is available covering computer basics and specific application programs. These methods provide the same detailed instruction by professionals as do courses. Other advantages of television and video include convenience and the self-paced nature of the instruction. Additionally, for the executive who does not have easy access to training opportunities, video instruction programs can be ordered by mail.

Books

Books offer even greater flexibility for self-paced learning than the methods considered thus far. The growth of the computer industry has been paralleled by a tremendous increase in the number of books that teach how to use computers and software applications. These books, many of which are now available at chain book outlets, attempt to cover the spectrum of users (most recently the ". . . For Dummies" series). Many publishers clearly label the target audience as novice, beginner, or "power user" or list the books as tutorial or reference in nature. The executive may easily be overwhelmed by the number of books on a single topic and by the size of the books themselves. Browsing is recommended. Many of the books often are also available from the local library. The executive should select a book that moves at a comfortable pace and is structured in a helpful way.

Application Software Tutorials

A final method to consider is the tutorial program that may be included with application software. Along with their application software, many commercial vendors (e.g., Microsoft, Borland, Novell) provide computer-aided instructional programs. These tutorials introduce the user to basic functions of the software through step-by-step instructions. As with books and videos, tutorials are self-paced and can be reviewed many times. Additionally, tutorial programs may be linked to functions within the software so that they can be called up and reviewed while running the application program. Finally, tutorials are free with the application software.

A wide variety of methods is available for training and instruction. All of these methods may be affected by accessibility and cost. The executive in a small community, without access to a wide selection of books or software, should be able to find training and instructional materials through mail order companies.

Rules of Thumb

The executive will see that ultimately, most instructional methods rely on an ability to teach oneself. The following are five rules of thumb to help guide the executive develop strategies for self instruction.

1. Familiarize yourself with an application. Browse or read the entire reference manual at a sufficient level of detail to understand what can and cannot be done with the software.
2. Identify a local guru. Selection of software may be guided by what everyone else is using. Choose something recommended by someone whose computer knowledge can be trusted. Ask this person if the software can accomplish specific tasks you need to accomplish. Find someone that can be consulted when really stuck.
3. Tackle a task that needs to be completed and requires the skills you are attempting to develop. Let the press of time drive the need to learn something that you may not otherwise find time to do. Be sure to give yourself enough time to accomplish the task, including extra time for learning more about the program. The payoff will come the next time you face the same task and are able to use the new found skills.
4. Make small contributions over time. Do not attempt to learn an entire program at once. However, having learned what the program is capable of (step 1, above), invest the time as the need arises (step 3, above) in learning a new feature that you don't already know how to use.
5. Avoid the temptation to memorize "the keystrokes." Instead, try to learn the process (the way the software "behaves") and the functions of the software that support the process. Without this understanding, a step-by-step list of keystrokes becomes meaningless if misread or if the context changes.

When Do I Know Enough?

In the end, time spent in computer training should be considered an investment and, consequently, managed like an investment. The executive should assess what will be the return on investment, not only short term, but long term. That investment should be balanced with what the executive must do personally and what can be delegated to others. This balance is changing. Computer literacy can be considered a competitive advantage because of its ability to "make you look good." For example, the literate executive can use a presentation graphics program to update a slide or an overhead transparency after hours, rather than wait for the assistance the next day. This capability can make a difference today. Increasingly, computer literacy must be considered a competitive necessity, not just an advantage. No longer does the executive have the freedom to ignore what the computer can do to make him or her "look good." Soon, the administrator who does not know how to use a computer will be a liability.

Application Software Programs

The remainder of this chapter addresses the second aspect of computer literacy by describing basic software tools. The computer is a tool for processing information, information required for daily business decision making. Various generalized application programs are available to the executive to assist in information processing, including spreadsheets, word processors, presentation graphics packages, database management systems, and electronic mail. These tools are described in some detail, and their capabilities are outlined.

Window Environments

Before the executive can even begin to use an application program, she will likely encounter the windowed operating environment (e.g., Apple System Software or Microsoft Windows). Because application programs for a window environment are designed to have similar visual characteristics and similar methods for performing basic functions, skills learned in one should be easily transferred to other. Whether using the Apple Macintosh or IBM-compatible personal computer, the executive should obtain a basic understanding of how to navigate in the windowed environment.

Necessary skills include an understanding of how to start an application program, how to open and how to save a file used by an application, and how to move about within an application. Additionally, the executive should know how to manipulate the command menus found in windows programs and provide information required to complete a task through use of "dialog boxes." More advanced skills such as working with more than one application program at a time or using keystrokes in place of mouse functions may make some tasks easier, but represent a reasonable boundary where not every executive need tread.

Spreadsheets

Perhaps the most useful software application for the executive is the spreadsheet. Electronic spreadsheets, such as Lotus 1-2-3, Excel, or Quattro Pro, permit the creation of electronic ledgers. Spreadsheets use mathematical formulas (in addition to exact figures) so that calculations do not need to be repeated and minor changes in one value automatically spread throughout a complex calculation.

Spreadsheet software also provides graphical presentation of numerical data, such as pie charts and line and bar graphs. As with formulas, graphics are updated automatically as a result of changes to values or formulas. More advanced spreadsheet features include "what if?" functions for decision making based on a range of values. Spreadsheet programs can also be used as simple databases. Data arranged in rows of entries with fields or properties arranged in columns can be sorted or filtered by their properties.

The executive should understand enough about spreadsheets to be able to find sums of a large number of figures and to be able to use simple functions for summing and averaging in place of adding machine calculations. The executive also should understand enough to be able to turn simple numerical data into basic graphical representations, such as bar or pie charts.

Word Processors

The next most important tool is likely the word processor. Because of the inherent ability to edit a document without printing it, programs such as Word, WordPerfect, MacWrite, and Ami Pro have nearly replaced the typewriter. Editable versions of documents, drafts, and frequently used letters can be kept for easy changes.

More sophisticated word processing functions permit merging of boilerplate text with personalized information, such as name and address. (This feature is often referred to as mail merge.) Many word processors also permit inclusion of graphic images and automatic formatting for footnotes, footers, and tables. Laser printers enhance the value of word processing with professional looking output.

Although word processing software may behave like an online typewriter, the executive will do well to learn the differences between word processing and typing. Perhaps the most important difference is that the word processing software controls the margins and new lines. The executive should understand how to use tabs, indentions, and automatic word wrapping to obtain a desired format rather than use spaces or the return key. If a document formatted using spaces and forced new lines is reformatted, the spaces and new lines may make the text appear irregularly formatted. Of course, every smart executive will learn how to use the spelling check feature found in most word processors and the grammatical check feature found in many.

Presentation Graphics

A large portion of an administrator's time is spent in making presentations. Today a number of presentation graphic tools provide support for electronic composition of presentations. These programs, such as PowerPoint, Persuasion, WordPerfect Presentations, and Harvard Graphics, provide simple templates for text-oriented information (titles, bulleted lists) and tools for creating graphic images. Many presentation graphic programs support output to a variety of formats, including kiosk-style computer display and 35mm slides. Increasingly more common are presentations with full stereo sound and animation made directly from the PC through use of special projection of the computer output.

The executive should know not only how to create simple text presentations but also how to print them. As with word processing, the executive should have confidence in her ability to turn hours of hard work on a presentation into usable hard copy, particularly on short notice and under pressure. This type of understanding comes mostly with experience.

Database Management

The fourth category of application programs is the database management system. A database management system provides tools for building and maintaining databases. In its simplest form, a database can be thought of as an electronic rolodex. However, most commercial database management systems provide mechanisms for very sophisticated databases, such as, for example, an inventory control system that links inventory to product to vendor accounts. Further, database management systems include tools for creating forms for entry of data and for formatting reports of data contained in the database.

In many cases, spreadsheets provide satisfactory database-like functions. However, as the amount of data grows, spreadsheets become too slow and cumbersome. The trade-off is that database programs often require more significant investment of time to learn and get started and may involve more effort to create something that can be used. Database applications include dBase IV, FoxPro, Access, and Fourth Dimension.

As the amount of data processed increases, executives turn increasingly to the use of database management systems. Formerly, executives could look to a technical assistant to set up a database for them. This, however, required that the structure of the data be relatively stable over time. Today, data are much more dynamic and often need to be analyzed in different formats. The executive that has an understanding of how to use a database management system to create a database and his own custom reports will have much greater control over his information processing.

Additionally, the executive who understands how to transfer data from another outside system to her database management system will be able to take much greater advantage of the wealth of data that already exist in other information systems. Much of the data that may be needed for critical decisions likely exists in an electronic form, but must be transferred from some other information system to the executive's personal computer for analysis. Formerly, if the data were available at all, the data processing department prepared the analysis of the data. Today, these data can be analyzed much more quickly if the executive knows how to move information from institutional information systems to her personal computer and how to manipulate it using a database management program.

Networks

The tools mentioned to this point all stand alone in that they can be run from a single computer and can be considered entirely self-contained. This means that all of the information may be carried around in a single laptop or notebook computer. However, the ability to share data is becoming increasingly more important. This need to share leads to the concept of network computing wherein computers are physically connected and able to communicate.

Having made the jump to the network, a new tool emerges that is growing in importance and popularity in the corporate culture—e-mail is the electronic transmission of messages between two computers attached to the same network. Many e-mail systems permit attachment of word processing or spreadsheet files so that work can be "mailed" to a fellow administrator. Electronic mail has the immediacy of the telephone because it is delivered immediately, although it does not require constant presence.

Many organizations have become highly dependent on electronic mail. In this type of environment, the executive should be as aware of the psychosocial factors of the medium as of any feature of the mail software. For example, electronic mail is not typically treated with as much formality as written hard copy communication. Spelling and grammatical errors are not only tolerated, but it is considered bad form to make note of them.

Many important social cues are absent in electronic communications. Lacking the verbal inflections, facial expressions, or the body language of personal or phone contact, an electronic message may be entirely misunderstood. Moreover, research has shown that many e-mail users are emboldened by the sense of anonymity resulting from the fact that they are not observed or immediately questioned, as in conversation. Thus, the executive must be cautious of the tone and intent of electronic communications.

Integrated Software

The software application programs described represent powerful additions to the arsenal of the administrator, either as personal tools or tools for the executive's assistant. However, today much of the power of these tools comes from the synergy of using them together. Already mentioned is the ability to send draft documents in the form of a word processing file or draft budgets in the form of a spreadsheet file to colleagues on Email. However, many of the applications described work together to create more powerful tools. Word processors now support tabular presentations that can be linked to spreadsheets. As the spreadsheet is updated, the contents of the table in the document are updated. In order to emphasize this interactive power, many of the applications are now marketed as bundled application or office productivity "suites." Advances in technology like MicroSoft's Object Linking and Embedding (OLE) and Apple's Publisher/Subscriber promise to enhance the interactivity of applications even further.

Decision Support Systems

One class of application has yet to be considered: decision support programs. As the use of computers in healthcare administration grows, so do niche applications. There are available specialized decision support systems. These systems may offer ease of use, functionality, or integration of functions not available through the combination of off-the-shelf application programs. The market for decision support tools is still maturing, and recently decision support applications have emerged in the healthcare market. It is important to recognize that these systems do not function in the absence of data and are often constrained to the preconceived questions and formats of their designers. The executive should consider carefully what she wants to accomplish and how the data required by these information systems will get into the decision support program.

Conclusion

The goal of becoming computer literate may seem overwhelming. No single book or chapter can describe all that needs to be known about personal computers. However, the executive can become literate by developing a personal strategy for obtaining, one step at a time, the knowledge of the computing tools at his/her disposal.

Questions

1. Discuss the role of self-assessment in developing and evaluating computer literacy.
2. Identify three different technology-based sources of information available to the executive for professional training.
3. Review the five rules of thumb for developing computer literacy.
4. List and describe briefly the capabilities of three or more software applications.
5. In your opinion, is the computer now a *required* personal productivity tool for the healthcare executive?

References

Andrews, D., & Reinhardt A. (1991). A PC & 1-2-3 in the palm of your hand. *Byte, 16,* 44–46.

Harlen, K.J., & Magraw, T.W. (1991). Computer literacy: An advantage to the administrator. In M.J. Ball, J.V. Douglas, R.I. O'Desky, & J.W. Albright (Eds.), *Healthcare information management systems: A practical guide* (pp. 173–177). New York: Springer-Verlag.

Williams G. (1982). A closer look at the IBM personal computer. *Byte, 7,* 36–68.

25
Technology-Assisted Training for the Clinical Nurse

PATSY B. MARR

To become part of a technologically advanced medical environment, nurses must master the new skills required to manage the computerized clinical information system. In most cases, nurses either have not used such systems before or have had minimal exposure to them. Yet nursing effectiveness is directly related to the speed and accuracy nurses bring to this core communications vehicle. The assimilation of nurses into the culture of the computer is essential not only to patient care but also to the well being of the caregivers themselves.

Understandably, many people approach new technology with apprehension. Any training program designed to help nurses learn to use a clinical information system must therefore be positive, based on sound adult learning theory and appropriate goal setting. The learning environment must encourage openness and self-pacing.

Nurses need to emerge from training with a grasp of the basics and an enthusiasm for learning more once they are back in the clinical setting. Further, nurses need to be sensitized to the issues of patient confidentiality, password security, and quality control. When fully experienced with such systems, nurses can become part of the change process itself, helping to enhance the use of such technology. In short, the training of system users needs to be as advanced as the system itself.

Training Theory

A sound training program is based on adult learning theories. Foremost among these concepts is that adults want to participate in their own learning process and want to help shape their own goals. Other considerations in designing the program are that adults want to learn in order to meet work needs and that they tend to relate new information to relevant experiences (O'Conner, 1986).

Accordingly, in the design of a clinical information system, computerizing the manually documented nursing process will help the nurse relate the familiar to the new and different communication technology. For example, a computerized patient record can be made to resemble a sample patient record from the manual era before the system. Similarly, other items can be made to resemble their earlier counterparts, such as supply or laboratory requisitions, medication administration forms, and nursing work documents like the patient kardex or nursing unit activity report. This enables the nurse to make the connection between day-to-day unit activities and the computer as a communication tool.

Certainly the most successful training programs are computer driven, with numerous pathways from which to select the level of detail a learner needs. This ability to manage diverse data interactively on the computer itself is a recent technological development popular with the adult learner.

Training Program Goals

At the conclusion of training, nurses should have a basic understanding of the relationship of the clinical information system to the functions of their specific jobs. It is not realistic to expect them to be fully skilled upon completing the training course. That comes only with practice in the clinical area. But the training goal has been achieved if the participating nurses understand the principal functions managed by the system and the essentials of how to use those functions.

System orientation and hands-on training should occur not more than two weeks before the nurses will put this learning to use on the job. Although the centralized course offers overall concepts that are reinforced through practice examples during training, it is through the daily use of the system in the clinical setting that computer skills and the finer points of system capabilities are learned. Some learning occurs through trial and error, but experienced nurses on the unit serve as the most valuable resource.

Training Environment

The ideal setting in which to learn basic computer skills is a room designed specifically for this purpose, a quiet environment with indirect lighting to prevent glare on terminal screens. A typing chair, with both back and height adjustments, is essential. The terminal is best positioned on a surface at a height that is comfortable for data entry as well as screen reading. Data entry and retrieval may be by touch screen, light pen, keyboard, or computer mouse, the small touch device with multidirectional arrows used for selecting specific functions or data.

It is helpful to have the training center both close enough to the clinical units to be convenient and separate enough to limit distractions. The right location will allow the trainer and trainee to focus on the concepts and content of the training program. A clinically trained instructor should be either in the room or readily available to answer any questions. Many hospitals have found that more questions are related to clinical content in the system than to the mechanics of using a computer.

Technology-Assisted Training

In recent years most computer training programs have moved from programmed instruction manuals to computer-based interactive learning modules. These modules present general concepts, specific examples, and immediate feedback, enabling the student to experience an environment that approaches real life. This method allows the adult learner to participate actively in the learning process at an individualized pace and provides opportunity to measure progress toward goals (O'Conner, 1986). Not only is this the method preferred by students, but it has added benefits. Institutions that have moved from programmed instruction manuals to computer-based training have reduced their training and instructor time and have improved training quality (Perez & Willis, 1989).

During the first training session the learner enters his/her name and social security number for identifying purposes. This becomes the basis of a tracking system for frequency of learner mistakes that in turn assists the computer-based training programmer in clarifying learner content. Training modules can be designed specifically for the various groups of users with the appropriate competency test. If a wrong answer is given, the module provides the right answer after the third try to prevent frustration in the learner and reinforcement of the right answer (Wedman & Stefanich, 1984). The training is self-paced and the individual can control the length of the training session based on attention span.

Internal learning processes can be triggered by using external instructional methods in a computer-based training program (Gagné, Wager, & Rojas, 1984). Some examples of these triggers are the use of color to highlight an important point for the learner, presenting the objectives at the beginning of each module to inform the learner the purpose of the exercise, and building the modules sequentially from simple to complex to allow the learner to apply prior information in proceeding through later modules. Pretests and posttests provide the learner an opportunity to assess his/her mastery of the training program. Allow the individual to review specific modules and to take the practice and review test at the conclusion of the training session as many times as desired.

Finally, it is important to create a learning atmosphere of trust, respect, and helpfulness. Nurses learn by connecting new information to past knowledge; a comfortable atmosphere allows the students freedom to express concerns, questions, or apprehensions they may have about the system (O'Conner, 1986). Training can encompass much more than the simple use of the system when nurses are taught by an experienced nurse instructor who has sophisticated clinical and organizational knowledge in addition to system expertise.

Quality Control in Training

The major areas of concern in maintaining quality control include accuracy in using a system, the timeliness of data entry, and completeness of system documentation. Depending upon the specific system, there can be predetermined program edits that prevent inaccurate or illogical data from being entered. In clinical information systems, however, the use of these edits is minimal because of information complexity. Most systems enable the user to view information as it is being collected and to correct the error at that time. Other systems offer only a final review of data immediately before entry, enabling verification and/or deletion and correction.

The importance of timely data entry is more difficult to convey to nurses than the importance of accuracy. Historically, except for medications, nurses have always charted at the end of their shifts rather than sequentially throughout the shift. With the installation of an information system, it is often expected that this will change. It seldom does. What usually happens is that whatever charting patterns existed prior to computerization are replicated when the system is installed. It is also difficult to monitor compliance with timeliness. Some systems accommodate data entry time guidelines that, when exceeded, produce management reports that can be used to help monitor timeliness. With the current trend of placing terminals at each patient bedside or in every patient room, there is some evidence that documentation is occurring at or nearer the time of the event (Marr et al., 1993).

The third area of quality control addressed in the training program is completeness of documentation. Even though the examples in the training modules emphasize documentation standards, it is daily follow-up by nursing leadership that addresses the completeness issue. This quality control item is so closely related to the standard of care delivery that only expert clinicians can do the monitoring.

Two more factors must be considered when addressing quality concerns in a training course. First, printed documentation carries a sense of finality and not-to-be-questioned accuracy. New practitioners must be specifically instructed to question a printed medical order entered by a physician just as they would a handwritten order. They should not assume that a computer-generated order is unquestionably accurate. The computer does not alter the nurse's professional obligation to question and to verify any order.

Second, new users of the clinical information system must be advised to go slowly in the system until their skills are well developed. When nurses finish the training program and begin to work with a seasoned user in the clinical setting, they often feel compelled to match the experienced user's speed. But speed will come. Training must emphasize accuracy rather than speed.

Maintaining Confidentiality

Converting the patient record from a handwritten document to a computer-generated document changes the procedures to be followed in maintaining patient confidentiality. Policy, however, does not change. The institution continues to be responsible for maintaining the confidentiality of the patient's health record.

With manually generated documents, there is only one copy of the data, located in the patient chart on the nursing unit. To access these clinical data, caregivers go to the unit and identify themselves as having approval to review and/or responsibility for caring for an individual patient. With computerized data, access is different. The information may be accessed from any terminal in the medical center. Patient records may be reviewed by any healthcare team member who has permission to access that category of data. Depending on the parameters of the user's sign-on code, a team member may be able to review data privately for any patient in the system at any given time, regardless of who is responsible for the care of that specific patient.

This makes it mandatory that users of the system never share their sign on code with anyone. Training must make it clear that each sign-on code uniquely identifies an individual to the system by name and title, gives the ability to carry out certain system functions, and provides access to patient data appropriate to the user's title and job function. It is the same as a handwritten signature, and attaches the person's name and title to all patient clinical data entered into the system. Because various groups of the healthcare team have access to this large clinical database, the professional obligation to maintain patient confidentiality must be reinforced with every individual.

Introducing Changes to Seasoned Users

Clinical information systems are never static. Drugs are added and deleted from the formulary, new radiologic procedures are developed while others become obsolete, and items obtained from central supply change with the current vendor. Because system programs have the capability to require specific information entry before the user proceeds through a given function, regulatory mandates can be met through system design. These mandates include the source of patient referral when a patient is admitted, clinical indication for doing invasive radiology procedures, and management reports for patients waiting for nursing home beds to become available.

If, in the initial design of the system, a standard protocol is followed for certain symbols and sequences of logic, then new capabilities added to the system can be readily communicated to users. Two major methods are used to inform staff of changes. The most common one is a system newsletter addressed to the affected user groups, including a description of the new function, an example of the change, and the date and time the change will become effective. The other method, which may be used in conjunction with the newsletter or as a stand alone, is to insert a message or help screen in the appropriate system module to tell users of the change they are about to encounter. This screen is left in the system only until all users have had an opportunity to become proficient in the new function, a process that usually takes two to four weeks. Only rarely is a change so complex that system instructors need to meet with users to demonstrate the added capability. An integral part of training should include information on how system changes are communicated.

Seasoned Users as Change Agents

Mature systems have seasoned users as change agents. They are a rich source of new ideas and creativity for system functions that uniquely benefit the user. Their involvement promotes system ownership, pride in contributions, and motivation for bigger and better system functionality. When this environment emerges, it must be nurtured and encouraged in order to take advantage of the added value (Marr, 1988).

Often, user committees are formed to create ideas. In most cases, the nursing committee proves to be the most dynamic in generating ideas. Nurses who are comfortable in hospital culture, knowledgeable in the practice of nursing, and skilled in the use of the system become proactive system users, not reactive users. In a real sense, such nurses become part of the institution's training and development process.

Clinical information systems are dynamic, changing communication tools. Nurses must, therefore, be students of the system, keeping abreast of its changes and even participating in them. Properly trained and actively encouraged, nurses can come to regard the system as a tool integral to their professional practice.

Questions

1. Name one or two adult learning theories that are useful in teaching nurses to master clinical information systems.
2. How soon before nurses use the computer on the job should they receive training?

3. Why is it important to have a nurse instructor available even when system training can be self-instructional?
4. What are two or three quality issues to be addressed in a clinical information system training program?
5. What is different about maintaining patient confidentiality in a computerized environment?

References

Gagné, R.M., Wager, W., & Rojas, A. (1984). Planning and authoring computer-assisted instruction lessons. In D.F. Walker & R.D. Hess (Eds.), *Instructional software: Principles and perspectives for design and use* (pp. 57–67). Belmont, CA: Wadsworth.

Marr, P.B. (1988). Successful implementation of a hospital information system. In T. Lochhaas (Ed.), *Nursing and computers; Third International Symposium on Nursing Use of Computers and Information Science* (pp. 781–786). St. Louis, MO: C.V. Mosby Company.

Marr, P.B., Duthie, E., Glassman, K.S., Janovas, D.M., Kelly, J.B., Graham, E., Kovner, C.T., Rienzi, A., Roberts, N.K., & Schick, D. (1993). Bedside terminals and quality of nursing documentation. *Computers in Nursing, 11*(4), 176–182.

O'Conner, A.B. (1986). *Nursing staff development and continuing education.* Boston: Little, Brown and Company.

Perez, L.D., & Willis, P.H. (July 1989). CBT product improves training quality at reduced cost. *Computers in Healthcare,* pp. 28–30.

Wedman, J.F., & Stefanich, G.P. (1984). Guidelines for computer-based testing of student learning of concepts, principles, and procedures. *Education Technology, 24*, 23–28.

26
Consulting in the Last Half of the 1990s

Bill W. Childs

The Marketplace

Change is the most common word of the 1990s when describing the world and our healthcare delivery system. In the last half of the 1990s and in preparation for our leap to the 21st century, again change will be the order of the day.

The president of the American Medical Association said in 1993 that "the constant change and the doubling of medical information every 3 to 5 years is placing incredible stress on our physicians and our healthcare delivery system." When one considers that a library full of everything we knew between the years 4000 B.C. and 1800 A.D. would double in size in the single century 1800 A.D. to 1900 A.D., because of the doubling of information, it boggles the mind. Add to this that information doubled again between 1900 and 1945 and again between 1945 and 1960 and then 1960 to 1970 and we are now in a doubling cycle every three to five years! Is it any wonder that we need consultants more today than we ever did before? (Figure 26-1)

Current Market Changes

"A Full Employment Act for Consultants" was the phrase often heard in 1994. The Clinton administration's declaration of a healthcare crisis and monumental changes needed sent health care into a mode of great soul searching and analysis. Consultants were called in all over the country to help figure out how we were going to look and act tomorrow. Medical and healthcare informatics were included in what needed to be done.

Add to this the frantic pace of mergers and acquisitions, firings, and lay-offs, and every available consultant was put on the line. But change is not easy. It became more complex when you add in hundreds of other factors, like the practice of medicine changing and the payor groups changing. It has almost become a sitcom for the old Abbott and Costello routine "Who's on First?"

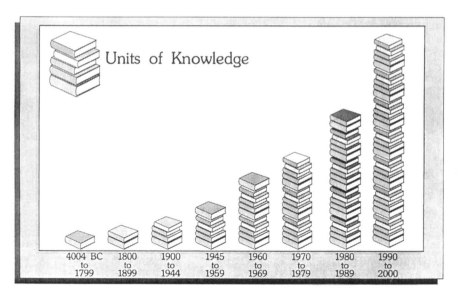

FIGURE 26-1. The Growth of information.

Market Size

Reported to be in excess of $400 million in 1994, the healthcare consulting market in the United States is big business. Estimates put this figure as exceeding $600 million in the year 2000. Why is this market so large and why has it drawn nearly every Big Six accounting firm into the business? Why also are there so many independent small and large firms in the business?

The answers to these questions are simple, and yet the reasoning behind most of the answers is quite complex. First, the answers. The buyers have demanded more and more consulting time. And the buyer community has changed to include HMOs, PPOs, clinics, and every other imaginable segment of the provider and payor community. Five years ago, the only buyers of consultants were hospitals. Today they remain strong purchasers of these services, but the need to determine how, what, where, and why, for now and into the future, has spread exponentially to hundreds of market segments within the healthcare bureaucracy. In 1994, several hundred consultants were used by the Clinton task force to develop strategy and policy for the U.S. Government. Consultants have done an outstanding job of marketing their services and convincing the states and the private sector of the need to understand what Washington would eventually do or require.

Almost all buyers have purchased systems in the past that did not meet their expectations after purchase. Several healthcare delivery systems have been absolutely burned by vendors who did not deliver as expected. Evidence the recent fall of Gerber Alley, plus the failures of several smaller vendors.

Because of this last item alone, it is no wonder that buyers are reluctant to make future purchase decisions without the assistance of outside experts to lessen their chance of making a mistake. After all, the cost of today's systems is high, and the potential for error is great.

The healthcare consulting market is actually divided into several segments and specialties. Some consulting firms offer a complete menu of services whereas others specialize in specific areas such as the clinical laboratory or perhaps the acquisition process only.

As shown in Table 26-1, there are many specialty areas for healthcare consultants. New areas not on the list continue to emerge. Consultants are quick to meet needs once they are identified. Also, it is fair to say that, with rapid change all about us, most healthcare delivery system management has problems and often lacks the exact expertise to arrive at good solutions. There are also healthcare managers who have already decided to go in a specific direction and are looking for a consultant to rubber stamp their decision and give it the seal of approval. After all, if the high-priced expert agrees that this is the path to take, then who can fault the buyer? When rubber stamps are needed or the risk for your company or your job is too high another phenomenon is often seen. This is the pass on hiring a small firm expert for a large firm whose name is known. The problem here is that often "big guns" at "name" firms sell the consulting deals, and then junior consultants are brought in to do the work. These big firms are smart if they hire knowledgeable outsiders to help them with the tasks. In recent years, firms like First Consulting and Superior Consultants have grown dramatically by retaining experts who have solid healthcare backgrounds and truly qualify as *senior* consultants. Of course, some of the Big Six firms and other consulting firms have done the same thing. There are also a lot of unknowns as we move into an era of great demand and less money. Still another reason for the significant growth in consulting over the last few years. We are indeed reinventing health care in America.

Choosing a Consultant

How should healthcare management choose a consultant? The answer to this question is fairly simple and straightforward. Consultants are and should be hired for the following reasons:

- They bring expertise that the healthcare executive does not currently have in-house. There may be several reasons why these people should not be permanently on staff. The expertise they have may not be needed

TABLE 26-1. Specialty Areas for Healthcare Consultants: A Partial Listing

The following represents a small list of issues facing our healthcare delivery system that consultants are being asked to help address

- Mergers and acquisitions
- Reengineering
- Integration
- New products and services
- Patient centered care systems
- Design, selection, and implementation
- Understanding what happens when:
  - In-patients move more and more to out-patients
  - Medical procedures increase or change
  - Downsizing occurs in the delivery system
  - Occupancy drops below 50%
  - Length of stay drops to 3 days
  - Capitation drives down prices for medical services
  - Medical staffs form their own groups
- General systems consulting
- Request for information (RFI) process
- Needs assessments
- Networking
- Staffing
- Hardware planning and acquisition
- Laboratory
- Radiology
- Development
- CHINS
- Marketing
- Downsizing
- General acquisitions
- Request for proposal (RFP) process
- Contracting
- Capital planning
- Facilities management
- Departmental systems
- Ambulatory care
- Other ancillaries
- Communications
- Planning
- Retrofitting

over the long haul, and it may not be within the executive's budget except for short durations.

- Consultants can be an addition to the hospital staff for short periods of time or for specific projects. When the need is over, the cost can be over.
- Politically a consultant may be needed to suggest or effect change where it just would not work if on staff employees or even executives suggested the same course of action.

Definition of the Consulting Task

Unless the task is predefined, some healthcare staffs can waste a lot of time and money on consultants. Of course, there is the case where a consultant is brought in to define the task or figure out the problem. These kinds of consulting engagements, by their nature, can be time consuming and costly. One should be prepared.

When consultants look at a potential engagement, they must consider billable hours. There is nothing wrong with this because they also need to understand how their engagement will fit in with other assignments. The point here is that the buyer needs to be aware that some consultants may create the largest, most comprehensive deal they can.

How Should Hospitals Use Consultants?

The Administrator's View

It should be obvious that there is no single view as to how consultants should be used. Consulting may not be the oldest known profession, but it certainly ranks right up there with other professions that are often lauded as the oldest.

After all, it was Moses some 5000 years ago that could not get his people moving to the promised land because of management problems. It was his father-in-law, Jethro, who suggested he needed rulers of tens and then hundreds and thousands because his span of control was too great. Even earlier, Job had several unwanted consultants give him advice on how to solve his many problems.

In preparation for this chapter, the author interviewed about 10 administrators for their words of wisdom regarding the use and misuse of consultants. Their varied responses are contained in the various sections of this chapter. They concurred in only a few areas: most could not have achieved their objectives without the help of the specialty consultants they brought in; they paid more than planned; the engagement took longer than intended; and 20 percent of their accomplishments fell short of what had been desired. Nonetheless, 9 out of 10 were relatively happy with their consultants' work, and all 10 indicated that they would be engaging another consultant within the year to address current or future problems. Five already had the same consultants working on new solutions to current problems. It should be noted that this small telephone study disclosed significant improvement in the perception of consultants by chief executive officers since the prior study for the first edition of this book.

In information systems, the largest use of consultants falls in to one of five categories: reengineering, systems integration, system selection, contract negotiations, and implementation. Consultants are offering services in other areas as well.

Buying into Consultants

A practice common among vendors is to bring in consultants to provide expert opinions in a given area. Many vendors select projects that the consulting community can work on and request that consultants provide their expertise.

Some things that should not go unnoticed are the obligations consultants set up when they perform vendor and hospital consulting. Some would say consulting for both is not a conflict of interest.

Some company executives that cannot afford to have consultants pass judgment on their systems believe they are often omitted from consideration for purchase. Several smaller vendors have told the author that in the last several years they have only won contracts when no consultant was involved in the selection process.

Educating the Consultant

How does one become a consultant? By what process does one become an expert? As with most things in life, there are multiple ways—hard work, brilliance, or luck (being in the right place at the right time). A few individuals even enter consulting when temporarily unemployed.

Over the years, how do consultants stay on top of developments in the marketplace? Some consulting groups do an outstanding job whereas others get by. Certainly a good question for any administrator to ask a potential consulting firm is, "What are the breadth and depth of your knowledge, and by what standards do you measure?"

A few consulting firms conduct annual educational seminars for their staffs. To these seminars they invite company spokesmen and experts in specific markets. Ernst & Young, for example, offers educational seminars characterized by information intensive formats. Other consulting firms only hire seasoned veterans out in the marketplace. Still others put their consultants through classes that range from three days to three weeks each year. Also, many consultants who have been in the marketplace for years have seen a lot of systems and situations.

Because the educational process is problematic, many vendors are hiring people to deal with the consulting community and provide them with the information they need to stay up with current products and services. This past year, this author's firm received videos from several vendors, explaining new directions, products, and services. Many vendors have started newsletters for consultants and other interested parties in the marketplace. These monthly or quarterly updates inform consultants about progress with specific systems or products. The key to successful newsletters is to keep the information short and relevant.

Another practice that is going on these days is the phenomenon of bringing knowledgeable experts out of places like California because of their early exposure to managed care, capitation, and the formation of new delivery groups or systems. In Denver alone, we have recently acquired three physicians out of California that are helping local groups define the future.

When selecting consultants, it is always prudent to ask, "Who will be working on my project?" and "What is that individual's background and expertise?"

A growing practice among the major consultants is the exclusion of start up and small vendors. The high costs of starting up and sustaining a product over time have driven many smaller companies out of the market. This phenomenon has made consultants much more conservative. Small companies complain that excluding them deprives customers of new technology. Although the pioneers know that leading edge technologies can become bleeding edge, there will always be visionaries that are willing to gamble on future rewards. It is also commonly believed that the largest of firms have become so busy meeting needs and solving problems among their current customers that they lack the skill or ability to develop new state of the art products. Smaller firms are quick to see this need and develop new products and services that are needed in this changing market.

Knowledge Couplers and Specialization

Information overload today brings both the blessings and problems inherent in specialization. In health care, specialization has been the norm for many years. Physicians began the separation of practice by specialty; nurses and hospitals followed. Inevitably, systems and consultants have had to specialize in order to remain expert in their fields. The problems with specialization are not on the surface, but appear when a given problem does not easily fit within a defined specialty or crosses over between specialties.

Background and specialization affect processes and decisions. The result may not be the best possible solution available but simply the best a given individual can come up with. Within companies and healthcare delivery systems, this phenomenon is often referred to as corporate culture. For certain companies, distinct cultures often come to mind, as shown in Table 26-2. It does not matter that these companies may excel elsewhere. Where they have made their mark is where they are remembered. Because of investments and expertise, they often have a difficult time moving away from these niche markets.

There is a theory saying, "If you have a hammer in your hand, everything looks like a nail." In health care, for instance, psychiatrists think first of the patient's mind, internists are likely to treat with medicine, and surgeons are predisposed to cut something out.

Specialists in any area tend to solve problems based on their specialties. As knowledge bases in health care get larger, this tendency becomes more obvious and the specialties grow narrower. Eventually computers will help

TABLE 26-2. Cultures and Niches Identified with Certain Companies

Company Name	Niche and Culture
Cerner	Laboratory based; moving out into the patient care system segment
SMS	Shared systems
HBO	In-house systems, microbased to mainframe
Systematics	Medical information systems
Cycare	Ambulatory systems
IDX	Ambulatory systems
Sunquest	Laboratory systems
HMDS	Microbased systems
Meditech	Minicomputer-based systems

to couple all of these knowledge bases together. For the moment, though, we rely on experts in the field who must do this knowledge coupling.

When selecting consultants, administrators should be aware of this phenomenon. The consultant educated on minisystems will find it hard to consider mainframe or microsystems. The consultant from a financial systems background will not be as much in tune with the subtleties of medical systems. Likewise, it is rare that someone who has always placed systems in-house can evaluate the advantages of time-shared, off-site systems. In short, the key question to ask in finding a good consultant is what that consultant's track record has been and why.

The Challenge

Consulting today is big business in the healthcare market. The complexities of health care and of information technology force potential buyers, managers, and systems to go to the market for help. The process is long and costly, and there are many places that it can go off track. Unfortunately, vendors and staff within hospitals often deliver less than originally promised. It's a very tough job.

It may be tempting to write this failure off as a problem in managing expectations. However, information systems, properly conceived, designed, developed, implemented, and managed, can go a long way toward saving money and improving the quality of care in health care. With an eye on service, a mind full of knowledge, and a heart committed to getting the job done, the consultant can provide invaluable assistance in this critical and demanding task.

We are quickly moving to an era when healthcare workers will not be able to function without a computer as an extension of their minds. The information is too great. The risk is too high. The change is ever present. And no one is an island unto themselves. It will take all of us working together to jump to the 21st Century. I look forward to seeing you there.

Questions

1. What are some significant reasons that a hospital should employ a consultant?
2. How should a hospital prepare itself prior to employing a consultant?
3. What are the advantages of employing a free-lance consultant as opposed to employing a large consulting firm? What are the advantages of dealing with a large consulting firm?
4. Should the hospital already have a solution to its problems predetermined and only employ a consultant to verify their solution or should a consultant be employed in order to determine the optimum solution?
5. Should a hospital employ a consultant who has been known to have close ties to a vendor bidding on the hospital system? Under what conditions might this be a good idea, under what conditions would this be a poor idea?

27
Maximizing the Benefits of Using Consultants

Elizabeth E. Concordia

Healthcare costs account for 14.4 percent of the United States' gross domestic product (GNP). As cost containment measures have been implemented to address the high costs of health care, acute care facilities have required speedy revenue recovery mechanisms to survive. To run more efficiently, hospitals are turning to information resources management and automating clinical and financial applications that provide administrators with the management information they need to make cost-effective decisions. The increased importance and cost of information resources management have spawned the growth of healthcare information systems (HCIS) consulting practices.

How Consulting Firms Work

Consulting firms make money by selling work. To keep their employees utilized and to command high rates, consulting firms must provide services that are of a high quality and caliber. Individual consultants have specialized skills and proven experience; established in their fields, they often have previously worked for a vendor, a hospital, or both.

The consulting firm's goal is to keep the client satisfied and to offer its clients the best services. It is important to realize that there is a finite number of hospitals in the country.

Although one survey notes that 41 percent of the hospital executives see consultants as necessary supplements, hospitals needing healthcare information system consulting services are only a fraction of this 41 percent.

If the consulting firm does not produce what its client requires, the firm will not sell any additional work. The dissatisfied client may look elsewhere; other hospitals may hear of the dissatisfied client. Future sales and utilization will suffer. To stay in business, the consulting firm must keep its clients. To do so, it must have employees who do high-quality work and make the firm stand apart from its competitors.

Services Provided by Consultants

Consulting firms rely on the inability of healthcare institutions to keep up with the latest innovations that affect information systems functionality and with developments in other acute care facilities. Consulting firms sell their ability to provide up-to-date product information and the benefit of experiences in other hospitals. Often the services of consultants protect the client from making the same mistake another institution has already made.

The services that a typical healthcare information systems consultant practice offers are:

- Selection and evaluation of information systems,
- Contract negotiations,
- Implementation support,
- Long-range information systems planning,
- System testing,
- Policy and procedure documentation,
- Project management,
- Telecommunications/networking,
- Quality assurance,
- Cost justification,
- Reorganization, and
- Interface support.

In retaining information system consultants, healthcare institutions may request the consultants to do any of the following.

Provide Specific Expertise

Often when healthcare institutions lack the specific expertise needed to get a job done, consultants have performed the required task numerous times at other hospitals and are familiar with the vendor or application. Hiring consultants to provide a service that the hospital is not capable of performing in-house is a common occurrence at acute care facilities.

Perform a Temporary Job

A hospital may have the need for a certain resource for four or six months but not for a full-time employee. In these instances it is more cost effective for the institution to pay for a trained individual for the duration of the temporary job or until the backlog is caught up. For example, when converting computer systems most applications are very labor intensive to install, and the hospital does not have the staff to perform all the necessary tasks. After the implementation, there is no longer a need for the resources. This is a common use of consultants.

Provide an Acting Information Systems Director

Hiring management information services directors may be a time-consuming process. Consulting firms often provide acting directors until an acceptable candidate is found. This service protects the hospital from the degradation of information service when the director leaves. It also takes the pressure off the hospital to hire someone immediately rather than taking the time necessary to recruit and hire the best candidate.

Review and Evaluate Organizational Structures or System Definition

Consultants are hired in this capacity for their objectivity and neutrality. When evaluating past work or current organizational structures, in-house hospital staff may be unable to assume an objective viewpoint. Again, because consultants are not biased by the political history or personalities within the hospital, they can make recommendations that are in the best interest of the hospital.

Ensure Successful Implementations

Stories of disastrous implementations are abundant. Administrators often hire consultants to prevent them from making the same mistakes other hospitals made and to protect the hospital from being taken advantage of by the vendor. Consultants are hired for their experience with implementations and to increase the chances for successful outcomes.

Do the Work No One Else Wants to Do

For example, the Joint Commission on the Accreditation of Health Organizations (JCAHO) requires hospitals to have written policies and procedures in place. Typically no one wants to write the policies and procedures, so consultants are hired to finish the job in compliance with JCAHO.

Meet Time Constraints

Time constraints are often the reason for hospitals to hire consultants. When a task needs to be completed in a tight time frame consultants provide the bodies to get the job done. For example, when looking for a new hospital information system, an institution may choose to expedite the process by hiring a consultant to assist in identifying the required functionalities and writing the request for proposal.

Assist in Project Management

Administrators may not have enough time to devote to project management or may fear that a project that they approved, or are responsible for, is not running smoothly. They may then hire consultants to assist or to warn of possible complications. On occasion, an administrator may hire a consultant as a security blanket or a scapegoat. If the project is a success, the administrator and the consultant both win. However, if the project fails, the administrator may place the blame on the consultant.

Avoid Making Costly Mistakes

As the financial portfolios of hospitals are becoming bleaker, hospitals cannot afford to make mistakes nor do they have the time to correct mistakes. As automation has become critical to an institution's ability to survive, hospitals are under pressure and must make decisions that are right the first time. Many hospitals hire healthcare information system consultants because they cannot afford to take the risk of making a mistake. More hospitals should.

Getting the Most Value from Consultants

Before hiring a firm, the hospital should arrange to meet the individual consultants from the firm who will be assigned to the project. The client should make sure those consultants are experienced and capable of discussing specific experiences with other hospitals. There should be no learning curve to prevent immediate results from the consultants. For example, if implementation assistance is required, the individual consultant should be familiar with not only the application but also the vendor. Checking references will also ensure that the most value is received from the consultants.

The hospital should stipulate deliverables with due dates and identify a series of continuing checkpoints before the project begins. Granting extensions for deliverables sets a bad precedent and should not be done. As clients, the hospital should clearly define the scope of the project and establish that the estimated hours will not exceed a certain dollar amount. The individual(s) directing the consultant should prepare a list of all items that are to be completed and share it with the consultant.

If the consultants are local, the hospital should request that they work on site at the hospital. There they will get more done for the client than they would at their own offices. The hospital should also ask the consultants for weekly status reports and make sure they know to alert the hospital immediately of any potential delays. To benefit from the engagement, the hospital must let the consultants know what its requirements and expectations are. This means, quite simply, that the hospital must function as a responsible client and present an organized account of what is to be accomplished by the consultants.

The Future for Healthcare Information Systems Consulting

In addition to the established trends toward decreased hardware costs and increased software costs, information resources management shows great increases in installation costs. Trends also suggest that the percentage of the total hospital budget devoted to management information systems will increase in the future.

Information resources management has become a critical factor in the ability of a hospital to survive. In order to survive in this era of cost containment, hospitals must be able to identify profitable services and growing markets. Without information systems, hospitals can neither run efficiently nor produce the information administrators need. Consultants are engaged to address many issues associated with information resources management.

The dependence of healthcare institutions upon their information systems and the increasing complexity of technology combine to make healthcare information systems consulting a growing and profitable market.

Questions

1. What reasons would you give to your administrator to justify using consultants?
2. What would you look for in hiring a consultant?
3. Name four services that healthcare information systems consultants provide.
4. What are the trends in making the best use of consulting firms and their employees?

28
Managing Consulting Services: A Guide for the CIO

AMELIA LEE MARLEY

CIOs have traditionally focused on computer hardware and software as the primary tools of their trade. Bringing the latest technology solutions to his or her organization often received high priority on the yearly list of CIO goals. Clearly, tremendous opportunities rest in the advanced technologies available today. Powerful relational databases, graphical user interfaces and the capabilities of current microchip technologies have opened information doors for organizations in all types of industries.

In an era labeled the "Information Age," technology alone will not solve the business problems faced by the healthcare industry, which, itself, is going through major transition. People resources will be equally important in ultimately supplying the right technology solutions for healthcare organizations. Consultants will be an important people resource and knowing how to manage consulting services will be an important skill for the successful healthcare CIO.

Of hospital executives surveyed, 41 percent saw consultants as necessary supplements to internal resources but only 29 percent believed consultants' fees are cost justified (Packter, 1987). Executives are leery of using consultants because they are an expensive resource and inappropriate use of consultants is extremely costly. When effectively used, consultants can greatly enhance the investment made in information systems, and it is critical that the CIO understand when, why, and how to use them. This chapter provides insights into how consulting firms work and gives practical guidelines for using consultants successfully.

Understanding How Consulting Firms Work

Consulting is a service industry in the purest sense. A consulting firm's primary assets are its personnel. These assets produce revenue by providing services to clients. Services are usually billed at a negotiated hourly rate. Within a practice, individual consultants are monitored in terms of their utilization rate, that is, the percentage of their time that is billed to clients.

A practice is monitored in terms of its revenue contributions. The consultant's goal is to stay utilized; the practice's goal is to contribute revenues at a level defined in the firm's business plan.

To meet these goals, consulting firms attempt to convince potential clients of needs that can be met by the personnel of the consulting firm. The marketing of consulting services is largely a process of needs identification. Needs identified are likely to be related to systems planning, systems selection, systems implementation, or systems use evaluation. It is during the consulting marketing cycle that the potential consumer can become quite confused. The CIO must discern the difference between the creation of a perceived need and a legitimate lack of resources to meet a stated goal.

Evaluating the Need for Consulting Services

There are five key questions the CIO should answer when determining whether or not to use consulting services.

How do the services being proposed fit into the overall information systems plan? The CIO should evaluate how the project being proposed by the consulting firm fits into the overall information systems plan. It may be that there is no plan. If so, the first and most critical step is to develop one. An information systems plan is essential, because without one a CIO has no way of knowing what the overall blueprint for change is. The plan can range from simple to complex and can be brief or bulky. Essentially, it depends on the culture of the organization as to how the mechanics of the plan should work. The important point here is that proposed services should be considered only if the services are relevant to the information systems plan.

Are the services being proposed critical to the implementation of the information systems plan? The CIO should evaluate how critical the proposed project is to the success of the information systems plan. If the project relates to the plan but is not essential to its success, then it probably is not worth pursuing. For example, a consulting firm might propose to conduct an extensive needs analysis prior to the selection of a radiology system. The selection of a radiology system might be part of the plan, but it may also be that the director of radiology understands radiology systems sufficiently that a needs analysis would be neither necessary nor welcome.

How aggressive are the dates incorporated in the information systems plan and how committed is the organization to these dates? It is important to consider how aggressive the organization is relative to the deadlines incorporated in the information systems plan. If the time lines are generous or the dates are flexible, there is less need to staff aggressively. If the organization is on a tight time schedule and the dates are inflexible, then adequate personnel resources must be quickly obtained. A consulting firm, being a provider of short-term manpower, is an appropriate resource to utilize in this scenario.

What risks are inherent in the information systems plan? The CIO should consider the degree of risk inherent in the institution's information systems plan. The implementation of new technology includes higher associated risks. It may be appropriate to involve consultants during the implementation of a pilot system to assist in managing the associated risks. For example, it would be appropriate to hire a consultant to perform extensive software testing on software that is newly developed. However, using a consulting firm to test mature software would probably not be critical to the success of the project.

Are there less costly resources available to accomplish the objectives to be met by the consulting firm? The CIO should also determine whether there is staff available, internal or third party, to perform the tasks of the project at a lesser cost. If so, these resources might be used in place of consultants. However, this involves the careful examination of the skill set of internal staff as well as a solid understanding of what contributions systems vendors can make. Consultants are a potential solution if internal personnel and vendor personnel cannot provide the resources needed to successfully meet the goals of the information systems plan (Gigiulio, 1984).

Selecting a Consulting Firm

Once it is determined that there is a need for consulting services, the next step is to select a firm. Answering the following questions should address the key areas to be considered:

- What kinds of experience and skills do the specific individuals assigned to the engagement have that are critical to the success of the project team?
- What resources are available to the project team from across the consulting firm that could be utilized as needed on the engagement?
- Has the consulting firm demonstrated a commitment to the potential client by providing services before a formal agreement is made?
- Does the consulting firm lend credibility at the board and departmental level?
- Does the executive consultant or partner who is marketing the engagement demonstrate a sincere interest in the success of the CIO's goals?
- Will the consulting staff assigned to the engagement blend well with internal staff and with any associated vendors?

In essence, the questions posed above relate to the experience, expertise, commitment, and compatibility of the consulting firm being evaluated. To be further considered, the consulting firm must have personnel available for the engagement who have the knowledge and skills to meet the demands of the project. If these criteria are met, it is simply a matter of cost and selecting the organization with which to do business.

In the final selection of a firm to engage, it is important that there is a positive business relationship between the client and the consultant. A variety of relationships should be considered between the organization's members and the consultant before engaging consultants. Key individuals in the executive suite, project members, and others within the user community will at some point be affected by the consultants. The more open and trustful all parties are, the more valuable the engagement will be to the organization (Williamson, 1993a).

Managing the Consulting Firm

A letter of agreement finalizes the understanding between the client and the consultant. In the letter of agreement, the scope, work plan, personnel, deliverables, and fees should be defined. If any of these items are missing from an engagement letter, the client should request that they be added. Each of these items is described below.

Scope: A general description of the project that sets forth the direction and boundaries for what will be included as part of the engagement. It is important that the scope be stated so that the consultant and client conceptually agree to what is included as part of the engagement. In the pace of today's rapidly changing business environment, the scope of the engagement may change. If a change in scope is proposed, the evaluation process is the same as that used for evaluating any prospective consulting services.

Work Plan: The definition of tasks to be performed and the associated dates of completion. The work plan is important to ensure that the engagement has been well thought out and to monitor progress once work begins.

Personnel: The identification and qualifications of specific individuals to be assigned to an engagement. It is important to state in writing that the individuals specified in the letter of understanding will not be substituted with other personnel unless expressly agreed to before the fact by the client.

Deliverables: Any product that will be produced during the course of the engagement. This would include any reports or other performance commitments stated in the letter of agreement. The due dates of deliverables should be outlined in the work plan.

Fees: Usually stated as an hourly rate. The key point here is that consulting firms have standard rates that are typically negotiated downward. The client might wish to establish an upper dollar cap for the project to protect against budget overruns. However, the hourly rate is generally not as negotiable when caps are incorporated in the letter of agreement. The client's negotiating strategy must be assessed on a basis specific to the needs of the organization.

Once the engagement begins, it is important to monitor progress. One of the best techniques for doing this is by regularly polling internal staff as to how they perceive the progress of the project. Also, discussing the engagement progress with consulting personnel and referencing the letter of agreement helps ensure that the project stays on track. A typical pitfall leading to a failed consulting engagement is to hand off responsibility for project completion to the consultant. The client (CIO) is *always* responsible for the project outcome and must *always* remain cognizant of that fact (Williamson, 1993b).

In managing consultants, the CIO must constantly evaluate the need for consulting services. The consulting firm should be discharged if the service does not meet expectations or is determined unnecessary to the successful implementation of the information systems plan.

Dealing with Future Trends

Technology is changing the information systems environment at a pace that challenges those in the industry to keep up. It makes sense to use outside resources, consultant or vendor, when lack of internal staff expertise prohibits an organization from using information as a competitive advantage. The rate of technology change will continue to accelerate resulting in the availability of new products. The major challenge will be how to assimilate these new products into the organization's culture in order to capitalize on new technologies. The fast pace of technology changes compounded by healthcare reform makes it likely that healthcare organizations will increasingly turn to consultants to help meet the challenge of implementing solid business solutions.

An editorial titled "The High Cost of Consulting" warned of the pitfalls in using consultants (Childs, 1989), and cost does make executives cautious in using consulting services. Difficult though it may be, knowing when and how to use consultants can greatly enhance the organization's utilization of information and literally mean the difference between success and failure. Guidelines for the CIO include the following:

- Recognize that consulting firms survive by keeping staff on engagements. Therefore, there is an incentive for the firm to identify a client need that can best be met by the consulting firm's resources.
- Evaluate the need for consulting firms in reference to an information systems plan. The services must be relevant and critical to the success of the plan.
- Select a consulting firm by assessing the skills of the consultants and determining the compatibility of the consulting firm with the CIO's organization.
- Manage the use of a consulting firm by establishing mutual expectations with the consultant and by monitoring, as client, the progress of the engagement.

Questions

1. Explain the importance of knowing how to be a prudent buyer of consulting services.
2. Describe why the marketing process used by consulting firms may lead to confusion on the part of a potential client.
3. What is the key reference that should be used in the evaluation of the need for consulting services?
4. Describe several key areas of consideration in the selection of a consulting firm.

References

Childs, B.W. (1989). The high cost of consulting, *U.S. Healthcare, 6,* 8.

Gigiulio, L. (1984). Who should plan for the implementation of a hospital information system? *Health Care Strategic Management, 2,* 28–31.

Packter, C.L. (1987). Executives wary of info systems consultants. *Hospitals, 61,* 91.

Williamson, M. (1993a). Strategic outlook: Consulting services, *CIO, 7,* 38.

Williamson, M. (1993b). Strategic outlook: Consulting services, *CIO, 7,* 32.

Index

Contributors

Lawrence B. Afrin, MD
Research Fellow and Physician Liaison, Medical University of South Carolina, Charleston, SC, USA (afrinl@honc.mhs.musc.edu)

James W. Albright
President and CEO, Rex Hospital, Inc., 4420 Lake Boone Trail, Raleigh, NC, USA

Edward L. Anderson, MD
Executive Medical Director, Bell Atlantic, Bell Atlantic Network Services, Inc., Arlington, VA, USA

Marion J. Ball, EdD
Chief Information Officer, Information Services, University of Maryland, Baltimore, MD, USA (mjb@umabnet.ab.umd.edu)

Bill W. Childs
Publisher and Editor in Chief, Healthcare Informatics, Evergreen, CO, USA

Elizabeth E. Concordia, MAS
Senior Director, Clinical Services, Johns Hopkins Bayview Medical Center, Baltimore, MD, USA

Glenn D. Crowe, PhD
President, Sirius Technologies Limited, Chairman, Healthcare Informatics Telcom Network (HITN), Norcross, GA, USA

Victor E. Del Bene, MD
Professor and Associate Dean for Students, College of Medicine, Medical University of South Carolina, Charleston, SC, USA (vic_del_bene@mac gate.musc.edu)

Judith V. Douglas, MA, MHS
Director, Information Services, University of Maryland, Baltimore, MD, USA (judy@umabnet.ab.umd.edu)

Karen DuBois, MSN, RNC
Project Coordinator, Special Projects Grant, American Journal of Nursing Co., New York, NY, USA (karen.dubois@ajn.org)

Michael G. Eckstein
President, EDI for Healthcare, Bryn Mawr, PA, USA

Martin Farber, MD
Executive Vice President, Medical Affairs, Bayfront Life Services, Inc., St. Petersburg, FL, USA

James M. Gabler
Manager, Health Care Information Services, The Analytic Sciences Corporation (TASC), Arlington, VA, USA (jmgabler@aol.com)

Charles F. Genre, MD
Chairman, Department of Pathology, Ochsner Medical Institutions, New Orleans, LA, USA

Joseph W. Hales, PhD
Assistant Research Professor, Division of Medical Informatics, Duke University Medical Center, Durham, NC, USA (hales002@mc.duke.edu)

Gary L. Hammon
Manager, Superior Consultant Company, Inc., San Antonio, TX, USA (gary_hammon@super.#u#dtw.ccmail.compuserve.com)

Gail Ann DeLuca Havens, MS, RN, C
Doctoral Candidate, School of Nursing, University of Maryland, Baltimore, MD, USA

Richard D. Helppie
President and CEO, Superior Consultant Company, Inc., Farmington Hills, MI, USA (richard_helppie@super#u#dtw.ccmail.compuserve.com)

Betsy S. Hersher
President, Hersher Associates, Ltd., Northbrook, IL, USA

Nancy M. Lorenzi, PhD
Associate Senior Vice President, University of Cincinnati Medical Center, Cincinnati, OH, USA (lorenzi@.uc.edu)

Laura A. MacFadden
Vice President, Corporate Facilities and Services, Bayfront Medical Center, St. Petersburg, FL, USA

Amelia Lee Marley
Vice President and CIO, Bayfront Life Services, Inc., St. Petersburg, FL, USA

Patsy B. Marr, RN, MSN
Director, Hospital Information Systems, New York University Medical Center, New York, NY, USA (patsy.marr@mchis.med.nyu.edu)

Mary N. McAlindon, EdD, RN, CNAA
Assistant to the Vice President, McLaren Regional Medical Center, Flint, MI, USA (mmcalindon@bix.com)

Mary Etta Mills, RN, ScD, CNAA
Chair and Associate Professor, University of Maryland School of Nursing, Baltimore, MD, USA (mmills@umabnet.ab.umd.edu)

W. Marcus Newberry, MD
Vice President for Academic Affairs and Provost, Medical University of South Carolina, Charleston, NC, USA (marc_newberry@ smtpgw .musc .edu)

Susan K. Newbold, MS, RN
University of Maryland School of Nursing, Baltimore, MD, USA (snew bold@umabnet.ab.umd.edu)

James I. Penrod, EdD
Vice President and CIO, University of Memphis, Memphis, TN, USA

Robert J. Pickton
Senior Vice President/CIO, Baylor Health Care Systems, Dallas, TX, USA

Robert T. Riley, PhD
President, Riley Associates, Cincinnati, OH, USA (rileyrt@uc.edu)

Mary Anne Rizzolo, EdD, RN
Director, Interactive Technologies, American Journal of Nursing Co., New York, NY, USA (ma.rizzolo@ajn.org)

Frances C. Seehausen
Director, IS Strategic Planning, EHS Health Care, Oak Brook, IL, USA

Roger H. Shannon, MD, FACR, FACMI
Director, Radiology Service, Department of Veterans Affairs, Durham, NC, USA (shannon.r@forum.va.gov)

Lawrence H. Sharrott
Corporate Chief Information Officer, AtlantiCare Health System, Pleasantville, NY, USA (lsharrott@acmcol.ccmail.compuserve.com)

Donald Simborg, MD
Chief Product Strategist, Medicus Systems Corporation, Alameda, CA, USA (Don_Simborg@medicus.com)

Donald M. Steinwachs, PhD
Professor and Chair, Johns Hopkins School of Public Health, Baltimore, MD, USA (dsteinwa@phnet.sph.jhu.edu)

Terrance T. Stretch
Senior Management Consultant, Superior Consultant Company, Inc., Marietta, GA, USA

Arlene J. Verona, MSN, RN
Formerly of Medicus Systems, Evanston, IL, USA

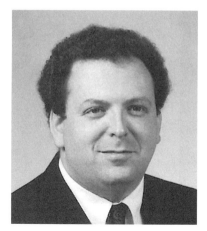

LAWRENCE B. AFRIN

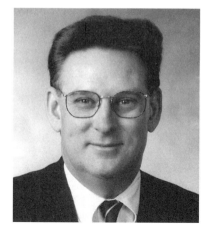

JAMES W. ALBRIGHT

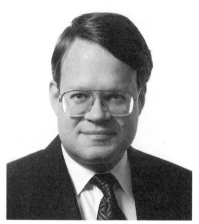

EDWARD L. ANDERSON

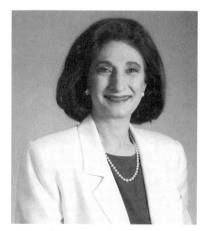

MARION J. BALL

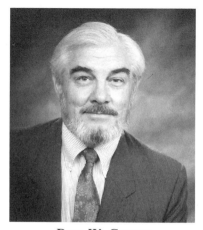

BILL W. CHILDS

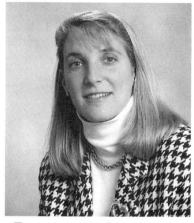

ELIZABETH E. CONCORDIA

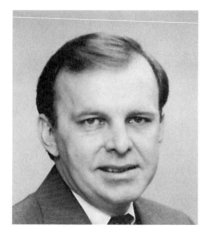

GLENN D. CROWE

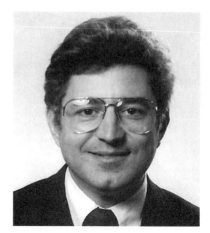

VICTOR E. DEL BENE

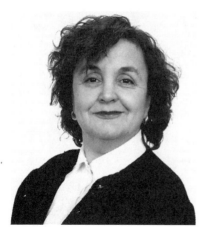

JUDITH V. DOUGLAS

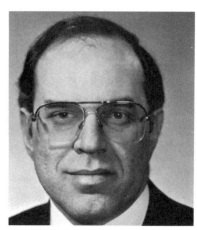

MICHAEL G. ECKSTEIN

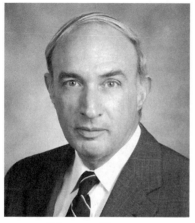

MARTIN FARBER

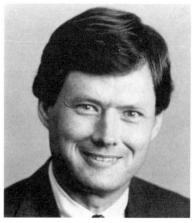

JAMES M. GABLER

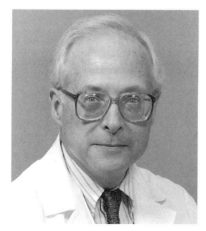

CHARLES F. GENRE

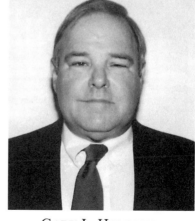

GARY L. HAMMON

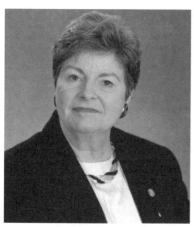

GAIL ANN DELUCA HAVENS

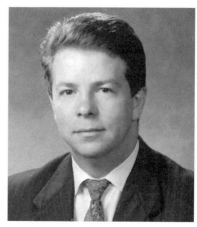

RICHARD D. HELPPIE

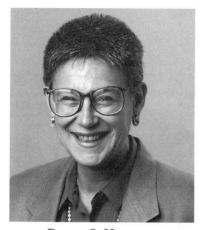

BETSY S. HERSHER

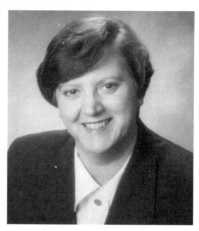

NANCY M. LORENZI

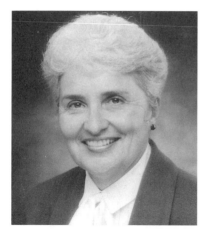

MARY N. MCALINDON

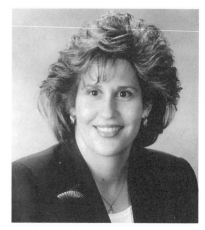

LAURA A. MACFADDEN

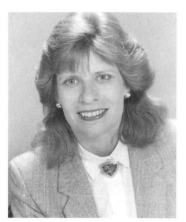

AMELIA LEE MARLEY

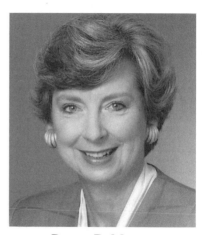

PATSY B. MARR

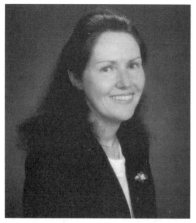

MARY ETTA MILLS

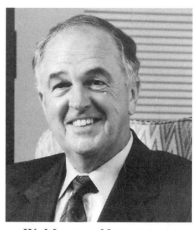

W. MARCUS NEWBERRY

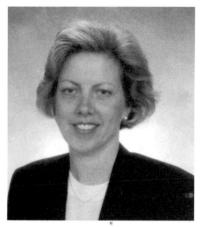

SUSAN K. NEWBOLD

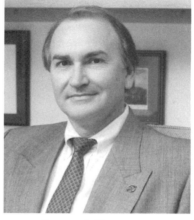

JAMES I. PENROD

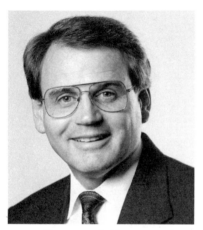

ROBERT J. PICKTON

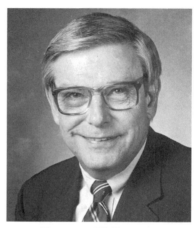

ROBERT T. RILEY

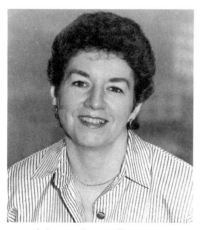

MARY ANNE RIZZOLO

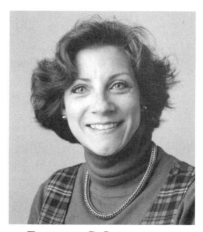

FRANCES C. SEEHAUSEN

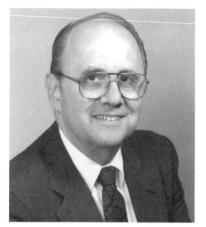

ROGER H. SHANNON

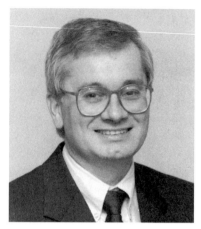

LAWRENCE H. SHARROTT

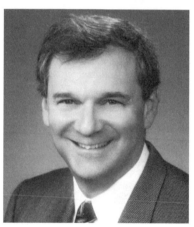

DONALD SIMBORG

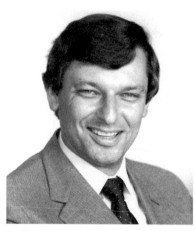

DONALD M. STEINWACHS

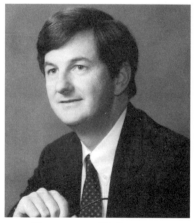

TERRANCE T. STRETCH

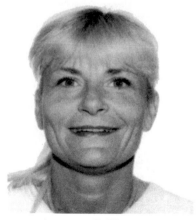

ARLENE J. VERONA